edexcel
advancing learning, changing lives

D0237604

BTEC National Health and Social Care

Book 1

Core and specialist units

Mary Crittenden
Sam Pope
Elizabeth Shackels
Alison Thompson
Douglas Thomson

S.E. DERBYSHIRE COLLEGE

R62642K0560

A PEARSON COMPANY

Contents

S. E. DERBYSHIRE COLLEGE
LEARNING CENTRE
362·1
L 060084

Introduction 4
How to use this book 6
Track your progress 8
Research Skills 13

Unit 1	Developing Effective Communication in Health and Social Care	14
	So, you want to be a...Health Care Assistant	15
	Grading criteria	16
1.1	Understanding effective communication and interpersonal interaction	17
1.2	Understanding factors that influence communication and interpersonal interactions in health and social care settings	27
1.3	Knowing how patients/service users may be assisted by effective communication	40
1.4	Demonstrating your own communication skills in a caring role	45

Unit 2	Equality, Diversity and Rights in Health and Social Care	48
	So you want to be a...Learning Disabilities Nurse	49
	Grading criteria	50
2.1	Understand concepts of equality, diversity and right in relation to health and social care	51
2.2	Understand discriminatory practice in health and social care	60
2.3	Understand how national initiatives promote anti-discriminatory practice	65
2.4	Understand how anti-discriminatory practice is promoted in health and social care settings	76

Unit 3	Health, Safety and Security in Health and Social Care	82
	So, you want to be a...Deputy Manager, residential care home	83
	Grading criteria	84
3.1	Understanding potential hazards in health and social care	85
3.2	Understand how legislation, guidelines, policies and procedures promote health, safety and security	99
3.3	Understanding roles and responsibilities for health, safety and security in health and social care settings	106
3.4	Dealing with hazards in a local environment	111

Unit 4	**Development through the Life Stages**	**116**
	So, you want to be an...Health visitor	117
	Grading criteria	118
4.1	Understanding human growth and development through the life stages	119
4.2	Understanding how life factors and events may influence the development of the individual	127
4.3	Understanding physical changes and psychological perspectives in relation to ageing	144

Unit 5	**Fundamentals of Anatomy and Physiology for Health and Social Care**	**150**
	So, you want to be a...Nurse	151
	Grading criteria	152
5.1	The organisation of the human body – overview	153
5.2	The role of energy in the body	162
5.3	How homeostatic mechanisms operate in the maintenance of an internal environment	179
5.4	Interpreting data obtained form monitoring routine variations in the functioning of health body systems.	189

Unit 6	**Personal and Professional Development in Health and Social Care**	**194**
	So, you want to be a...Midwife	195
	Grading criteria	196
6.1	The learning process	197
6.2	Planning, monitoring and reflecting on your development	207
6.3	Understand service provision in health or social care sectors	217

Unit 7	**Sociological Perspectives for Health and Social Care**	**228**
	So, you want to be a...Social Worker	229
	Grading criteria	230
7.1	Understand sociological approaches to study	231
7.2	Be able to apply sociological approaches to health and social care	242

Unit 8	**Psychological Perspectives for Health and Social Care**	**258**
	So, you want to be a...Mental Health Nurse	259
	Grading criteria	260
8.1	Understand psychological approaches to study	261
8.2	Be able to apply psychological approaches to health and social care	280

Why choose a career in health and social care?

Health care careers include:

- **Doctors** – e.g. consultants, registrars, house officers and associate specialists
- **Nurses** – e.g. nurses, midwives and health visitors
- **Scientific, therapeutic and technical staff** – e.g. art, music and drama therapists, chiropodists/podiatrists, dietitians, occupational therapists, orthoptists, physiotherapists, and radiographers, pharmacists, speech and language therapists
- **Ambulance staff** – e.g. ambulance paramedics
- **Support staff** – e.g. nursing assistants/ auxiliaries, nursery nurses, health care assistants, clinical and administrative staff (medical secretaries/records officers, and maintenance and works staff)

One of the biggest employers in the UK

- Around **2 million** people are employed in the health sector, with approximately 1.3 million of these employed by the NHS
- Around 1.2 million people work in the social care sector – around **5%** of the UK workforce.

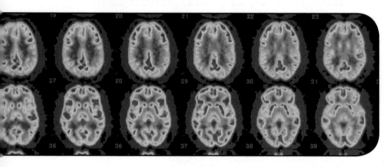

A growing sector

- Between 1999 and 2004, the number of jobs in the health care sector increased by 34,000, (an increase of 13%), and the number of jobs in the social care sector **increase by 14%**.
- Over the same period the number of jobs in the economy as a whole increased by 4%.

A diverse sector

- There are over 300 different careers available in the NHS
- There are over 360 different organisations within the NHS
- There are 60,000 employers in the social care and children's workforce

Social care and children's care careers include:

- children's homes and care homes
- domiciliary care and support services
- day centres and services
- social work
- fostering agencies and services
- foster carers
- nurse agencies
- adoption services
- nursery and early years work
- childminding
- voluntary youth services
- Connexions
- day nurseries
- voluntary and charitable care

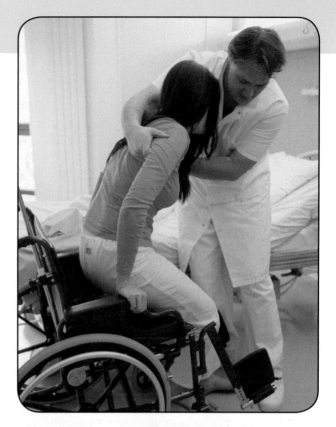

Did you know...

Employees

- More than ¾ **of employees within the health and social care sector are women**, and 1/3 are aged between 35 and 44.

- 73% of the health care sector employees work within the public sector. 21% work in the private sector, and 2% in the charity or voluntary sector. The remainder are employed by local authorities or other organisations

- 65% of social care workers are employed outside the public sector

- Nearly **50% of social care workers work part time**, and nearly 40% of health care workers.

- The average salary of staff in the NHS is **£22,300**. The average salary of a consultant is £74,600. The average salary of an assistant is £13,800.

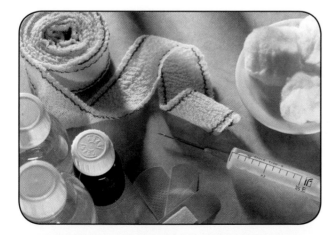

Service users

- Every day, the NHS is in contact with over **1.5 million patients** and their families

- In a typical day for the NHS:

  - Over 835,000 people visit their GP practice

  - Almost 50,000 people visit accident and emergency departments

  - 49,000 outpatient consultations

  - 94,000 people are admitted to hospital as an emergency admission

  - 36,000 people are in hospital for planned treatment

  - 28,000 sight tests are carried out

  - 18,000 calls to NHS Direct

[source: Department of Health]

How to use this book

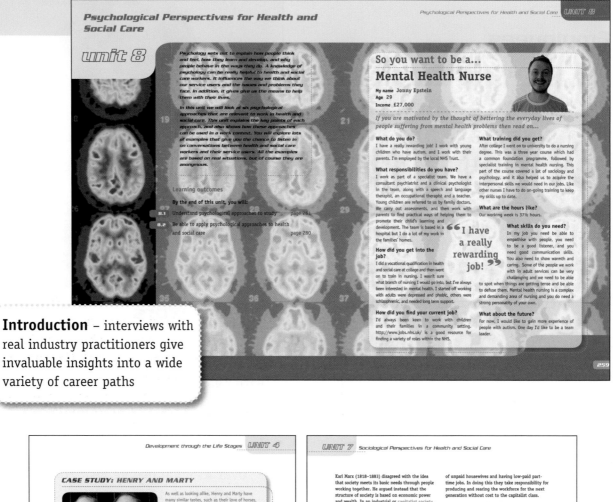

Introduction – interviews with real industry practitioners give invaluable insights into a wide variety of career paths

Case studies – in-depth focus on industry-specific scenarios show you how the theory works in real-life situations

Key words – easy to understand definitions of key industry terms

Grading criteria – learning outcomes and grading criteria are located at the beginning of every unit, so you know right from the start what you need to do to achieve a pass, merit or distinction

UNIT 8 *Psychological Perspectives for Health and Social Care*

Grading criteria

The table shows what you need to do to gain a pass, merit or distinction in this part of the qualification. Make sure you refer back to it when you are completing work so you can judge whether you are meeting the criteria and what you need to do to fill in gaps in your knowledge or experience.

In this unit there are six evidence activities that give you an opportunity to demonstrate your achievement of the grading criteria:

page 37	P1
page 38	P2
page 39	P3
page 40	P4
page 43	P5, M1
page 44	M2, D1

To achieve a pass grade the evidence must show that the learner is able to…	To achieve a merit grade the evidence must show that, in addition to the pass criteria, the learner is able to…	To achieve a distinction grade the evidence must show that, in addition to the pass and merit criteria, the learner is able to…
P1 describe the application of behaviourist perspectives in health and social care	**M1** analyse the contribution of different psychological perspectives to the understanding and management of challenging behaviour	**D1** evaluate the roles of different psychological perspectives in health and social care
P2 explain the value of the social learning approach to health and social care service provision	**M2** analyse the contribution of different psychological perspectives to health and social care provision	
P3 describe the application of psychodynamic perspectives in health and social care		
P4 describe the value of the humanistic approach to health and social care service provision		
P5 explain the value of the cognitive perspective in supporting individuals		
P6 describe the application of biological perspectives in health and social care		

Evidence activities – short activities are spread throughout the unit giving you the opportunity to practice your achievement of the grading criteria in small steps

Think – questions help you reflect on your learning and to think about how it could be applied to real-life working practice

Care UNIT 7

Research tip

The Kings Fund website has a useful section about health inequalities. http://www.kingsfund.org.uk/ resources/briefings/health.html

Example

Middlehampton is a large town in the UK with a diverse population spanning the whole range of socio-economic groups. Some areas are very affluent, whereas others have many properties in bad condition. The Links housing estate mainly contains poor housing stock, occupied disproportionately by single older people, with young unemployed couples and minority ethnic groups making up the rest of the residents. In contrast, Cavendish Park is a highly desirable housing development occupied by professional families, some of whom have children educated at boarding school or university. The Broadlands is a new development under construction with a proportion of affordable housing. Some young families have already bought or rented properties in this development, but, because of health and safety considerations, it has no play facilities for the young children living there.

Think How could the artefact, social selection, cultural and behaviourist approaches help to explain the differences?

Research tip

You can find *Saving Lives: Our Healthier Nation* at the TSO website. www.official-documents.co.uk

EVIDENCE ACTIVITY

P5 – M3 – D2

1. a. Compare patterns and trends of health and illness in three different social groups. Make sure that you keep a list of the sources that you use when getting your information.

b. Display your findings for the three different groups.

c. Compare the differences between the different groups. (P5)

2. Explain the possible sociological reasons for the differences in the three groups (M3)

3. Using the four sociological explanations for health inequalities evaluate their strengths and weaknesses in explaining the patterns and trends in the three different groups. (D2)

Research tips – direct you to useful websites and key organisations to help you take your study further

Developing Effective Communication in Health and Social Care UNIT 1

Example

Leon is a youth worker. He has a large group of teenagers who visit the youth centre each Saturday night. The group has split into several different groups and there are signs of tensions growing between them. He has suggested that they should all try to put on a play together which involves music and drama. This has been met with enthusiasm as a number of the young people see themselves as good musicians and actors.

Think How might communication between the groups be improved by putting on such an event?

Arts and crafts

In the same way that music and drama can provide a means of communication, so may the use of arts and crafts. They are used as therapeutic activities in many care settings. Children, clients with mental health problems and those with learning disabilities may particularly benefit from such activities in aiding communication. Psychologists may use pictures drawn by children as a basis for understanding family relationships that a child cannot express in words.

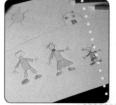

Figure 1.2 A child's depiction of t…

Communication using technology

The use of technology for communication is increasing all the time. Many records are now stored electronically. The NHS has begun a massive project to introduce an electronic patient-record system. This will not only keep details of individual patients, but allow GPs to book appointments with hospital consultants and give the patient a choice of which hospital to attend.

Technology is also used to diagnose patients and communicate findings. For example, X-rays can be viewed by consultants working in a different hospital without the need for bulky pictures to be sent manually from one centre to another. Technology also enables individuals to overcome an impairment which affects their ability to communicate orally; for example through the use of hearing aids or voice-recognition systems.

TYPES OF INTERPERSONAL INTERACTION

Communication in care settings usually takes place as part of an interaction between individuals or in a group. There are many different types of interpersonal interaction that occur every day when working with people. For example, someone working in an early-years setting may interact with children, staff, parents, visitors or contractors. Those working in a care setting may interact with clients, other professionals, staff, voluntary workers, family and friends of service users.

Think Think of as many different people as you can with whom a care worker might interact during the course of the working day.

With all of these different people, a range of different types of interpersonal interaction takes place in the workplace, including speech and language, non-verbal communication and listening. You may also observe variations between different cultures in the way that individuals…

Examples – industry-specific examples show you what the theory looks like in practice

Track your progress

This master grid can be used as a study aid. You can track your progress
by ticking the level you achieve. The relevant grading criteria can also
be found at the start of each unit.

To achieve a pass grade the evidence must show that the learner is able to...	To achieve a merit grade the evidence must show that, in addition to the pass criteria, the learner is able to...	To achieve a distinction grade the evidence must show that, in addition to the pass and merit criteria, the learner is able to...
Unit 1		
P1 describe different types of communication and interpersonal interaction, using examples relevant to health and social care settings		
P2 describe the stages of the communication cycle	**M1** explain how the communication cycle may be used to communicate difficult, complex and sensitive issues	
P3 describe factors that may influence communication and interpersonal interactions with particular reference to health and social care settings		
P4 identify how the communication needs of patients/service users may be assisted, including non-verbal communication	**M2** explain the specific communication needs patients/service users may have that require support, including the use of technology	**D1** analyse how communication in health and social care settings assists patients/service users and other key people
P5 describe two interactions that you have participated in, in the role of a carer, using communication skills to assist patients/service users		
P6 review the effectiveness of own communication skills in the two interactions undertaken	**M3** explain how own communication skills could have been used to make the interactions more effective	**D2** analyse how communication in health and social care settings assists patients/service users and other key people

To achieve a pass grade the evidence must show that the learner is able to...	To achieve a merit grade the evidence must show that, in addition to the pass criteria, the learner is able to...	To achieve a distinction grade the evidence must show that, in addition to the pass and merit criteria, the learner is able to...
Unit 2		
P1 explain the benefits of diversity to society		
P2 use recognised terminology to explain the important of promoting equality, recognising diversity and respecting the rights in health and social care settings		
P3 explain the potential effects of discriminatory practice on those who use health or social care services		
P4 describe how legislation, codes of practice, rules of conduct, charters and organisational policies are used to promote anti-discriminatory practice	**M1** explain the influences of a recent or emerging national policy development on organisational policy with regard to anti-discriminatory practice	**D1** evaluate how a recent or emerging policy development influences organisational and personal practice in relation to anti-discriminatory practice
P5 explain how those working in health and social care settings can actively promote anti-discriminatory practice	**M2** explain difficulties that may be encountered when implementing anti-discriminatory practice	
P6 describe ways of reflecting on and challenging discriminatory issues in health and social care	**M3** analyse how personal beliefs and value systems may influence own anti-discriminatory practice	**D2** evaluate practical strategies to reconcile own beliefs and values with anti-discriminatory practice in health and social care
Unit 3		
P1 use work placement experiences to explain a minimum of six potential hazards in a health or social care setting		
P2 describe how key legislation in relation to health, safety and security influences health and social care delivery		
P3 using examples from work experience describe how policies and procedures promote health, safety and security in the health and social care workplace	**M1** explain how legislation, policies and procedures are used to promote the health, safety and security of individuals in the health and social care workplace	**D1** using examples from work experience evaluate the effectiveness of policies and procedures for promoting health, safety and security
P4 examine the roles and responsibilities of key people in the promotion of health, safety and security in a health or social care setting		
P5 carry out a health and safety survey of a local environment used by a specific patient / service user group	**M2** assess the risk associated with the use of the chosen local environment and make recommendations for change	**D2** justify recommendations made for minimising the risks, as appropriate, for the setting and service user groups.
P6 demonstrate basic first aid skills	**M3** demonstrate first aid skills on a critically injured individual.	

To achieve a pass grade the evidence must show that the learner is able to...	To achieve a merit grade the evidence must show that, in addition to the pass criteria, the learner is able to...	To achieve a distinction grade the evidence must show that, in addition to the pass and merit criteria, the learner is able to...
Unit 4		
P1 describe physical, intellectual, emotional and social development through the life stages		
P2 describe the potential influences of five life factors on the development of individuals	**M1** discuss the nature-nurture debate in relation to individual development	**D1** evaluate the nature-nurture debate in relation to development of the individual
P3 describe the influences of two predictable and two unpredictable major life events on the development of the individual	**M2** explain how major life events can influence the development of the individual	
P4 describe two theories of ageing	**M3** use examples to compare two major theories of ageing	**D2** evaluate the influence of two major theories of ageing on health and social care provision
P5 describe physical and psychological changes due to the ageing process		
Unit 5		
P1 describe the functions of the main cell components	**M1** explain the physiology of three named body systems in relation to energy metabolism	**D1** use examples to explain how body systems interrelate to each other
P2 describe the structure of the main tissues of the body and their role in the functioning of two named body organs	**M2** explain the probable homeostatic responses to changes in the internal environment during exercise	**D2** explain the importance of homeostasis in maintaining the healthy functioning of the body
P3 describe the gross structure and main functions of all major body systems	**M3** analyse data obtained to show how homeostatic mechanisms control the internal environment during exercise	
P4 describe the role of energy in the body and the physiology of three named body systems in relation to energy metabolism		
P5 describe the concept of homeostasis and the homeostatic mechanisms that regulate heart rate, breathing rate, body temperature and blood glucose levels		
P6 measure body temperature, heart rate and breathing rate before and after a standard period of exercise, interpret the data and comment on its validity		

To achieve a pass grade the evidence must show that the learner is able to...	To achieve a merit grade the evidence must show that, in addition to the pass criteria, the learner is able to...	To achieve a distinction grade the evidence must show that, in addition to the pass and merit criteria, the learner is able to...
Unit 6		
P1 explain key influences on personal learning processes of individuals	**M1** analyse the impact of key influences on personal learning processes and on own learning	**D1** evaluate how personal learning and development may benefit others
P2 describe own knowledge, skills, practice, values, beliefs and career aspirations at the start of the programme		
P3 produce and monitor an action plan for self-development and the achievement of own personal goals		
P4 describe own progress against action plans over the duration of the programme	**M2** explain how the action plan has helped support own development over the duration of the programme	**D2** evaluate your own development over the duration of the programme
P5 produce and reflect on own personal and professional development portfolio	**M3** reflect on own experiences and use three examples to explain links between theory and practice	
P6 describe one local health or social care service provider and identify its place in national provision		
P7 describe the roles, responsibilities and career pathways of three health or social care workers		
Unit 7		
P1 use sociological terminology to describe the principal sociological perspectives		
P2 describe different concepts of health	**M1** use two sociological perspectives to explain different concepts of health	
P3 describe the biomedical and socio-medical models of health	**M2** explain the biomedical and socio-medical models of health	**D1** evaluate the biomedical and socio-medical models of health
P4 describe different concepts of ill health		
P5 compare patterns and trends of health and illness in three different social groups	**M3** explain the biomedical and socio-medical models of health	**D2** evaluate the four sociological explanations for health inequalities in terms of explaining the patterns and trends of health and illness in three different social groups.

To achieve a pass grade the evidence must show that the learner is able to...	To achieve a merit grade the evidence must show that, in addition to the pass criteria, the learner is able to...	To achieve a distinction grade the evidence must show that, in addition to the pass and merit criteria, the learner is able to...
Unit 8		
P1 describe the application of behaviourist perspectives in health and social care		
P2 explain the value of the social learning approach to health and social care service provision		
P3 describe the application of psychodynamic perspectives in health and social care	**M1** analyse the contribution of different psychological perspectives to the understanding and management of challenging behaviour	
P4 describe the value of the humanistic approach to health and social care service provision	**M2** analyse the contribution of different psychological perspectives to health and social care provision	**D1** evaluate the roles of different psychological perspectives in health and social care
P5 explain the value of the cognitive perspective in supporting individuals		
P6 describe the application of biological perspectives in health and social care		

Research Skills

Before you start your research project you need to know where to find information and the guidelines you must follow.

Types of information

Primary Sources

Information you have gathered yourself, through surveys, interviews, photos or observation. Ensure that you ask the appropriate questions and people. You must get permission before including someone's photo or interview in your work.

Secondary Sources

Information produced by somebody else, including information from the internet, books, magazines, databases and television. You need to be sure that your secondary source is reliable if you are going to use the information.

Information Sources

The Internet

The internet is a useful research tool, but, not all the information you find will be. When using the internet ask yourself if you can trust the information you find.

> Acknowledge your source! When quoting from the internet always include author name (if known)/document title/URL web address/date site was accessed.

Books, Magazines and Newspapers

Information in newspapers and magazines is up to date and usually researched thoroughly. Books have a longer shelf life than newspapers so make sure you use the most recent edition.

> Acknowledge your source! When quoting from books, magazines, journal or papers, always include author name/ title of publication/publisher/year of publication.

Broadcast Media

Television and radio broadcast current news stories and the information should be accurate. Be aware that some programmes offer personal opinions as well as facts.

Plagiarism

Plagiarism is including in your own work extracts or ideas from another source without acknowledging its origins. If you use any material from other sources you must acknowledge it. This includes the work of fellow students.

Storing Information

Keep a record of all the information you gather. Record details of book titles, author names, page references, web addresses (URLs) and contact details of interviewees. Accurate, accessible records will help you acknowledge sources and find information quickly.

Internet Dos and Don'ts

Do ✔

- check information against other sources

- keep a record of where you found information and acknowledge the source

- be aware that not all sites are genuine or trustworthy

Don't

- assume all the information on the internet is accurate and up to date

- copy material from websites without checking whether permission from the copyright holder is required

- give personal information to people you meet on the internet

Developing Effective Communication in Health and Social Care

unit 1

Communication is central to working in health and social care. Health and social care professionals need to be able to communicate effectively to carry out their roles in caring for others. Understanding how to communicate underpins the practical work you will do during work experience and provides good preparation for future work and study in health and social care.

Communication and interaction with people can take different forms and use different methods. In this unit you will look at the different types in order to gain knowledge and understanding of the ways in which communication can occur. You will also explore the factors that influence communication and interpersonal interactions in health and social care settings. You will see what can help communication, or make it difficult.

The ways in which service users can be helped by effective communication is examined by reviewing the role of support services including other professionals, technology, alternative languages such as Braille or sign language, and support through the promotion of individual rights.

Having looked at the principles of communication you will be expected to develop your own skills and demonstrate them. You should be able to reflect on your performance and that of others by evaluating them against the principles you have studied.

Learning outcomes

In this unit you will:

1.1 Understand effective communication and interpersonal interaction   page 17

1.2 Understand factors that influence communication and interpersonal interactions in health and social care settings   page 27

1.3 Know how patients/service users may be assisted by effective communication   page 40

1.4 Be able to demonstrate own communication skills in a caring role   page 45

So you want to be a...

Health Care Assistant

My name Kathy Robinson
Age 19
Income £5.50–£6 per hour

Working with elderly people can be demanding, but if you've got what it takes, you could find it an emotionally rewarding and satisfying career.

So, what do you do?

I work in a residential home as care assistant working in a team to provide care for older people.

What does a typical day look like?

I work with a group of the residents and help them with their personal care. This includes helping them to wash, bath, get dressed and go to the toilet. The most important part of my job is talking to the residents and making sure they are happy. I have reports fill in at the end of each shift and I take part in the handover to the staff coming on duty.

What made you decide to work in a residential home?

I did two weeks of work experience at a home whilst studying for my BTEC National Diploma. At the end of my time there the manager asked me if I would like to work for them at weekends. I have gradually increased my hours and now work even more over the holidays. It's been great.

How useful has the BTEC been in your work?

The experience I gained helped me with my course and at the same time, the topics we studied also gave me confidence at work. Communication skills are the single most important thing that I have needed, and what I learned in college has really helped me.

What sort of training do you need?

Before we started our work experience placements we did some preparation in college. For example, we discussed such things as confidentiality. At the care home I was given an induction. This covered health and safety and information about the running of the home, as well as my role.

What advice would you give to someone thinking of doing this sort of job?

You need to be able to relate to different people easily. Some of the tasks you need to do are very personal, so you need to be sensitive to the clients and treat them with respect at all times. Working as part of a team is important and rewarding; you also need to be reliable and punctual, and a sense of humour is always useful!

> **"Working as part of a team is rewarding"**

Any future plans?

I've actually now got a place to do nursing training. The experience of working as a health care assistant, as well as my BTEC National Diploma, made a huge difference at my interview. My employer's been brilliant - I can continue to work here part-time when I start my degree in nursing. It will give me even more experience and help with my college expenses.

Grading criteria

The table shows what you need to do to gain a pass, merit or distinction in this part of the qualification. Make sure you refer back to it when you are completing work so you can judge whether you are meeting the criteria and what you need to do to fill in gaps in your knowledge or experience.

In this unit there are 6 evidence activities that give you an opportunity to demonstrate your acheivement of the grading criteria:

page 25	P1	page 44	P4, M2, D1
page 35	P2, M1	page 47	P5
page 39	P3	page 47	P6, M3, D2

The evidence for this unit should be drawn from experience in a health or social care setting. You may also see examples of communication by watching appropriate videos or undertaking role play. Make sure that confidentiality is maintained throughout your writing.

To achieve a pass grade the evidence must show that the learner is able to...	To achieve a merit grade the evidence must show that, in addition to the pass criteria, the learner is able to...	To achieve a distinction grade the evidence must show that, in addition to the pass and merit criteria, the learner is able to...
P1 describe different types of communication and interpersonal interaction, using examples relevant to health and social care settings		
P2 describe the stages of the communication cycle	**M1** explain how the communication cycle may be used to communicate difficult, complex and sensitive issues	
P3 describe factors that may influence communication and interpersonal interactions with particular reference to health and social care settings		
P4 identify how the communication needs of patients/service users may be assisted, including non-verbal communication	**M2** explain the specific communication needs patients/service users may have that require support, including the use of technology	**D1** analyse how communication in health and social care settings assists patients/service users and other key people
P5 describe two interactions that you have participated in, in the role of a carer, using communication skills to assist patients/service users		
P6 review the effectiveness of own communication skills in the two interactions undertaken	**M3** explain how own communication skills could have been used to make the interactions more effective	**D2** analyse the factors that influenced the interactions undertaken

1.1 Understanding effective communication and interpersonal interaction

In order to develop good communication skills it is important to understand how communication and interaction between people works. We will do this by looking at

- types of communication

- types of interpersonal interaction

- the communication cycle.

TYPES OF COMMUNICATION

Every day most individuals experience a huge range of different types of communication.

> **Think** What types of communication have you experienced today? For example, how have you communicated with your friends, your parents or with people you don't know on your way to school or college? What about other forms of communication, such as advertising?

The next section will explore lots of these different types of communication.

One-to-one communication

Conversations between two individuals are used to convey information. Sometimes the information itself is unimportant, but the fact that the two people are communicating can suggest interest and support for each other. At other times the information communicated is very important.

Example

Danny is a psychiatric nurse. Every morning when he comes on duty he goes round all the rooms to chat to each patient individually. He talks to them about things like football and what they watched on television the night before. His line manager has questioned whether this is a good use of his time.

Makeda is a community midwife. She has an appointment to see a woman who is expecting her first baby. Makeda needs to talk to her about the pregnancy and the birth. There are tests to explain and some important decisions the woman needs to take. She will see her in the clinic at the medical centre.

> **Think** These are both examples of one-to-one communication. What do you think are the purposes and outcomes of each?

All care practitioners will, at some point, communicate with clients on a one-to-one basis. In these situations they will need to use a wide range of verbal and other skills to make sure that the communication is effective. We will look at these skills later in the unit.

Group communication

Communication can also take place in group settings. Individuals often react in a different way when they are part of a group, than they would on a one-to-one basis. Some groups will be made up of individuals who know each other well. Other groups will be made up of people who do not meet very often or who have come together for the first time. Within the group there may be a number of different roles. The structure of a group will influence the way communication happens.

Example

At the local hospital a group has been formed to discuss the proposed building of a new surgical ward. The group consists of the senior surgical consultant, the ward manager and a patient, as well as managers responsible for finance and facilities.

Think In this group who do you think will have the most influence and why? How might this affect communication within the group?

Theorists have looked at the way in which groups form. One of the most well known is Bruce Tuckman. In 1965, he outlined the way that small groups form:

- **Forming** – the group members come together. They ask questions about the purpose of the group and what roles are expected. At this point, individuals are not fully committed to the group. Some individuals may feel anxious. Sometimes one person emerges as a possible leader of the group.

- **Storming** – this second stage in the formation of a group can be a period of conflict. There may be arguments between group members about the purpose of the group and who should take various roles. Some groups may fail as individuals drop out.

- **Norming** – the group develops a set of shared values and beliefs. Roles are agreed. The group starts to work together.

- **Performing** – because the group has developed a set of values or norms it is able to work effectively. A sense of group purpose enables the individuals to work together.

Think Think about what happens in your class or when you work in small groups. What are some of the roles that individuals take on in these groups?

Because so much communication takes place in groups many people have studied how groups work. The interaction that happens within groups is known as group dynamics. One of the most well known studies is the work undertaken by R.F. Bales in 1970. He analysed the behaviours of group members and suggested that they fell into certain categories:

- behaviours that focus on the task

- behaviours that maintain the group

- behaviours that block communication in the group.

Table 1.1 gives examples of these different types of behaviour.

Table 1.1 Different types of behaviours

Behaviours	Examples
Task focused	• giving suggestions • giving opinions • giving information, e.g. clarifying points, confirming ideas • asking for information • asking for opinions • asking for suggestions
Group maintenance	• agreeing • supporting • relieving tension, e.g. with humour • including all members
Communication blocking	• disagreeing • being aggressive in attacking or defending a point of view • dominating • excluding members or 'pairing off'

Example

Here is a transcript of a meeting, in which four carers are planning a day out for their clients.

Carlos – I think that we should go to the cinema.

Henry – No, I think that's a rubbish idea. Who wants to be stuck indoors for three hours?

Parvati – I think there are good reasons for suggesting the cinema, but let's look at what other options there are.

Henry – Well, I was thinking we should go to the seaside for the day. I've taken people there before and they've really enjoyed it. If Carlos doesn't want to come with his clients, that's fine by me. We can still go.

Kate – I can just see you, Henry, with candyfloss and a kiss-me-quick hat! (*Everyone laughs*) Anyway, let's look at what the various options are, including the costs. Also, we must ask our clients what they would like best.

Carlos – Yes. I was only making a suggestion. How about making a list of all the possible outings and then asking our clients? We could meet again next week and see what has come up as the favourite.

Parvati – Good idea. Right, let's get down to that list. All ideas on the table.

Think What are the different behaviours illustrated in this transcript?

Formal communication

Formal communication can use a range of different methods. There are many occasions when it is necessary to make sure that information is shared formally. This may be because of legal requirements, such as health and safety information, or because treatment or a diagnosis may depend on the correct facts being communicated. Teaching and training are often undertaken using formal communication methods. Formal communication can occur verbally or in writing, either in a letter or by email, for example. In some instances several different methods may be used to convey the same information to ensure that there is full understanding.

Think In what instances might people be asked to sign to confirm that they have understood what has been explained to them?

Informal communication

Informal communication happens whenever we are in contact with others. Working in health and social care provides constant opportunities for informal communication, including short conversations and chats. Informal communication is often unplanned and therefore it is important that care workers always act in an appropriate manner in order that the highest standards are maintained.

The basis for all care is the care values. These values must be applied to all communication, including any informal communication. The five main areas of care values are:

- promoting anti-discriminatory practice

- maintaining confidentiality

- promoting and supporting individuals' rights

- acknowledging individuals' personal beliefs and identities

- promoting effective communication.

Key words

Care values – the set of values and principles that should underpin all practice in health, care and early-years settings

Example

Lisa works in a day nursery. It cares for children from a wide range of different ethnic backgrounds. She is responsible for a group of three- and four-year-olds. Every day she chats to them as she plays with them. They sometimes share stories about their home lives. She notes that there are several different religions among the children and they follow different practices.

Think How should Lisa ensure that her informal communications with the children do not contradict the care-value base?

Text

Written communication is used often in care settings. This not only includes handwritten information, but the increasing use of email and other electronic forms of communication. Lots of different types of information are communicated using text, including patients' records, policies and procedures, letters and memos, and care plans. Care workers frequently have to spend time ensuring that records are up to date and relevant.

> **Think** Choose a care setting. What examples of text-based communication might be used in that setting?

Oral

The basis of oral communication is spoken language. However, it is not only through words that oral communication takes place. The cycle of speaking and listening can also be affected by the way in which the words are spoken. The **tone** of voice used by the speaker can affect how the information is received. If someone sounds bored or angry it influences how the listener reacts. If the **pitch** or volume is high or low it may give the impression of shouting or whispering, either of which may convey an inappropriate message. The **pace** of speech needs to ensure that it is clear and easily understood. **Styles** of speech may reflect the community from which the speaker comes. For example, different terms of affection, such as 'pet' or 'love', are used in different parts of the country.

> **Think** In what different ways are older people addressed by their carers? Do any of these ways make communication more difficult? If so, why?

Communication does not rely only on speech and language. A lot of information is communicated visually and sometimes does not need words to explain the message (see Figure 1.1). This includes the visual messages conveyed by facial expressions and body language. The use of visual techniques to communicate can be very powerful. Advertising companies develop brand identities that no longer rely on words to convey their messages. The use of a certain colour or design is enough to communicate the message.

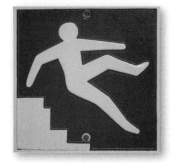

Figure 1.1 Hazard signs communicate warnings visually

Touch

The acceptability of touching another person varies from situation to situation. Different cultures have different norms regarding the role of touching as a method of communication. In addition, there may be different 'rules' about how close people should be in relation to each other. In the UK, individuals tend to stand further apart and touch each other less than in some other parts of the world.

Used appropriately, touch can convey messages of support, caring and affection. In other circumstances touch may be seen as suggesting dominance or sexual interest. Care workers need to take care to ensure that any circumstance in which they use touch to communicate is appropriate, welcomed and understood by the client.

Music and drama

Music and drama can be used as a way of communicating and expressing a range of feelings. They can be used when individuals are having difficulty in expressing themselves in other ways. Music can be used to calm and soothe, and to promote relaxation. It can also be used as an opportunity to promote communication within groups.

Example

Leon is a youth worker. He has a large group of teenagers who visit the youth centre each Saturday night. The group has split into several different groups and there are signs of tensions growing between them. He has suggested that they should all try to put on a play together which involves music and drama. This has been met with enthusiasm as a number of the young people see themselves as good musicians and actors.

Think How might communication between the groups be improved by putting on such an event?

Arts and crafts

In the same way that music and drama can provide a means of communication, so may the use of arts and crafts. They are used as therapeutic activities in many care settings. Children, clients with mental health problems and those with learning disabilities may particularly benefit from such activities in aiding communication. Psychologists may use pictures drawn by children as a basis for understanding family relationships that a child cannot express in words.

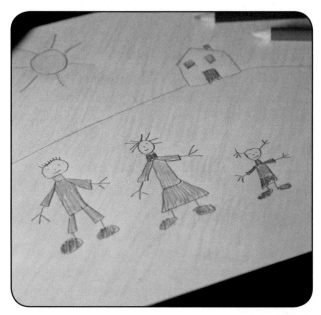

Figure 1.2 A child's depicition of their family life

Communication using technology

The use of technology for communication is increasing all the time. Many records are now stored electronically. The NHS has begun a massive project to introduce an electronic patient-record system. This will not only keep details of individual patients, but allow GPs to book appointments with hospital consultants and give the patient a choice of which hospital to attend.

Technology is also used to diagnose patients and communicate findings. For example, X-rays can be viewed by consultants working in a different hospital without the need for bulky pictures to be sent manually from one centre to another. Technology also enables individuals to overcome an impairment which affects their ability to communicate orally; for example through the use of hearing aids or voice-recognition systems.

TYPES OF INTERPERSONAL INTERACTION

Communication in care settings usually takes place as part of an interaction between individuals or in a group. There are many different types of interpersonal interaction that occur every day when working with people. For example, someone working in an early-years setting may interact with children, staff, parents, visitors or contractors. Those working in a care setting may interact with clients, other professionals, staff, voluntary workers, family and friends of service users.

Think Think of as many different people as you can with whom a care worker might interact during the course of the working day.

With all of these different people, a range of different types of interpersonal interaction takes place in the workplace, including speech and language, non-verbal communication and listening. You may also observe variations between different cultures in the way that individuals communicate and interact.

Speech and language

The words 'speech' and 'language' are often used interchangeably to describe the interaction of people talking to each other. However, speech is linked with *how* we say words while language defines *what* we say.

Different people have different styles of speaking. These styles may be influenced by their cultural backgrounds or communities. Regional or national accents can be very distinctive and sometimes difficult to understand outside the immediate geographical area. As we have already seen, the tone of voice used, including pitch and volume, can convey a meaning quite separate from the words that are being used. A warm and friendly tone of voice with the words spoken in a calm, clear and well-paced manner can convey reassurance and support.

> **Think** What celebrities or other well known people can you think of who have different styles of speaking? How easy is it to fully understand them?

Children start to develop language skills very early in life. The use of words follows a period of 'babbling' as babies interact with their care givers. The first clear words are usually heard some time after a baby is a year old. From then onwards language develops quickly.

It has been demonstrated that children under the age of 11 years are very receptive to learning, not only their own language but other languages as well. Most people have a first language. A few people are completely bilingual as two languages are spoken equally at home. A person's first language is usually the language that he or she is most comfortable using. In the UK it is assumed that most people have English as their first language, but this may not always be the case.

Key words

First language – the language that is the first one a child learns or the language spoken at home

Regional influences may affect speech and language. There may be differences in vocabulary, grammar and pronunciation. This is known as a **dialect**. Sometimes the differences are only slight, but in other instances they are so marked as to make communication difficult.

> ### Example
>
> The following is a quote from a research project published by Mildred Blaxter in 1982. She asked women to describe health and disease.
>
> *'I dinna think their surroundings has onything to dee wi'it. I mean, you could have ony God's amount of money and the best of everything to give them, and you could hae the most unhealthiest child in the world. An' you could have nothing, an' hae to work an' bring them up yourself, an' you'll find you've got the healthiest kids.'*

> **Think** Why might it be important to ensure that you fully understand what is being said by an individual who is describing their health?

Slang refers to words that are used in informal language. They are not part of standard English expressions and are not expected to be used in formal situations. Slang words often change as new ones come into fashion, and they may be particularly linked with certain groups. The use of slang can exclude individuals from a particular group. Other expressions may be seen as belittling. Some slang expressions eventually become accepted into formal language.

Jargon is the technical or specialised language used by professionals. Although jargon is very important to ensure accurate communication between professionals, it can be very confusing for service users. Care workers need to take particular care to ensure that information has been fully understood by their clients.

Example

The following are commonly used medical terms or jargon. Try to match them to their meanings.

aphasia	abnormally low body temperature
rhinitis	loss of ability to speak or understand speech
dyspepsia	inflammation of the inside of the nose
hypertension	abnormally fast heartbeat
tachycardia	indigestion
hypothermia	high blood pressure

Non-verbal interaction

Interactions do not only occur through talking to other people. They can happen in a number of non-verbal ways.

Posture and body language

We send messages through the positions of the body. Sometimes the messages these convey are subconscious, but in other situations a decision could be made to convey or reinforce a message by adopting a particular posture or using certain body language.

The way an individual sits or stands can reveal what he or she is feeling and communicate this very clearly to others. If someone is standing or sitting very rigidly it may convey he/she feels serious or anxious about the situation. However, if someone is sitting in a very casual manner it may suggest a relaxed approach. Leaning forward can indicate interest in what is being said. People's hands and what they are doing with them can also give messages. Are they sitting with their hands still or are they fidgeting and showing anxiety? The muscle tension in the body can also be a good indicator of a person's state of mind. Care practitioners need to be able to read the messages coming from the individual with whom they are interacting and also be aware of the messages that they themselves are conveying.

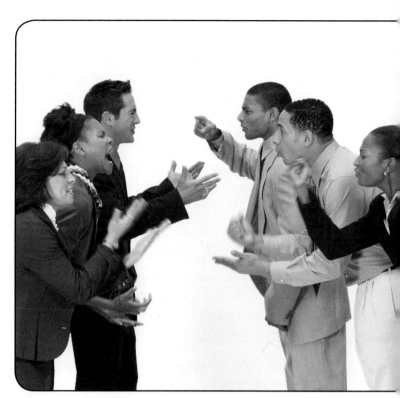

Figure 1.3 Your body language can say a lot about how you feel

> **Think** Look at Figure 1.3. What messages are being communicated through body language and posture?

Facial expression

Facial expressions and the type of eye contact that is made are a useful indication of what another person is feeling. We subconsciously take in what is being shown through facial expressions and eye contact. However, some people may try to hide their true feelings by controlling their expressions.

A lot can be expressed through someone's eyes. The eyes may be open wide or narrowed. The length of any eye contact can have different meanings. A long fixed stare is often interpreted as an angry look, while a long contact which then becomes a smile may indicate a friendly approach. Narrowed eyes might suggest suspicion. A look away might be because of boredom or embarrassment. However, it is important to remember that eye contact is also culturally influenced.

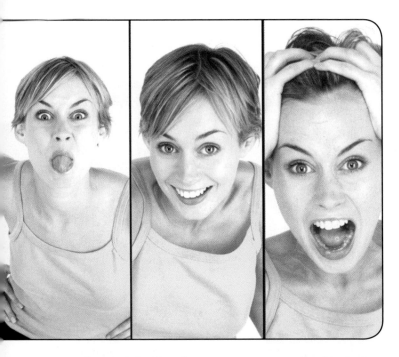

Figure 1.4 *Facial expressions are a good indicator of a person's mood*

Gestures

Hand and arm movements can be used to convey a meaning. Some people use their hands frequently when they are talking to illustrate or emphasise a point. Some gestures carry a particular meaning of their own, such as a thumbs-up sign, although there may be variation in meaning from country to country.

Touch

Touch is frequently used in care settings to convey messages of support or care. However, used inappropriately it can be misunderstood as indicating a sexual interest or as a way of having power over an individual.

Silence

It may sound strange, but silence can convey a message in an interaction between people. A space between words can give a sense of calm and an unrushed approach. Counsellors often allow periods of silence in which their clients are given space to think and consider. On the negative side, a silent reaction may indicate anger or disagreement and lack of co-operation.

Proximity

The physical space between people is known as their proximity. Like touch, it can convey different meanings and be interpreted in different ways. Sometimes it is very appropriate to move closer to an individual. At other times it may be seen as invading an individual's personal space and may make him or her feel uncomfortable.

Reflective listening

Non-verbal interactions can also indicate that the carer is listening to the service user. This can be done in a number of ways. Nodding the head encourages a speaker to continue and expand on what they are saying. Sounds like 'Mmm' are frequently used. In 1986 Gerald Egan suggested the following as a reminder of the non-verbal actions that can be taken to help communication:

Face the other person	**S** quarely
Adopt an	**O** pen posture
	L ean towards the other person slightly
Maintain good	**E** ye contact
Try to be	**R** elaxed while paying attention

Variation between cultures

We have already suggested that there may be significant variations between different cultures. These variations may be in attitudes, as well as in language and non-verbal communication. Certain cultures have expectations of who in the family should be spoken to and who will make the decisions. In some cultures it would not be acceptable for a woman to be seen by a male doctor or nurse. There may be obvious differences in language, but some are more subtle. For example, both British people and Americans speak English, but use some of the same words very differently with different meanings. Care needs to be taken that not only is the meaning clear, but unintentional messages are not inadvertently conveyed.

Example

Many common gestures used in the UK have a very different meaning in other cultures.

- Beckoning using your index finger: this can be insulting or an obscene gesture in some cultures including Spain, and the Middle and Far East.
- Pointing using your index finger: it is not acceptable to point with an index finger in the Middle and Far East.
- Sitting with the sole of your foot or shoe showing: this is a sign of disrespect in some cultures, particularly in Thailand.
- Nodding to indicate agreement: in Greece nodding means 'No'.
- Patting a child on the head: this is not acceptable in parts of Asia. The head is seen as the most important part of the body in some religions.
- Forming a circle with thumb and first finger – while in the UK this gesture is taken to indicate that something is 'OK' or 'perfect', in Germany it is regarded as obscene and in France means 'zero'.

Listening and reflecting back

Communication is a two way process. It requires that messages are listened to. There are several aspects that affect the listening process: the **linguistic** or spoken aspects, the **paralinguistic** aspects, such as tone and accent, and the **non-verbal** aspects.

Care workers listen to, and communicate with, service users in a range of different situations. They may be giving or collecting information, providing help and support, building relationships or checking understanding. There are various practices that can help in ensuring that listening is effective. These skills include:

- showing **empathy**
- checking for **understanding**
- asking **open questions**.

Showing empathy means demonstrating the ability to understand the feelings of others. It does not necessarily mean agreeing with their point of view, but it means showing an acceptance of them and a non-judgmental attitude. Empathy can be demonstrated by the listener repeating or reflecting back a statement made by the service user. For example, the listener might say, 'from what you are saying it sounds as if you are very anxious about …'.

It is sometimes important to ensure that there is a clear understanding of an issue. It may be important to check that the service user has fully understood what has been communicated. The listener can check understanding by asking questions that seek to **clarify**, **paraphrase** or **reflect** what has been said. Clarifying might mean repeating or recapping the information. Paraphrasing involves repeating the information in a summarised way to ensure that it is all fully understood. Reflecting means repeating back some of the words directly, sometimes in a questioning manner.

There are different types of questions. **Open questions** are those that require more than a 'yes' or 'no' answer. They give an opportunity for the speaker to give a longer answer; for example, 'how are you feeling today?'. The service user is able to cover a number of different aspects of how they are feeling in their answer. However, a closed question, such as 'are you feeling better today?' gives little opportunity for any description as it asks for a short, one word answer.

Evidence activity

P1

1. Before you go on work experience make a list of all the types of communication and interpersonal interaction. Keep a record of the types of communication and interaction you experience during your work experience. (P1)

2. Using your list and the record of your work experience describe the different types of communication and interpersonal interaction and give examples of what you have observed. (P1)

THE COMMUNICATION CYCLE

Communication occurs between a sender and a receiver, who in turn sends feedback to the original sender. This process therefore goes round in a circular manner and is known as the communication cycle (see Figure 1.5).

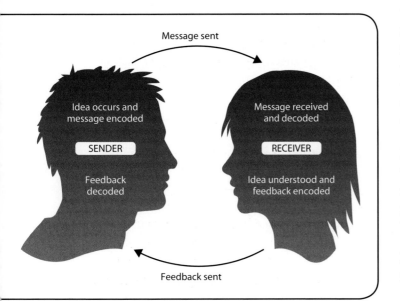

Figure 1.5 Communication cycle

The stages in the communication cycle can be described as follows:

- ideas occur
- message coded
- message sent
- message received
- message decoded
- message understood
- feedback to sender.

The first stage is when the idea or thought occurs as to what information needs to be communicated and to whom. The sender then **encodes** the message by putting it into a form that can be understood by the receiver. This may mean making a choice of appropriate language or images. The message is then sent. Alongside any verbal communication is the non-verbal communication conveyed through the posture, facial expressions, touch or proximity of the sender. The message is received through listening, looking or reading. The receiver then **decodes** the message, interpreting the meaning of the message and gaining understanding. By taking in all the information that has been received, both verbal and non-verbal, the message is **understood**.

Most interpersonal interaction involves a two-way communication. The original receiver of the message **feeds back** to the sender. This process is then repeated and a pattern of speaking and listening is established.

Inevitably there are factors along the way that can influence the effectiveness of the communication cycle. We will look at some of these in more detail in section 1.2.

Example

Fei Yen is a nursery nurse. She has responsibility for the eight three-year-olds who attend the day nursery. She works with her colleagues Latoya and Jayanta, who have recently qualified. The children have been getting very bored as they have been indoors because of the wet weather. Today is looking much brighter and there might be a chance of going outside.

Think What communication cycle might Fei Yen use to change the routine, communicating with both the children and the staff?

1.2 Understanding factors that influence communication and interpersonal interactions in health and social care settings

This section will explore some of the factors that influence communication and interpersonal interactions, particularly in health and social care settings. By being aware of these factors you will be able to recognise any steps you could take to help communication and identify factors that might be a barrier to good communication.

COMMUNICATION AND LANGUAGE NEEDS, AND PREFERENCES

Although language is the most common method of communication, it cannot be assumed that all communication should take place by using the most common language of a country, for instance, English in the UK. There are other ways of communicating that may be more appropriate for certain individuals or situations.

Example

Mr and Mrs Khan have lived in the UK for over 30 years since coming from Pakistan to study at university in the UK. Their parents remained in Pakistan and they used to visit them every few years. Mr Khan's father has now died and they have brought his mother over to England to live with them. Mrs Khan senior is very frail and needs to visit a doctor for a full medical examination. She does not speak any English. Mr and Mrs Khan can interpret for her, but are aware that some things may be difficult to explain to her. If she has to go into hospital they cannot be with her all the time as they are both at work.

Think
What communication problems are there likely to be for Mrs Khan senior and anyone who may be caring for her?

The individual's preferred language

It may not always be possible to speak to someone in their preferred spoken language, but carers should try to ascertain what an individual's preference is. There should not be an assumption that everybody living or staying in the UK is able to or prefers to communicate in English. Some people speak very little English, while others may be able to speak enough to 'get by', but may struggle with jargon or specialist terms. At times of stress it may be particularly difficult for individuals to communicate in anything other than their preferred spoken language.

In certain areas of the UK, the numbers of non-English speakers may be so significant that language support is well developed. Strategies to ensure that the language needs of individuals are met include providing letters and leaflets translated into the most common languages used in the locality, multilingual signposting, and access to staff who are able to speak the language.

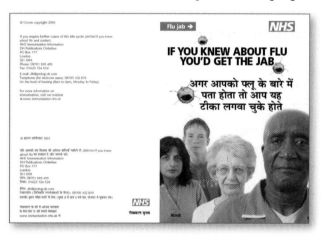

Figure 1.6   Information published by the NHS in Hindi

When speaking to someone who does not share the same language it is important to speak clearly and avoid using jargon. Sentences should ideally be short. It may be necessary to reword information to make it more easily understandable. The Red Cross produce an emergency multilingual phrasebook. Based on a questionnaire covering essential information that might be required by health professionals in an emergency, it is available in 36 languages.

Research tip

You can download copies of the multilingual phrasebook from www.dh.gov.uk/publications.

Signs, symbols, pictures and writing

The appropriate use of signs can be an effective way of communicating. Some gestures or signs can help to convey a message. Perhaps the best known example is the use of sign language for those who have hearing impairments. The sign language used in the UK is known as **British Sign Language** (BSL). In addition to the finger spelling chart shown in Figure 1.7, there are a range of gestures that allow words to be communicated.

In addition to the signs made in interactions between individuals, organisations can ensure that appropriate printed signs and symbols are used to give information to service users, for example, directions to clinics, to fire escapes or to toilets, etc. Many symbols are recognised internationally while others may be used to convey specific information in a particular situation.

Research tip

There are many websites that demonstrate British Sign Language, including www.britishsignlanguage.com/.

Think Can you think of any other symbols related to health or social care that are universally recognised?

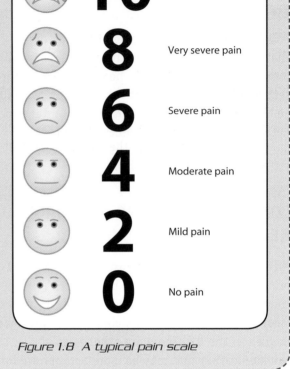

Figure 1.8 A typical pain scale

Pictures and writing can also help support communication. Cards depicting various activities or needs can be shown to clients. Children may be asked to describe how they are feeling by pointing to a cartoon face depicting different emotions. Patients who are in pain may be asked to point out the level of their pain on a pain scale (see Figure 1.8).

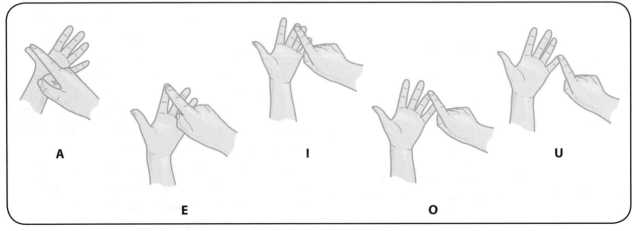

Figure 1.7 The two-handed manual alphabet used by many sighted deaf people

Objects of reference

Objects that symbolise an activity or idea and which therefore become associated with it can be used instead of words. For example, a towel might be used to symbolise having a bath. Meal times may be symbolised by a spoon. Objects of reference can be used with children or with adults with communication difficulties. An individual who is blind and deaf could use the feel of a towel to know that it was time to have a bath. The use of objects of reference promotes choice as the individual can indicate what they want to do by pointing to or selecting the object of reference. The object needs to be chosen with care with the individual so that there is no confusion as to its meaning.

Example

Roberto has learning difficulties and cannot communicate verbally. He likes to go swimming, and uses a pair of goggles as an object of reference.

Communication passports

The idea of a communication passport was first developed by Sally Millar, a specialist speech and language therapist at the Communication Aids for Language and Learning (CALL) Centre, University of Edinburgh in 1991. She suggested that children with a range of communication difficulties could be given better support if the information about their needs and preferences was readily available to all those who care for them (see Figure 1.9).

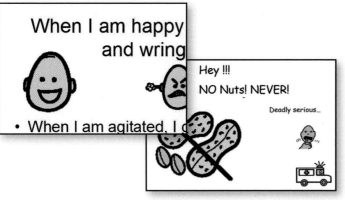

Figure 1.9   Pages from a personal communication passport [Source: Personal Communication Passports by Sally Millar PCS © Mayer-Johnson Inc.]

The passports aim to:

- present the child positively as an individual, not as a set of problems or disabilities

- pull together key information, both past and present, from different sources

- describe the most effective means of communication with the child

- present the information in an attractive and easy to understand way.

> **Think** What are the advantages of developing communication passports for children with communication difficulties?

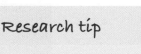

Research tip

More information about communication passports can be found at www.communicationpassports.org.uk.

Human and technological aids to communication

Other people can help in communication between service users and carers in a formal or informal manner. A service user's relatives may be more familiar with his/her mannerisms and expressions and will therefore be able to make helpful suggestions relating to what the service user is trying to communicate.

There are also formal services that may be used, such as interpreters, signers or note takers. The use of an interpreter for a client who does not have English as their first language can greatly benefit the care of that patient. Some organisations keep a list of people who are qualified to act as interpreters and who can be called upon even in an emergency. When using an interpreter it is important that the client and interpreter are given an opportunity to get to know and understand each other. Questions should be directed to the service user, not the interpreter. Speech needs to be slow, clear and in short sections so there is time for the interpreter to translate while they can remember what has been said. For those who have a hearing disability a signer can be used to interpret what is being said. A note taker may be needed if an individual needs to concentrate on watching a signer or lip reading the speaker, as they will not be able to make their own notes at the same time.

Technological aids are improving all the time in availability and sophistication. Hearing aids have been in use for many years, but are becoming more effective and much less bulky. They amplify sounds so that they can be heard more easily. Cochlea implants can be used to directly stimulate the auditory nerve using a microphone, speech processor and transmitter to send messages to the brain. Voice-recognition systems, synthesisers and computer-aided communication have opened up communication for individuals with speech disabilities.

CASE STUDY: STEPHEN HAWKING

The most well known person to use these systems is Professor Stephen Hawking, who speaks, writes and lectures, despite having severe physical problems caused by the degenerative Motor-Neurone Disease. Here is an extract from his website www.hawking.org.uk.

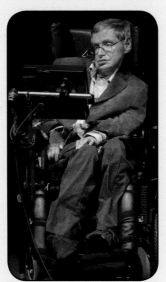

'In 1985 I had to have a tracheotomy operation. After this, I had to have 24-hour nursing care.

Before the operation, my speech had been getting more slurred, so that only a few people, who knew me well, could understand me. But at least I could communicate. I wrote scientific papers by dictating to a secretary, and I gave seminars through an interpreter, who repeated my words more clearly. However, the tracheotomy operation removed my ability to speak altogether. For a time, the only way I could communicate was to spell out words letter by letter, by raising my eyebrows when someone pointed to the right letter on a spelling card. It is pretty difficult to carry on a conversation like that, let alone write a scientific paper. However, a computer expert in California, called Walt Woltosz, heard of my plight. He sent me a computer program he had written, called Equalizer. This allowed me to select words from a series of menus on the screen, by pressing a switch in my hand. The program could also be controlled by a switch, operated by head or eye movement. When I have built up what I want to say, I can send it to a speech synthesizer.

David Mason, of Cambridge Adaptive Communication, fitted a small portable computer and a speech synthesizer to my wheel chair. This system allowed me to communicate much better than I could before. I can manage up to 15 words a minute. I can either speak what I have written, or save it to disk. I can then print it out, or call it back and speak it sentence by sentence. Using this system, I have written a book, and dozens of scientific papers. I have also given many scientific and popular talks. One's voice is very important. If you have a slurred voice, people are likely to treat you as mentally deficient.'

QUESTIONS

1. What changes have there been in how Professor Hawking communicates as his disease has progressed?

2. What has been the role of technology in helping him to communicate?

ENVIRONMENT

The environment in which communication takes place can determine its effectiveness and quality. The main environmental factors to be considered are the setting, noise level, seating and lighting.

Example

Sunita is the staff nurse in charge on a ward for older people. She receives a phone call from the daughter of one of the patients, Mrs Jones. She tells Sunita that Mr Jones has been taken seriously ill overnight and that neither she nor her father will be in at their usual visiting time. She asks Sunita to inform Mrs Jones of the situation. Mrs Jones is currently in the day room with the other patients waiting for her lunch. The television is on. All the chairs around the outside of the room are full. A number of staff are in the room chatting to the patients and having a laugh with them. Mrs Jones is slightly deaf.

> ***Think*** What would you do if you were Sunita? What issues in the environment might affect her communication with Mrs Jones?

Setting

The setting in which communication takes place can have a major effect. It is important to try to assess whether or not the setting is appropriate for the type and content of communication that is going to take place. If there are personal or sensitive matters to discuss, a private setting should be found. If there is to be a talk to a group of people then an appropriately sized room is needed. Trying to communicate when there are frequent interruptions, such as phone calls or visitors, causes

disruption. All care professionals should be aware of the importance of communicating information only in appropriate settings. For example, it would be inappropriate to talk to parents about their child's progress at nursery if you met them casually while out shopping.

Noise

Different people are able to tolerate different amounts of noise. Many young people happily work with loud music in the background. Televisions and radios are often left on permanently during the day in residential care homes. Traffic noise may also be particularly intrusive, especially in the summer months when windows are left open. Any type of noise may affect communication. However, noise may particularly affect older people. Physical changes associated with the ageing process cause difficulties in hearing. There is a gradual loss in the ability to hear high- and low-pitched sounds, which is made worse in the presence of high levels of background noise.

Seating

The way that people are seated in relation to others can influence how they communicate. The position may give an immediate impression of what type of communication is going to take place. A lecture hall that has rows of chairs facing the front and where there is a place for a tutor to stand behind a desk tells the participants that this is a formal occasion when they are likely to be 'talked to' and will only contribute when invited to do so. In group work it may be important to have contributions from all members of the group, and so seating should be arranged to facilitate this. The way the seating is arranged in one-to-one situations may be important, depending on the purpose of the meeting. Sometimes it can be appropriate to have a space between the participants.

Think Look at the photos in Figure 1.10. What sort of communication do you think is occurring in each one? Is each participant contributing equally? How does the seating reinforce this type of communication?

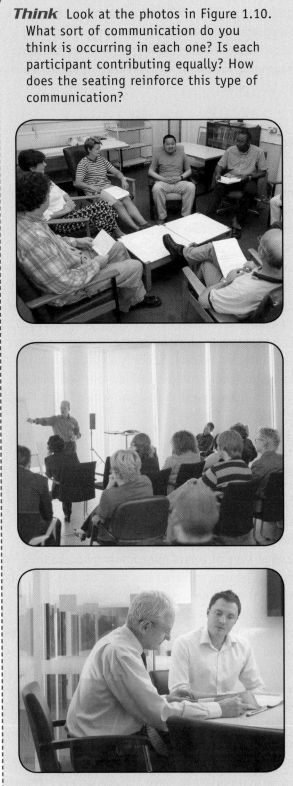

Figure 1.10 Different kinds of communication

Lighting

Because we often rely on non-verbal communication to fully understand what is meant, lighting can be important. Poor lighting may mean that clues from facial expressions or body language are missed. Anyone relying on being able to lip read the speaker needs good lighting to see their mouth. Sometimes glare from the sun or certain types of artificial light may cause reflection. If there is strong light behind a speaker then their face may be obscured.

BEHAVIOUR

The behaviour of both the speaker and receiver of information can affect communication. All communication is best undertaken in a 'good' atmosphere. This enables people to concentrate on the message rather than being distracted by other issues.

Attitude

Individuals' beliefs, feelings, values and tendencies can cause them to respond in certain ways. People are sometimes described as having a negative or positive attitude. Knowing what attitude someone holds may influence the way in which any communication is undertaken. The attitude of both the speaker and recipient can affect the content and the manner of the communication.

Example

Mrs Stewart is 92 years old. She has always been very independent and has lived on her own since her husband died 10 years ago. She has always said that she wants to die in her own home. She has had a number of falls recently. Her daughter and her GP think she should consider going into a residential home. They are going to talk to her about it shortly.

Think What sort of attitude do you think Mrs Stewart has about residential care? How might her attitude affect the communication between herself, her daughter and her GP?

Assertiveness

Assertive behaviour is where individuals are able to stay in control of their own emotions and to stand up for themselves. Being assertive enables them to express their own feelings and needs to ensure that their personal rights are respected. Assertiveness skills can be developed and are linked with an individual having a positive self concept. The characteristics of assertive behaviour are:

- showing respect for others
- negotiating with others
- trying to solve problems
- ability to express own needs
- listening to others.

Non-verbal behaviour associated with assertiveness includes a warm and relaxed tone of voice, open and varied eye contact, relaxed facial expressions and a posture that conveys a sense of being in control.

Aggressiveness

If individuals are determined to get their own way, even at the expense of others, they may show aggressiveness. This is dominant behaviour that seeks to humiliate or 'put others down'. Aggressive individuals very often express anger. The characteristics of aggressive behaviour are:

- determination to get one's own way
- not being interested in others' needs
- making demands
- humiliating others
- not listening
- shouting or talking very loudly.

Non-verbal behaviour associated with aggressiveness includes an angry, cold and demanding tone of voice, cold, narrowed and fixed eye contact, a tense and angry facial expression, and a stiff and rigid posture with arms folded or with clenched fists, pointing fingers, etc.

Submissiveness

Submissive behaviour is shown when an individual is willing to carry out the wishes of others. Sometimes those who are submissive do things that are against their own good because they are frightened or unwilling to stand up for their own wants or needs. It is the opposite of aggressive behaviour, and is sometimes a response to aggression. The main characteristics of submissive behaviour are:

- not expressing own views or wants
- agreeing with others
- letting others win
- being afraid.

Non-verbal behaviour associated with submissiveness includes a quiet tone of voice, not making eye contact or looking away, frightened or anxious facial expression and tense and submissive posture.

Think Look back at the example of Mrs Stewart on page 32. How might she have responded to the suggestion of going into a residential home in an assertive manner, an aggressive manner and a submissive manner?

Responses to behaviour

These different types of behaviour provoke different responses from the person on the receiving end. This is part of the interaction that occurs during communication. The feedback from the receiver often influences the way in which the communication cycle continues. For example, if someone has a negative attitude to a proposal, much more effort may be required to persuade him or her to agree, while a positive attitude may allow the conversation to move more swiftly. Assertive behaviour encourages negotiation and is a good basis for ensuring that the views of all parties are expressed. The response to assertive behaviour can therefore be positive, as each person feels valued and respected. Aggressive behaviour can cause either an aggressive response in reply or a submissive response. Neither response is satisfactory in ensuring effective communication.

Effects on identity, self-esteem and self-image

How people are treated may affect their identity, and how they view both themselves and others. Self-esteem is determined by how much someone likes, accepts, and respects him or herself as a person. Someone with low self-esteem feels undervalued and can easily be influenced by others. Those with high self-esteem feel independent and capable of taking decisions and influencing others. Behaviour can cause or reinforce feelings associated with self-esteem and self-worth.

BARRIERS

Barriers to effective communication can exhibit a range of different forms, some of which have already been discussed.

Example

Hajar has been admitted to hospital for tests. She is in a busy and noisy ward with a number of other women. She arrived in the UK as an asylum seeker two months ago. She speaks little English and her husband is detained in their country. She is very worried about him and the other family members that she has left behind. She is a devout Muslim. The doctor thinks that she may be pregnant and that there may be complications which could endanger her unborn child. It is against her culture to be examined by a man, however all the local consultants are male. It is important that decisions are made soon before her health and that of any baby are put at risk.

> **Think** What barriers might there be to communicating with Hajar? How might these be overcome?

Type of communication

People working in health and care settings are frequently called on to communicate difficult, complex or sensitive information. These types of communication may present barriers to effective communication and may need careful consideration and planning in order to overcome them.

There are a variety of reasons why the information to be communicated may be difficult. For example, the issue itself may be difficult for the individual to accept or discuss, such as the closure of a residential home or jobs that are due to be lost. Difficulties may also arise from a personality clash or conflict between two individuals.

Some information can be complex for the recipient to understand. It may be the responsibility of a care worker to explain medical, financial or social issues to individuals. Professional terminology may make the information even more difficult to understand. It is important that care is taken to ensure that complex information is fully understood, particularly if decisions need to be based on it.

Sensitive information may be linked to very personal issues. It may relate to the individual or to members of their family. At times, people may suppress knowledge that is too difficult to face, yet it may need to be raised in certain circumstances; for example, the paternity of a child who has a life-threatening genetically inherited disease.

Evidence activity

P2 – M1

1. Draw a diagram of the communication cycle and describe each stage. You could illustrate the cycle by describing an interaction that you have witnessed. (P2)

2. Identify a difficult, complex or sensitive issue that has been communicated at your work placement. Explain how the communication cycle is used in these circumstances. (M1)

Language needs and preferences

Failure to recognise the language needs or preferences of an individual creates a barrier to effective communication. Sometimes information can be shared without an interpreter, but other more complex issues will require the more specialised help of an interpreter. If possible the preferences of an individual should be explored.

Disability

Disabilities that can cause barriers to communication can result from physical, mental or learning disabilities. Some are associated with the ageing process, but others are the result of disabilities that have been present from birth or have been caused by illness or accidents. Some disabilities affect the ability to speak, but others affect the way in which non-verbal communication takes place.

> *Think* What different types of disability can you think of that might cause a barrier to communication?

Personality

People's personalities affect their behaviour and thinking, making them different from each other. Some people are more receptive to other people and to receiving information. This means that the personality of an individual may either help or hinder effective communication.

Environment

Environmental barriers to effective communication include noise, lighting and the physical space in which the communication is taking place. If difficult, complex or sensitive information needs to be shared, an unsuitable environment may create even more of a barrier. For example, if a care worker wants to discuss particularly personal issues the physical surroundings may be very important. Nobody would want such discussions to occur in the middle of a crowded day room.

Time

The amount of time that is available for any communication may be a barrier to communicating effectively. Rushed explanations can lead to misunderstandings. A brief consultation may leave many unanswered questions. There may be times in the day when it is most appropriate to discuss certain issues. Talking to people about difficult issues close to the time they are going to bed may cause them to worry throughout the night.

Self-esteem

Self-esteem is affected by how individuals view themselves and their worth. Both high and low levels of self-esteem can cause a barrier to communication. An individual with particularly high self-esteem may be very self-confident and unwilling to listen to advice or other information that they do not consider relevant. If individuals have low self-esteem they may be easily influenced and might find it difficult to express their own views and thoughts.

Anxiety and depression

Emotional factors, such as anxiety or depression, can be a barrier to communication. When anxious about something individuals may only hear what they want to hear. This may mean that they do not hear the full story and fail to understand additional information given once their anxiety has been either relieved or confirmed. For example, a person may be anxious about a diagnosis, expecting to hear they have cancer. If a doctor were to say, 'There is no sign of cancer but ...' the patient may only remember that they have not got cancer, rather than taking in the further information which is just as important. Individuals who are depressed may be withdrawn and unwilling to communicate. They may also not be prepared to believe any positive news.

Assumptions

We frequently make assumptions about people and situations. This can affect communication and in some circumstances can be a barrier. If you assume that an individual has already got a good understanding of an issue, you may not take the trouble to give a full explanation. For example, it might be assumed that people who are medically qualified have appropriate knowledge about their own condition. Assumptions about different age groups are also sometimes made. For example, don't assume that all older people have hearing and memory problems or that children cannot understand difficult issues, such as illness and death.

Research tip

Look at the website www.winstonswish.org.uk to explore suggested methods of communication with young people who are experiencing grief.

Cultural differences

When communicating with someone from a different culture it is important to identify any factors that might be a barrier to good communication. Many care practitioners follow the behaviour of the dominant culture. This risks causing offence and creating a barrier to communication. Even within cultures, there may be differences such as how individuals like to be addressed. Older people may not be used to being called by their first names. In some cultures touching is less acceptable than in others.

Value and belief systems

In addition to the values and beliefs associated with different cultures, individuals may personally hold particular values and beliefs. These may have an effect on communication as individuals might find it difficult to accept any information that goes against their values or beliefs. For example, someone who does not believe in having a blood transfusion for religious reasons would find it difficult if faced with a doctor recommending one to save the life of a close relative.

Stereotypes

When making assumptions about people and individuals, people sometimes use stereotypes. Stereotypes are certain beliefs about groups of people and may be used to put individuals in a category. It makes it less likely that we will recognise and accommodate differences between individuals. Stereotypes can have positive or negative attributes. Negative stereotypes may be held about older people, those with disabilities or people from certain cultures. Barriers are caused when stereotypes limit the communication possibilities because of the assumptions made about what is, or is not, possible or appropriate.

Use and abuse of power

Those working in health and social care settings may very often find themselves in a position of power over service users. This may be the case with a nursery nurse working with children, a medical professional treating a patient or a care worker providing personal care to someone with a disability. This unequal situation can cause a barrier to communication. The service user may feel disempowered and unable to fully communicate his/her needs. Communication will not be truly effective if the barriers are not recognised and addressed. Power can be abused which can lead to individuals being intimidated and too frightened to express their own needs.

Example

Mrs Wu has just started to receive care in her home. The care worker gets her out of bed each day and does her shopping. Her meals are provided by a commercial service. Mrs Wu likes to choose her meals and is confident enough to ring up to complain if they are not satisfactory. A cleaner comes twice a week to ensure that the flat is kept clean. Mrs Wu ensures that her cleaner does a good job. However, she is not happy with the way in which her personal care is delivered. She does not feel able to complain or express her thoughts to her carer. Her daughter has offered to talk to the carer for her, but Mrs Wu has not agreed to this because she is worried about how she might be treated.

Think Why might Mrs Wu feel unable to complain to the carer?

THE INTEGRATED WORKFORCE AGENDA

Working in health and social care involves working with and alongside a wide range of other people. These include professionals and people from other agencies. Multi-professional working involves arrangements whereby different categories of professionals work together to meet the needs of a service user. Multi-agency working involves different organisations working together to provide care.

Example

On 25 February 2000 an eight-year-old child named Victoria Climbié died in St Mary's Hospital, London. The pathologist who examined her body found 128 separate injuries and scars. He described it as the worse case of child abuse that he had encountered. A public inquiry was set up under Lord Laming. His report has had far-reaching implications for the protection of children.

Victoria Climbié had been seen by a number of different professionals during the year prior to her death. The report heard that there were 12 points at which professionals could have acted on the evidence before them. These professionals included social workers, police, paediatric consultants and other care workers. She had also not been attending school. Four local councils, the NHS, the police, the NSPCC and the government's own Social Services Inspectorate were all involved in her case and failed in their duty of care. Poor communication between professionals and agencies was one of the problems identified.

The Government's response was to publish a White Paper called *Every Child Matters*.

Research tip

You can read the summary of the Every Child Matters paper to find out how information sharing is to be improved. You will find it at www.everychildmatters.gov.uk.

Communication with professionals

Communicating with other professionals is central to the jobs of people working in the health and social care sector. However, individuals do not always have the appropriate skills to ensure that this communication is effective. There is now a greater awareness that all professionals should develop their skills in this area and increased emphasis is put on communication skills when recruiting individuals to work in health and social care. There are sometimes official channels and protocols that must be followed in order to make contact with a professional. For example, in the UK a patient is expected to be referred to a consultant by their GP, while in other countries individuals can make direct contact.

Multi-agency working

For some service users with complex needs several different agencies may be involved in their care. These can be statutory organisations, such as the NHS or Social Services, private organisations, such as care-service agencies, or voluntary organisations, such as support groups. In addition, individuals may receive informal care from friends and relatives.

Many of these organisations will have their own structures and methods of communication. This can sometimes cause problems due to overlaps or gaps in care. Multi-agency working therefore requires good collaboration between the different agencies. In some situations this has become more formalised. For example, many Mental Health Trusts are a partnership between the NHS and Social Care Partnership Trusts. This recognises the overlap between health and social care responsibilities in meeting the needs of individuals with mental health problems.

Example

Gary has had mental health problems since his early twenties. He has been arrested by the police, who recognise him as a patient of the local mental health services. Instead of taking him into custody they contact his social worker. She takes him back to the supported housing unit in which he lives, which is run by a housing association. She reminds him that he has promised to attend the local meeting of MIND, the mental health support group.

Think Identify the different agencies that are supporting Gary. Why is communication between them important?

Multi-professional working

Care practitioners working in different areas have different skills and knowledge. The expertise of several different practitioners may be needed to provide the full range of care that an individual requires. For example, a person with physical disabilities may need medical, nursing and social care as well as specialist care from a physiotherapist, occupational or speech therapist. It is important that all these practitioners work together and communicate effectively so that they are working to common goals. This is usually accomplished by the creation of a care plan. This is a method of planning for the treatment for an individual by assessing, planning, implementing, monitoring and reviewing care. By this involvement with, and coordination between, all the professionals involved, more effective care and treatment is delivered. Communication between professionals and with the service user is of huge importance.

Think Think about your work experience placement. What different professionals contribute or have contributed to the care of the clients? How have they ensured good communication between them?

CASE STUDY: THE LIMES

Anne has recently taken over as manager of The Limes, an adult resource centre. It provides a range of services for individuals with disabilities. Situated on the outskirts of a large city it has clients from a number of different ethnic groups, many of whom do not have English as their first language.

Anne qualified as an occupational therapist after leaving school. Before taking over as manager of The Limes, she had gained experience of working in a number of different settings.

Anne is keen to make a number of changes. She would like to get the service users more involved in running the centre. She would like to introduce some different activities which she believes would be more appropriate for their needs.

The centre is currently run by a management committee. This is a group of professionals, such as social workers, occupational therapists and physiotherapists. They will need to be persuaded of the need to make changes. Anne would also like to promote the centre by making it more widely known in the local community.

One of the people who attend the centre is Mark. He is 21 years old. He has to use a wheelchair following a motorbike accident when he was 17. He sustained a head injury that affected his sight and he is paralysed from the waist down. Another service user at the centre is Becky. She has Down's Syndrome. She has a part-time job packing bags at the supermarket on Saturdays. Both Mark and Becky would like to contribute to the running of the centre.

Anne is aware that she will need to communicate with many people to get her ideas implemented. She is considering how best she should address this challenge.

QUESTIONS

1. Who are the different groups and individuals with whom Anne will need to communicate?

2. What barriers might there be to good communication with each of these groups or individuals?

3. How could Anne plan to overcome these barriers?

Evidence activity

P3

1. Write down a list of factors that influence communication and interpersonal interactions.

2. For each factor give examples of how and why the interactions were influenced. (P3)

1.3 Knowing how patients and service users may be assisted by effective communication

Service users can be assisted in communicating in a variety of different ways. Some of these methods rely on additional help from other people, but others use technology. The range and variety of technical assistance is changing and developing all the time.

SUPPORT SERVICES

Advocates

An advocate is someone who speaks on behalf of someone else. If service users are unable to speak for or represent themselves an advocate will sometimes speak for them. This may occur if a person has a learning disability or an illness, such as dementia. The advocate might be a family member or someone who works closely with the client. At other times a lawyer might be responsible for acting as an advocate. Using an advocate means that the service user's wants and needs can be communicated and their rights protected.

Interpreters

An interpreter will ensure that individuals who speak different languages can communicate effectively with each other. He or she will be able to speak and understand both languages. Skilled interpreters have an in-depth knowledge of the language and idioms used by both parties. For particularly important discussions it may be essential to have an interpreter present, for example, for hearings under the Mental Health Act when an individual's freedom is at stake. Most NHS Trusts have a list of suitable interpreters who can be called on.

Translators

Translators are responsible for interpreting the meaning of a written text from one language to another. This is a highly skilled activity if complete accuracy is to be achieved. There are several websites that can translate the most common words and phrases, but it is important that professional services are used if a service user is unable to fully understand an important written communication.

Signers

Signers are used to communicate with service users who have a hearing impairment. In the UK, deaf and hearing-impaired individuals use British Sign Language (BSL). The British Deaf Association estimates that BSL is the first or preferred language of approximately 250,000 people in the UK.

Research tip

Visit www.signcommunity.org.uk to learn more about sign language and to see videos of people using BSL.

Other people who assist communication

Other professionals who assist communication include the following:

- **Speech therapists** assess, diagnose and treat individuals with speech, language or other communication problems.

- **Counsellors** work with an individual or group to provide guidance and support in tackling personal problems or difficulties in relationships. Clients are encouraged to develop skills that will help them to communicate their own needs more effectively.

- **Mentors** support an individual. They can help individuals to achieve something by discussing their needs with them.

- **Befrienders** act as a friend. It may be an informal relationship that gives support at a specific time or in a particular circumstance. In other situations a befriender, or buddy, might act as an advocate or take on a more formal role by supporting individuals and assisting them to communicate.

- **Psychologists** specialise in various fields of psychology. They are concerned with different aspects of the human mind or behaviour. Clinical psychologists work in mental health care using individual or group techniques to provide treatment. Psychologists can help individuals to understand issues about communication and enable them to communicate more effectively.

Example

The Media Trust is a charity that works in partnership with the media industry and charities to build effective communication in the voluntary and community sectors. In February 2007 it launched a youth mentoring scheme. In this scheme, people who work in the media are partnered with young people aged 14 to 25 at risk of becoming involved in antisocial behaviour. The mentors share their knowledge of communication skills. You can read more about the charity at www.mediatrust.org.

TECHNOLOGY

The use of technology to assist communication is continually developing. Communication aids are becoming more sophisticated and less visible. It is no longer always obvious when an individual is wearing a hearing aid. This has helped to ensure that individuals are not labelled or marginalised. However, there are still examples when the presence of an aid or adaptation causes people to speak to the carer rather than to the individual.

Aids and adaptations

Aids for the hearing impaired

Hearing aids have changed significantly in recent years. The use of digital technology means that they are now more accurately linked to an individual's specific requirements. They can be worn behind or in the ear. Induction loops improve the ability of individuals to pick up signals from a microphone or other sound source. Other aids that help hearing-impaired people include smoke alarms, phone alerts and alarm clocks adapted to use light or vibration to catch the attention.

Aids for the visually impaired

Glasses and contact lenses are the most common aids used by those who have problems with eyesight. Other aids include magnifiers and objects such as telephones with big numbers. Clocks and watches can have a speaking facility which reads the time. Books and other written materials are produced in large print, or on tapes or CDs as talking books. Screen readers are software programmes that can turn onscreen text into speech or Braille.

Computer adaptations

There is a wide range of adaptations available to meet the communication needs of the physically disabled as well as those with hearing and sight impairments. For example, a computer's mouse and keyboard can be adapted to be used by those with little or no limb use through a pointer controlled by head movements.

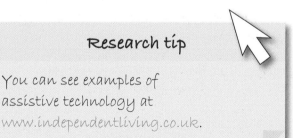

Research tip

You can see examples of assistive technology at www.independentliving.co.uk.

Text facility on mobile phones

Text messaging allows short messages to be passed between mobile phones, fax machines or email addresses. It is a very popular way of communicating and has developed its own language. Health and social service providers have realised that this technology offers opportunities for communicating with their service users, for example by texting reminders about appointments.

PREFERRED LANGUAGE

In addition to spoken languages used by individuals for whom English is not their first language there are other programmes that have been developed to meet the needs of individuals with disabilities.

Makaton

Makaton is a language programme that combines spoken words with signs (see Figure 1.11) and symbols. It is used as a way of communicating by children and adults with learning disabilities and is also increasingly used by people in mainstream settings.

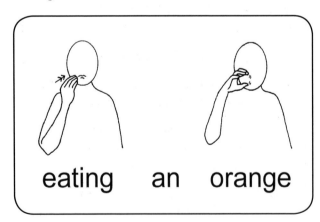

Figure 1.11 A Makaton reading sign in use
Source www.makaton.org

Research tip

For further examples of signs and symbols visit

www.makaton.org/docs/events-posters.pdf.

Signing

British Sign Language (BSL) is the preferred language of the deaf community in the UK. It is a language in its own right, but uses hand gestures and signs instead of speech. There are regional variations in different parts of the country. Sign languages from different countries differ from each other as much as spoken languages.

Braille

Braille is named after its inventor, Louis Braille, a Frenchman who became blind at the age of six. It is 'read' by passing the fingers over characters made up of an arrangement of one to six raised dots (see Figure 1.12). It has been adapted to almost all languages.

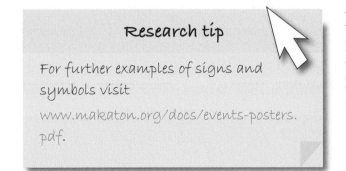

Figure 1.12 Braille alphabet

First language

An individual's first language is almost always their preferred language of communication. However, it is not always possible to ensure that this is possible when living in another country. Interpreters and translators are often used to allow people to communicate in their first language.

SUPPORTING

We have already seen that factors related to the identity of an individual, such as self-esteem, can affect communication. Care practitioners have an important role in supporting their clients by empowering them, ensuring that their rights are promoted and by maintaining confidentiality.

Empowerment

Empowerment is the process of increasing individuals' power or authority to allow them to make decisions for themselves. This means encouraging choice, promoting an individual's self-esteem and allowing them to take control. If service users are empowered, they should feel able to express their needs and wants rather than having decisions imposed on them. If decisions are taken away from service users they can become dependant or 'institutionalised'. If this happens individuals can lose confidence and will not be able to make decisions for themselves.

Example

Compare these two scenes, which show how communication can be used to empower service users.

Scene 1

Carer – Morning Youri. Time to get up. I have run the bath, so off we go.

Youri – Alright. You're the boss.

Scene 2

Carer – Morning Youri. Are you ready to get up yet? Would you like to have a bath or not this morning?

Youri – Good morning. I'm just listening to the end of this piece on the radio, so perhaps you could come back in half an hour. I had a bath last night so just some help to wash will be fine today.

Promotion of rights

The care-value base in the health and social care sector lays down the rights of service users. In 2002 the General Social Care Council published a Code of Practice for Social Workers which identifies some of the rights of service users. Care practitioners are expected to adhere to the codes of practice and respect the rights of service users.

These rights include:

- treating each person as an individual

- respecting and, where appropriate, promoting the individual views and wishes of both service users and carers

- supporting service users' rights to control their lives and make informed choices about the services they receive

- respecting and maintaining the dignity and privacy of service users and carers

- promoting equal opportunities for service users

- respecting diversity, different cultures and values.

Social workers are expected to 'strive to establish and maintain the trust and confidence of service users' by:

- being honest and trustworthy

- communicating in an appropriate, open, accurate and straightforward way

- respecting confidential information and clearly explaining policies about confidentiality to service users.

[Source: General Social Care Council, Codes of Practice 2002]

Think How would the promotion of these rights help to support effective communication?

Maintaining confidentiality

The maintenance of confidentiality is key to establishing trust between individuals. Any information that is given with the expectation that it will not be passed on to other people inappropriately should be kept confidential. In the health and care sector, private and personal information may be available to a care practitioner that an individual would not want to be shared with others. For example, a woman who has had an abortion would expect only her doctor and appropriate medical and nursing staff to be aware of the fact. The information should not be shared with anyone else unless she wishes. There are legal requirements under the Data Protection Act 1998 that cover information contained in personal records.

Confidentiality does not mean never sharing any information. It is about using information appropriately. Members of the care team need to know information about their clients in order to provide continuity of care. Permission can be sought from an individual to share information; however, there are certain situations when the right to confidentiality is overridden, including:

- if there is a significant risk of harm to the service user or to another person

- if a court of law requests information

- if a criminal act has taken place or is planned

- if it is required in the wider public interest.

If confidentiality is not maintained, trust is eroded and communication affected. The principle of ensuring that only the information that someone needs to know is passed on should underpin the sharing of any information.

> **Think** What effects might there be if the confidentiality of a service user's personal information is not maintained?

Evidence activity

P4 – M2 – D1

1. Produce a presentation showing how the communication needs of service users can be assisted. This could take the form of a poster, leaflet or PowerPoint presentation. (P4)

2. Either from your work experience or from research, identify specific communication needs. You should describe at least one technical aid. Explain the working of the aid and how it helps in communication (M2)

3. Review how communication assists not only the service user but also other key people.

a) You need to identify the key people and give examples of the interactions between them and the service user.

b) You should discuss the strengths and weaknesses in terms of the support that is given to the service user. (D1)

1.4 *Demonstrating your own communication skills in a caring role*

This section is all about how you can put into practice some of the principles of communication that you have explored in this unit. As part of your assessment for this unit you will be expected to undertake two interactions in the role of a carer in which you must demonstrate your communication and interpersonal skills.

COMMUNICATION SKILLS

Now is your opportunity to review all that you have learned about communication and to develop your own skills. It might be worth observing some examples of effective communication, either by using role play or by watching a video. This will help you to identify the skills that are being used. You may want to practice your skills in role plays before undertaking the interactions on which you will be assessed.

When planning for your assessed interactions you will need to think about:

- who is receiving the communication – you will be expected to have one interaction with a group and one with an individual

- what the topic is

- where it is to take place.

Verbal skills

These are some of the verbal skills you need to develop:

- ensuring that communication is in an appropriate language and at a level that is understood

- using active listening skills, e.g. encouragement, reflection, use of prompts, open questioning, clarification, paraphrasing, checking understanding

- respecting individuality and diversity through use of appropriate language

- conveying feelings of warmth, empathy and interest

- maintaining the pace of conversation

- ensuring that all members of a group are involved and can contribute

- defining the boundaries of confidentiality

- being prepared to listen.

Non-verbal skills

You need to be able to critically assess your own non-verbal skills in interactions. Think about the messages that you send through some of the following non-verbal behaviours:

- dress and appearance

- posture and angle of the head

- proximity and touch

- eye contact

- facial expression

- tone of voice

- use of hands and arms.

Remember also to think about the quality of the environment in which the communication is due to take place, including the layout of the room, the need for privacy, lighting conditions and any background noise.

> **Think** Remember SOLER? If not, revisit page 22 to check what it stands for and make sure you practice it!

EFFECTIVENESS

Look back at the ways in which patients and service users can feel supported. These include:

- empowering them

- promoting their rights

- maintaining confidentiality.

Make sure when planning your interaction that you consider how you are going to support the service user. You should think about what might make them feel more empowered, what are the rights of the service user and how they could be promoted. Confidentiality must be maintained at all times. Ensure that you understand your responsibilities for this and how you are going to ensure that it is preserved.

KEY PEOPLE

As well as communicating with the service user, there are other key people who may be involved and who may also need to be part of any communication. These can include relatives, friends, and other health and social care workers.

The most important principle is to remember the needs of the service user. It is important to consider confidentiality when having any contact with other key people. You need to ask the questions:

- do they need to know, and if so, what?

- do I need permission from the service user to share the information?

Relatives and friends

Relatives and friends usually want the best for their loved one, but this is not always the case. In most circumstances it is important to ensure that the service user has agreed to any sharing of information with relatives and friends, whether it is face to face or over the telephone. It is important to discreetly check who someone is before giving or receiving any information.

On some occasions, relatives and friends may be particularly upset because of the circumstances in which they find the service user, for example, if they are very ill or unlikely to recover following an accident. In these situations care workers may need to use their communication and interpersonal skills to provide them with support and help. If communication with a service user takes place with relatives or friends present, the care practitioner must remember that their responsibility is to the service user and ensure that it is their rights that are promoted.

> ***Think*** When discussing the possibility of a patient moving into a residential home, why might the views of relatives or friends differ from those of the service user?

Health and social care workers

Care is often delivered by a team of health and social care workers. Communication between the team of workers is important in order to ensure that there is continuity of care and that care is delivered to the highest standards. This communication can be verbal, written or electronic. The style and content of any communication will vary depending on who you are contacting. Sometimes it is important that any information discussed is formally recorded and forms part of the service user's record.

The people who may be involved in giving care to service users may include:

- GPs

- social workers

- occupational therapists

- physiotherapists

- nurses

- care workers

- community psychiatric nurses

- staff providing recreational activities.

You will need to identify the key people in your workplace and observe how communication takes place between them and the service users.

> ***Think*** For your work experience placement, list all the key people who are involved in providing care. What is the policy on communication or maintaining confidentiality?

Evidence activity

P5

1. You must take part in and record two interactions in which you have participated. You should take the role of the carer and use your communication skills to support the service user. One should be on a one-to-one basis and the other in a group setting. At least one of the interactions must be observed by your course tutor or your workplace supervisor. They should write a witness statement or check list which you can use as evidence. (P5)

Evidence activity

P6 – M3 – D2

1. Write a review of your own communication skills in the two interactions. You may wish to do this against a check list. (P6)

2. Explain how the interactions could have been more effective by reviewing your own skills. Identify what you could do to improve. (M3)

3. Explain what factors influenced your interactions. Identify the strengths and weaknesses and draw conclusions. (D2)

REVIEWING YOUR INTERACTIONS

You may find it helpful to get feedback from others on your communication skills and interpersonal interactions. In addition, it is good practice to be able to critically analyse your own performance.

Type of communication	Marks out of 10	Comments, including how skills could be improved and what factors influenced the interaction
Verbal communication skills • listening skills • •		
Non verbal skills • dress and appearance • •		
Environmental issues • • •		
Assistance for communicating • • •		
Use of care values • • •		

Table 1.2 Communication skills chart

Equality, Diversity and Rights in Health and Social Care

unit 2

This unit investigates how equality, diversity and rights are central to the effective operation of health and social care services. It explores key terms and concepts such as confidentiality, empowerment and examines discriminatory practice and the potential effects it can have on patients/service users. The unit also investigates how health and social care organisations have developed specific strategies such as policies and procedures to help them combat the worse effects of discrimination. In addition you will also be introduced to the different pieces of legislation which government has introduced to help promote and safeguard the rights of those most vulnerable in our society.

The knowledge and understanding gained from this unit will underpin many other units in this qualification and help prepare you for you future careers in the health and social care sectors.

Learning outcomes

In this unit you will:

2.1 Understand concepts of equality, diversity and rights in relation to health and social care — page 51

2.2 Understand discriminatory practice in health and social care — page 60

2.3 Understand how national initiatives promote anti-discriminatory practice in health and social care — page 65

2.4 Understand how anti-discriminatory practice is promoted in health and social care settings. — page 76

So you want to be a...

Learning Disability Nurse

~~My name~~ Claire Reeve
~~Age~~ 29
Income £19,500

If you are a good listener who is able to communicate with people from a variety of backgrounds this rewarding job could be for you.

What do you do?

I work with clients with learning disabilities. I assess their needs and draw-up care plans and then make sure my recommendations are put into place. My aim is make sure my clients lead as 'normal' a life as possible.

What are your day to day responsibilities?

I work with other health and professionals to assist clients with basic living skills and social activities. I assess the needs of clients and draw up care plans, risk assessments and make recommendations on other issues, such as housing, I co-ordinate client care programme reviews and attend doctors appointments with my clients to monitor their progress

What skills do you need for the job?

Many of my clients have physical or sensory impairments, mental health needs and sometimes challenging behaviour. You need to be calm, sensitive and empathetic. You must be able to talk to and gain the trust of people from a range of backgrounds. Some days having a thick skin can really help!

> ❝ I really enjoy daily contact with my clients ❞

What qualifications do you need?

I took the usual route into nursing, a 3 year degree course, and then chose to specialise in learning difficulties.

What's the pay like?

I started on around £19,000, as I gain more experience my salary will improve. Top level Learning Disability Nurses earn as much as £31,000.

How are the hours like?

They are pretty standard although I do occasionally have to work outside the usual nine to five when needed.

What does the future hold?

Once I have completed my two years' post-qualification and gained more experience I can aim for promotion. If I want, with further study and training, I can move into health management or residential care management. At the moment though, I am really enjoying daily contact with my clients and I would like to work in the prison service in specialist secure units for offenders with disabilities.

Grading criteria

The table shows what you need to do to gain a pass, merit or distinction in this part of the qualification. Make sure you refer back to it when you are completing work so you can judge whether you are meeting the criteria and what you need to do to fill in gaps in your knowledge or experience.

In this unit there are 6 evidence activities that give you an opportunity to demonstrate your acheivement of the grading criteria:

page 55	P1	page 75	P4, M1, D1
page 60	P2	page 77	P5, M2
page 64	P3	page 81	M3, D2

To achieve a pass grade the evidence must show that the learner is able to...	To achieve a merit grade the evidence must show that, in addition to the pass criteria, the learner is able to...	To achieve a distinction grade the evidence must show that, in addition to the pass and merit criteria, the learner is able to...
P1 explain the benefits of diversity to society		
P2 use recognised terminology to explain the important of promoting equality, recognising diversity and respecting the rights in health and social care settings		
P3 explain the potential effects of discriminatory practice on those who use health or social care services		
P4 describe how legislation, codes of practice, rules of conduct, charters and organisational policies are used to promote anti-discriminatory practice	**M1** explain the influences of a recent or emerging national policy development on organisational policy with regard to anti-discriminatory practice	**D1** evaluate how a recent or emerging policy development influences organisational and personal practice in relation to anti-discriminatory practice
P5 explain how those working in health and social care settings can actively promote anti-discriminatory practice	**M2** explain difficulties that may be encountered when implementing anti-discriminatory practice	
P6 describe ways of reflecting on and challenging discriminatory issues in health and social care	**M3** analyse how personal beliefs and value systems may influence own anti-discriminatory practice	**D2** evaluate practical strategies to reconcile own beliefs and values with anti-discriminatory practice in health and social care

2.1 *Understand concepts of equality, diversity and rights in relation to health and social care*

HEALTH AND SOCIAL CARE SETTINGS

Within health and social care there are many different types of settings that you will either work in or encounter during your professional life.

- **Residential care** – covers a number of services, both formal and informal, is provided for people who require a level of care that cannot be provided in their own homes. Residential care can be provided for all client groups – children, adults and older people.

- **Day care facilities** – have been developed for people who are at risk or have a condition that would benefit from interaction with others. Facilities focus upon rehabilitation or respite and include hospital day procedure units, drop-in centres for older people or those with mental health problems, community resource centres, crèches and play groups.

- **Nursing care** – is provided within a specialist facility for people experiencing a range of illnesses, problems or disabilities.

- **Domiciliary care** – personal care services provided to help service users achieve daily living tasks and remain independent within their own homes and community.

Provision will be accessed by a range of client and service user groups, including:

- children – 0-18 years

- adults with sensory, physical, learning and mental health problems – 19-65 years

- older people – 65 years plus.

Clients will access these services because they have a range of health and social care needs, such as:

- physical needs

- sensory needs – hearing, sight, speech

- learning needs

- mental health needs.

The provision of such services will be provided by a range of providers:

- central/local government

- private organisations

- voluntary providers

- informal carers – family and friends.

CASE STUDY: CARE PLANS

Maggie is 78 years of age and lives on her own. Six months ago she suffered a stroke which left her with little mobility. To help her recover, Maggie moved into a nursing home temporarily and a physiotherapist from the local hospital visited her once a week to help her regain her mobility. She recently left the nursing home and has returned home. Maggie's social worker designed a care plan that allows Maggie to live independently. It includes domiciliary care, meals on wheels, day care at the local Age Concern centre once a week and a visit from the district nurse once a week to ensure that she is taking her medication and doing her exercises.

QUESTIONS

1. Identify the different settings Maggie has used.

2. Identify which Client Group Maggie belongs to.

3. Identify Maggie's different health and social care needs.

TERMINOLOGY

There are many terms and concepts that you will need to understand if you are to develop the underpinning knowledge required for this unit.

Equality, equity and diversity

Equality – being the same or having the same value.

Equity – people with greater needs are treated more favourably than people with fewer unmet needs. In doing so, 'outcomes' are equalised.

Equality of opportunity – equal access to the chance of obtaining society's prizes – education, jobs, income etc on the bases of merit rather than social background.

Diversity – within health and social care, diversity means promoting the individual's own sense of identity. It involves recognising that the values, beliefs, tastes and preferences of individuals must be supported, nurtured and encouraged.

> **Think** Can you think of ten ways in which other people differ from you in terms of personality, appearance, religion, ability/disability, sexual orientation, gender, age, race/ethnicity, health status and socio-economic status?

Empowerment

Empowerment is the process of giving greater power to clients. Empowerment promotes the idea that the individual has independence and control over their lives. It is closely associated to concepts such as social exclusion. Empowerment can refer to self-help, community action or an involvement in a political process. Within health and social care empowerment is achieved by care professionals working with a client in an open and transparent manner, and by the care professional attempting to increase the service user's abilities to help them deal with their own problems.

Disempowerment

Disempowerment occurs when individuals are not given the opportunity to have any say in their care and so become reliant or dependent on their carers for support. It should be noted, however, that disempowerment does not necessarily originate with health and social care agencies. Disempowerment may be due to client or service users' low levels of education, poor literacy, and a lack of confidence or low self esteem, which means they are unable to make decisions for themselves.

Beliefs and values

All individuals have values and attitudes that are developed within the culture they are socialised into. The culture of a society is the set of values and ways of acting that mark that particular society. Our culture is learnt through the process of socialisation. Socialisation is the process by which the individual learns the norms, values and attitudes of the society in which they live.

Norms are accepted patterns of behaviour. Values underpin how an individual acts by providing the moral framework within which decisions are made. Values are based on beliefs that some things are good or desirable. They define what is important, worthwhile and worth striving for. Attitudes are firmly held beliefs that cause an individual to respond in a particular way. Beliefs are general opinions held about the world and about the nature of society and can influence action.

> **Think** Why do you think health and social care practitioners need to understand about how norms, values and attitudes are formed?

Disadvantage

Because the UK is a multi-cultural, diverse society, individuals or groups may have different values, attitudes and beliefs to our own. Although this diversity can enrich society it can also lead to friction and problems. Socialisation can, in some cases, lead to the development of attitudes, prejudices and stereotypes that are inaccurate, which in turn may lead to disadvantage and discrimination.

Prejudice, stereotyping and labelling

Inequality, discrimination and malpractice within care practice occurs for many reasons but perhaps the most common is the fact that because people are different it can be easy to think that some people are better than others, or that some views are right but others wrong. Socialisation, culture and life experience may lead to assumptions being made about what is right or normal. Anyone who is different is then seen as 'not right' or 'not normal', and discrimination a result.

Prejudice – making assumptions about an individual or group of people based on myths or stories which are not factual and generally inaccurate.

Stereotype – attributing specific characteristics to members of particular groups and expecting them to behave in specific ways.

Label – a name, phrase or word assigned to an individual or group of people from a particular background that can have a negative impact upon that individual or group.

Overt discrimination

To understand the way in which people can be treated unequally, denied access to services, have their choices limited and their rights as an individual undermined and infringed, care workers should be aware of the different ways in which negative discrimination can occur. This can happen quite overtly, in the form of direct discrimination, where an individual could be ridiculed, verbally humiliated or snubbed.

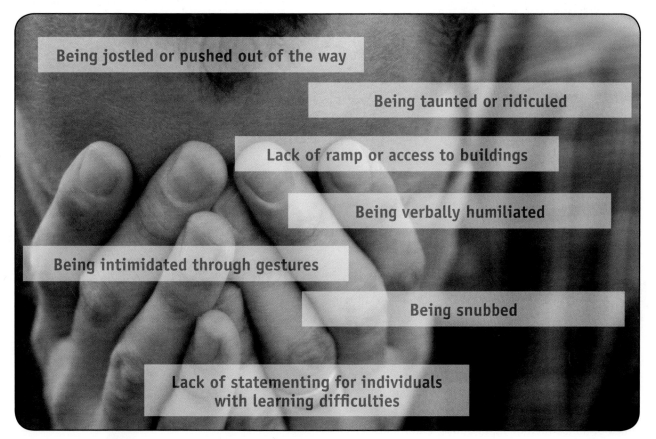

Figure 2.1 Examples of overt and direct discrimination

Covert discrimination

Indirect or covert discrimination is much more subtle that direct discrimination. It can be difficult to detect and insidious because it does not manifest itself with the outward show of physical violence, obvious intimidating gestures and language; however, it can be very easy to feel. For recipients of such treatment the effects can be profound; they may not be believed, they may be ridiculed when they make a complaint, they may even doubt their own experience.

Racism

This is the idea that each ethnic group has particular characteristics or attributes, and that therefore some ethnic groups are superior to others. Racism can originate from personal belief (individual racism) or from wider society influences (institutional racism).

Sexism

This is the belief that one gender is superior to another. Sexism is the negative treatment of a person by virtue of their sex or gender. Like Racism, sexism can develop from personal belief or from wider social forces.

> **Think** Have you ever been treated in a negative way because of your gender?

Homophobia

Is an intensely negative feeling about homosexuals and homosexuality. It originates from a lack of understanding or possibly a hatred of homosexuals and their lifestyle.

Abuse

Abuse is a generic term used to cover a range of negative and intentional behaviours designed to hurt or damage an individual. Commonly reported types of abuse include child abuse, elder abuse and domestic violence. Different types of abuse include:

- physical abuse, e.g. hitting, biting or kicking

- sexual abuse – forcing a child or adult to participate in sexual acts either knowingly or unknowingly

- emotional abuse – belittling or humiliating an individual

- financial abuse – stealing, withholding or tricking money from an individual

- institutional abuse – a lack of choice over decisions an individual should have the right to make.

Vulnerability

Vulnerable people are individuals or groups in society who are at greater risk to themselves or from others due to a physical, sensory or learning disability, age or mental health problem. They may need continual, supervised care to protect them either within their own homes or in specialist facilities such as nursing care homes or hospitals.

Independence

Independence is closely associated with empowerment, in that when a service user has been empowered they will have greater independence and control over their lives and the decisions they make. A key outcome of good care practice is promoting service user independence.

Interdependence

Some service users have very complex needs and rely on different agencies working together to promote their health and well-being. In health and social care the term refers to different agencies working together to promote the independence of a service user through multi-disciplinary working.

CASE STUDY: UNEQUAL TREATMENT

Jamilla is 26 years old and is a single mother of three children. Jamilla came to the UK from Nigeria with her parents when she was 4 years old. Neither she nor her parents spoke any English. Jamilla attended local schools but didn't progress well as the schools did not provide any support to help Jamilla communicate with her teachers. At secondary school she found the classes boring and failed her GCSEs.

When Jamilla left school she worked in a number of jobs but found some employers hostile and difficult to work for. At 18 she left home and went to live with her boyfriend. Jamilla then became pregnant and her relationship broke down due to the stress of the pregnancy. She went to the local housing authority and has been living in a damp and run down council flat for the past 6 years. When Jamilla complained she was told "be grateful, it's better than what you came from." She is now unemployed and living on benefits.

BENEFITS OF DIVERSITY

Care practitioners should be aware of and value diversity within society. In order to learn about other people's culture and beliefs, it is necessary to listen to and watch what other people say and do. Learning about diversity can be interesting and exciting, but some people find this learning process stressful. They may feel that their own culture and beliefs are being challenged.

Skilled carers have to get to know the people that they work with in order to avoid making any false assumptions. In getting to know an individual, carers will also need to understand the ways in which class, race, age, gender and other social categories influence the person.

There are many different ethnic groups, religions and cultures in the world. Two individuals may belong to the same ethnic groups yet belong to different religions or social classes. Knowing someone's religion will not necessarily reveal everything about that person's beliefs or general culture. It is possible to gain background knowledge on different ethnic and religious customs, but it is impossible to study all the differences that might exist for individual clients. The best way to learn about diversity is to listen to and communicate with people who lead different lives from our own.

EVIDENCE ACTIVITY

P1

Using the case study above, answer the following questions.

1. Identify three ways in which Jamilla has been treated differently from other people.

2. Explain why she may have been treated unequally.

3. Explain the effect this may have had on her life to date and future life chances.

4. Using recognised terminology explain the benefits of diversity for society. (P1)

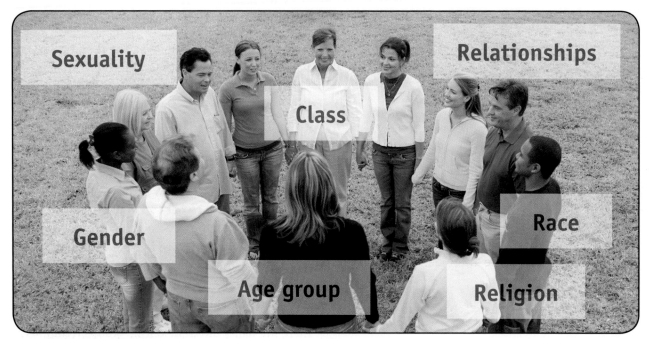

Sexuality

Relationships

Class

Gender

Race

Age group

Religion

Figure 2.2 Diversity in action

Social and cultural benefits of diversity

Valuing diversity can be enriching. Being able to understand other people's life experiences and differences may help you to become more flexible and creative in your thinking, because you can empathise with other people's views. It may result in the development of a wider range of social skills through meeting different people. Learning about different cultures may offer new experiences – such as new foods or places to visit. Understanding other people's lives may also help you to adapt your own lifestyle to cope with change.

Other benefits of celebrating diversity include:

- developing greater social cohesion
- cultural enrichment
- expanding your own range of foods and tastes
- educating yourself
- developing new languages
- greater tolerance
- developing the economy of the nation further.

Economic benefits of diversity

Employers are likely to want to employ people who value diversity because:

- effective non-discriminatory care depends on staff valuing diversity
- people who value diversity are likely to be flexible and creative
- people who value diversity may make good relationships with one another and with clients
- diverse teams often work together effectively. If people have different interests there is more chance that the team will cover all the work and enjoy working together.

ACTIVE PROMOTION OF EQUALITY AND INDIVIDUAL RIGHTS

Principles of the care value base

Health and social care professionals are guided by a set of values called the care value base that influence how they interact with service users to promote access and equality in service provision.

These values include:

- empowerment

- confidentiality/privacy

- effective communication

- support of individual rights and choices

- respect of beliefs and identity.

When you are on your placement see if you can identify examples of when you have applied or when you have observed others applying the care value base principles. You might want to use a chart similar to the one in figure 2.3 to help you record examples.

CVB principle	Examples
Empowerment	
Confidentiality / privacy	
Effective communication	
Supporting individual rights and choices	
Respecting client beliefs and identity	
Anti-discriminatory practice	

Figure 2.3 Recording of care value base principles

Putting the service user at the heart of service provision

Within care settings every individual should receive services of an equal quality that meet their personal needs. This is not the same as every individual receiving the same service. Treating people as individuals with different beliefs, abilities, likes and dislikes is at the heart of caring for others. In care settings there are policies to help protect individuals against discrimination. Equal opportunity policies help both clients and staff by establishing standards that must be adhered to.

Promoting individuals' rights

All care service providers have a responsibility to accept people as unique individuals, to respect them and to treat them with respect and dignity. They have a responsibility to enable individuals and groups to obtain rights and services to which they are entitled. However, individuals may wish to pursue and exercise rights (such as free speech, personal characteristics); that infringe the rights of others (because they constitute discrimination), or lead to self-harm. In such instances, the care worker and agency have a responsibility to balance the conflicting rights, within the health and welfare of those concerned.

All agencies and care workers should ensure that service users are aware of their rights and responsibilities and also that they understand how exercising these may have an impact on the rights of others. The rights of an individual include:

- the right to be respected – in terms of religion, gender, political opinion, sexual orientation

- the right to equal treatment – in how care and services provided

- the right to be treated as an individual – in religion, gender etc

- the right to be treated in a dignified way – i.e. personal care

- the right to privacy – e.g. having own room, a key to the room

- the right to be protected from danger and harm – having policies designed to protect individuals

- the right to information about themselves

- the right to communicate their needs using their own preferred method of communication and language – e.g. by using an advocate or interpreter

- the right to be cared for in a way that meets their needs – e.g. ensuring religious observances are respected

- the right to have their choices and preferences taken into account – in terms of food, dress and care

All agencies providing care services should have guidelines or codes of practice setting out how individuals' rights will be fostered and promoted, and how the agency will support them. Care workers should be familiar with them, as they outline the type of service they should be delivering. Services users should also be aware of them, to enable them to understand how their rights will be met.

Example

Carer: Come on Bill, it's time for lunch.

Bill: What time is it?

Carer: 12 o' clock – come on Bill, look lively!

Bill: But it's too early for lunch and I'm not hungry.

Carer: Well I'm sure that will change when you see your lunch – you'll change your mind when you're in the dining room.

Bill: What's for lunch anyway?

Carer: You got the menu yesterday – there will be something nice that you will like – you're not fussy anyway.

Bill: I'll not eat pork or that sweet corn stuff – it's chicken feed! I want some decent food!

Carer: Fine! Look – sit over there. If you don't like the dinner then leave it.

Bill: But I don't sit there.

Carer: Well it's all change today – the change of seating will do you good.

> **Think** What is wrong with the above scenario? How might the carer promote Bill's rights and choices?

Providing active support

Active promotion of equality and individual rights means treating people equally and supporting them in the choices they make regarding their care. It also involves promoting privacy and confidentiality and being aware of the practical implications of confidentiality.

It also involves effective communication. Sometimes clients/service users are unable to communicate effectively for themselves and in such circumstances it is essential that an advocate is provided who can represent their interests. Because the UK is a multi-cultural society some service users may not speak English as their first language so it is important that an interpreter is provided who can speak on behalf of the service user and communicate with them. This also has implications for information that is provided, which must be in a format easily accessible for all clients.

Empowerment

Care service providers have a responsibility to empower individuals and groups to increase their range of choices, and exercise their preferences.

Example

Josh is 21 years of age. He is a wheelchair user following a car accident he had when he was 10 years of age. For the past year Josh has been attending the Willows Adult Resource Centre, which provides day care for adults with physical, sensory and learning disability. Josh really enjoys his time at the day centre as the day care workers support him in developing new skills and encourage all the service users to be actively involved in the running of the day centre. Josh has recently been invited to join the centre's management forum and is really enjoying his new found responsibility.

> **Think** How is the centre empowering Josh and the other service users? What effects might this have on Josh's physical, social, emotional and intellectual development?

Dealing with tensions and contradictions

Although the goal is to promote equality and greater access, sometimes conflicts and tensions do occur between the service provider and service user and their families. This could be as a result of resource shortages, finance, lack of human resources, or inability to provide a particular service (e.g. as a result of a risk assessment). In such situations the care practitioner must always work in the best interests of the client/service user and communicate clearly to them the reasons for a particular course of action.

Staff development and training

As a practitioner it is essential that continual staff development and training is undertaken to keep abreast of current developments, issues that are arising and good practice that aims to promote greater access and reduce discrimination.

> **Think** Where are rights clearly identified in the policy? Are there any rights not included in the policy? If so, which ones? Could the policy be improved in any way?

Practical implications of confidentiality

To appreciate how service users might feel about personal information being shared, think about the information you share with others:

- information you give out regularly
- information you give to close friends only
- information you give out rarely
- information you give out only when asked.

> **Think** Would it bother you if any of the information you give is given openly to others? What information would you object to others having access to? What information would you not object to others having access to?

Research tip

Obtain a policy from your placement such as a confidentiality or advocacy policy

CASE STUDY: RESIDENTIAL CAR

John Wilkins is 78 years old. Three months ago he suffered a stroke, which has left him with little mobility. John's ability to communicate is good and he can feed himself but he needs help with personal care and can't walk without aid. He has moved into a residential unit to help him recover and for his own safety. He has been living in the Elms Residential Care Home for two months.

The home cares for 48 residents. On John's arrival he was taken to her room and left alone for over an hour. No nursing staff came to check on him. Although the nursing staff are diligent in their work, they never talk or interact with the residents and few activities are planned for them. John would like to visit his family from time to time but is afraid to ask. She would like his local church minister to call on a Sunday but no religious observances are organised in the home. John likes to go to bed around 10.30 pm each night and when in bed he likes to read or do the crossword. However, the nursing staff insist that he goes to bed before 9 pm, just before the night staff start their duty. He also gets annoyed at the lack of privacy he is given and is feeling very lonely and depressed.

EVIDENCE ACTIVITY

P2

Use the case study on page 59 to:

1. Identify six weaknesses in the way the Elms Residential Home cares for its clients.

2. Identify which aspects of the Care Value Base the Elms Residential Care Home has failed to integrate into its daily practices.

3. Explain how the home could improve their day to day practices in a way that would make John feel happier.

4. Using recognised terminology explain the importance of promoting equality, diversity and rights in a care home such as the Elms. (P2)

2.2 Understand discriminatory practice in health and social care

BASIS OF DISCRIMINATION

Each society is characterised by differentiation (the way in which different groups or individuals differ from one another), which in turn creates the social structure of that society. Unfortunately this does not mean that each of us will be treated equally. Sometimes differentiation can lead to some groups or individuals experiencing low self-esteem, loss of opportunities or even discrimination and marginalisation. Before examining the negative effects of differentiation it is worthwhile identifying some of the ways in which each of us differ.

Age

There are several commonly recognised age groups, i.e. children, teenagers, young adults, middle aged and old aged. There is a risk of discrimination if some age groups are seen as being more valuable than others, or if assumptions are made about the abilities of different groups e.g. older people.

Gender

In the past men often had more rights and were seen as more important than women. Assumptions about gender can still lead to discrimination.

Race

People may identify themselves as being Black, White, European, African or Asian. Many people have specific national identities such as Polish, Nigerian, English and Welsh. Making assumptions about racial characteristics may lead to discrimination.

Class

People differ in their upbringing, the kind of work they do and the money they earn. People also differ in the lifestyles they lead and the views and values that often accompany different levels of income and spending habits. Discrimination against others can be based on their class or lifestyle.

Religion

People grow up within different religious (or non-religious) traditions. For some people spiritual beliefs are at the centre of their understanding of life. For others, religion influences the cultural traditions that they celebrate, for example Christmas. Discrimination can take place if people assume that their customs or beliefs should apply to everyone else.

Sexual orientation

Many people see their sexual orientation as very important to understanding who they are. Gay and lesbian relationships are often discriminated against, where their relationships are judged as 'wrong' or abnormal.

Cognitive and physical ability

Assumptions may be made about what is 'normal'. People with physical disabilities or learning difficulties may be labelled or stereotyped.

Health

People who develop illnesses or mental health problems may feel that they are valued less by other people and discriminated against.

Family status

People choose many different lifestyles and emotional commitments, such as marriage, cohabitation, having children, living in a large family, living a single lifestyle but having sexual partners, or being single and not being sexually active. People live within different family and friendship groups. Discrimination can happen if people think one lifestyle is 'right' or best.

Presentation and dress

People express their individuality, lifestyle and social role through the clothes, hairstyle, makeup and jewellery they wear. While it may be important to conform to social expectations at work, it is also important not to stereotype individuals.

Through the process of socialisation we develop attitudes, prejudices and stereotypes which very often can be inaccurate and can lead to discrimination. The problem with prejudices, stereotypes and labels is that they can also lead to discrimination which can be direct and indirect.

> **Think** From your own knowledge and experience identify one prejudice, stereotype and label that is common in our society.

DISCRIMINATORY PRACTICE

Infringement of rights

Discrimination whether overt or covert is an abuse of power. Very often when an individual has experienced discrimination it also leads to an infringement of rights. This refers to an individual or group being denied the right to participate in society fairly and equally in areas such as education, employment, politics, housing etc.

Abuse and bullying

Two other forms of discrimination worth mentioning are abuse and bullying. Abuse and its various forms have already been covered. Bullying refers to harassment, threats, intimidation or physical violence shown by one person or more towards another person. Although most reported cases of bullying involve children or adolescents bullying can occur in any environment. Acts of bullying may involve name-calling, text-messaging or simply ignoring the individual.

The effects of bullying can however be devastating, as the individual can feel powerless, de-valued, distressed and scared. It will affect their ability to lead a normal life and can be evident in a change of behaviour, loss of appetite, loss of sleep and poor motivation. Many organisations have developed policies on bullying; because it is often hard to detect, allegations of bullying must be taken seriously and procedures for its investigation followed rigorously.

EFFECTS OF DISCRIMINATORY PRACTICE

The feelings experienced by individuals who have had their rights denied are shown in figure 2.4

Marginalisation

People who have been discriminated against are more likely to be marginalised or socially excluded. From a health and social care perspective it means that individuals or groups in society are less likely to have the same opportunities in areas such as education, employment, housing etc as others in society. They are disadvantaged by factors such as age, gender, ethnicity, social class or disability. The term marginalisation is often used interchangeably with the term 'social exclusion', which refers to a process whereby individuals or groups in society are cut off, disadvantaged or deprived of resources that the majority of people in society have access to.

> **Key words**
> ---
> Marginalised – literally means to be on the margins

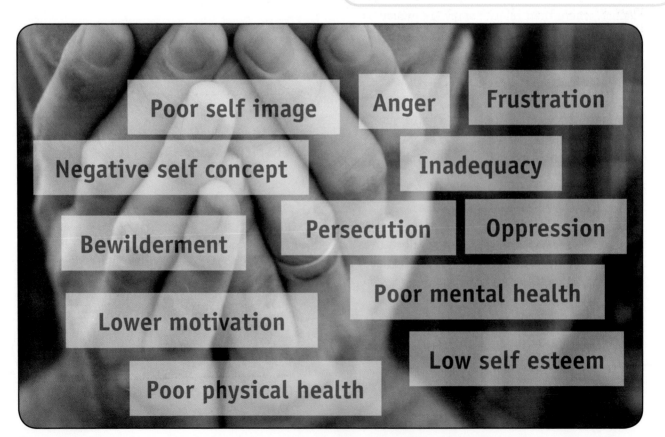

Figure 2.4 The feelings individuals experience as a consequence of having their rights denied to them

Negative behaviours e.g. aggression, criminality

Marginalisation and social exclusion tends to originate in poverty and low income. One of the consequences of marginalisation and social exclusion is that individuals who experience it are more likely to be involved in negative behaviours such as increased levels of aggression and criminality.

Example

In response to this the government set up a Social Exclusion Unit in 1997 (now the Social Exclusion Taskforce). One of their current projects is entitled the Multi-Systemic Therapy Pilots which is a family and community based treatment for young people with complex clinical, social, educational problems including violence and anti-social behaviour.

Restricted opportunities

When individuals or groups in society face discrimination it very often results in those individuals having restricted or fewer opportunities than the majority of people in society. This could mean fewer opportunities to do well at school, achieve good results in exams, get a good job, earn a good wage or salary, or live in decent accommodation etc.

Low self esteem and self identity

Restricted opportunities can also affect individuals by negatively affecting their self esteem or self identity. Self identity refers to how individuals perceive themselves in terms of gender, sexual orientation, ethnic background etc. Self esteem means how highly individuals think of themselves. Individuals with low self esteem may feel worthless, useless, frustrated etc.

One of the simplest ways of discussing the effects of discrimination is to break it down into three levels.

Personal level

In other words, how does it affect the individual? Over the course of a life time each individual develops a self concept that is a combination of self image and self esteem. Individuals will rate their self concept as either positive or negative, depending on how highly they value themselves (self esteem) and how they think they are perceived by others (self image). If an individual has encountered or experienced discrimination it is more likely that their self concept will be negative and will result in feelings of insecurity, lack of confidence or low self worth. Within health and social care settings this can occur when individuals are not fully involved in the decisions relating to their care, making them feel disempowered.

Organisational level

If an individual has experienced discrimination by an organisation very often it will be evident through restricted opportunities or by the denial

of the individual's rights. The individual may be refused any choice, may have their identity and beliefs ignored or denied and will generally feel excluded.

Societal level

Individuals or groups who face discrimination on a regular basis experience a cycle of oppression. The cycle of oppression illustrates the way in which discrimination and oppression can be adopted and replicated by the very individual who has encountered discrimination and unequal treatment.

The cycle occurs in the following way:

- A person, group begins the cycle by treating others in a discriminatory way, which ignores the individual's right to be treated with respect, dignity and value.

- The discrimination can occur in a variety of ways – humiliation, belittling, ignoring the individual or threats. Such behaviours not only oppress but also generate mis-information and ignorance. The individual becomes stereotyped and this becomes justification for further mistreatment.

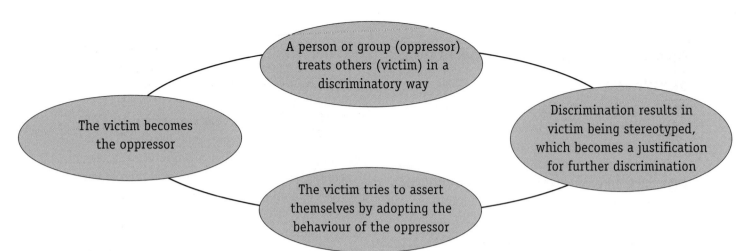

Figure 2.5 The cycle of oppression

- Consequently the individual who is experiencing such discrimination feels the only way to assert themselves is to adopt similar behaviour patterns as the individual or groups who is discriminating against them. This creates a **self-fulfilling prophecy**.

- Adopting such behaviours turns the victim of the discrimination into the oppressor and the cycle begins again.

Key words
Self-fulfilling prophesy–something a person causes to happen by saying and expecting it to happen

The effect of the cycle of oppression is that individuals can become marginalised or socially excluded from mainstream society. Not only can this damage an individual's self concept but it can also have the effect of leading to other negative behaviours such as aggression and anti-social behaviour and criminality.

LOSS OF RIGHTS

Loss of rights means being denied the same rights as those of others such as the right of choice over services, right to dignity, right to be respected with regard to culture, religion etc.

Breaking discrimination and a commitment to change

To begin breaking the cycle of oppression there needs to be a commitment to change by the individual, the group, organisation and society. Policies, procedures and practices will reflect this change. Organisations will need to address their policies, procedures and practices to ensure that care workers understand their responsibilities when promoting equity and diversity.

Sometimes this will mean that care workers will have to proactively change their attitudes and beliefs. It may also mean challenging others who persist in continuing the cycle, which may be difficult.

EVIDENCE ACTIVITY

P3

1. For each of the following statements, identify the individual or group who could be offended by it and explain how they may feel.

a) not inviting a disabled individual to an event because it may cause inconvenience

b) writing a job advert that excludes for reasons some individuals that are not relevant to the job

c) use of language which excludes the participation of others

d) inappropriate use of language to gain power over others.

2. Explain the potential effects of discriminatory practice on those who use health and social care services.

2.3 *Understand how national initiatives promote anti-discriminatory practice*

CONVENTIONS, LEGISLATION AND REGULATIONS

Over the past 40 years UK society has become more multi-cultural and as society's values and attitudes have changed, (for example, more women are now in the work place), government has felt the need to introduce legislation to provide protection from direct and indirect discrimination, to develop greater equality in the workplace and in society in general, and to protect vulnerable and/or minority groups.

A number of Acts and Orders have been passed to make discrimination on the basis of gender, race, age and disability illegal. These include:

- The Sex Discrimination Act 1975
- The Race Relations NI Order 1997 / Act 2000
- The Disability Discrimination Act 1995 / 2005
- Human Rights Act 1998

Research tip

You can get the full text of all the legislation covered in this section by visiting http://www.opsi.gov.uk/acts.htm.

Factors that have influenced the development of equality legislation

There are a number of different factors that have influenced the development of equality legislation over the past 30 years:

- greater participation of women in the work place
- recognition that we live in a multi-cultural society

- the Welfare State – access to services depends on all services being open, transparent and accessible to all sections of society
- the education system has provided greater access to qualifications and employment opportunities for groups who previously would have been denied such access
- the development of the European Union
- the development of Human Rights legislation.

Although different legislation addresses different, specific areas of equality, all legislation shares some common goals. Legislation aims to provide a means of redress for individuals who feel their rights have been infringed, to outlaw direct and indirect discrimination, to promote good practice within the work place and to promote positive action. All laws follow a similar format in what they cover:

- defines the key terms of the legislation – e.g. gender, race, discrimination, direct or indirect
- outlaws direct and indirect discrimination
- outlines the areas covered by the law – access to public services, housing and education, and terms and conditions of employment etc.
- identifies employers' responsibilities under the law
- provides guidance on how employers can promote good practice and guard against indirect discrimination
- identifies forms of redress and complaints procedures
- emphasises and promotes the concept of positive action
- outlines the responsibility of the Equality Commission or other agencies.

Sex Discrimination Act 1975 (Amended Regulations) 1988

In the field of employment, the Sex Discrimination 1975 (Amended Regulations) 1988 Act is an important piece of legislation designed to eliminate discrimination and promote equal treatment between men and women.

The Sex Discrimination Act deals with and outlaws discrimination in the areas of:

- education

- housing

- provision of goods, facilities and services to the public.

In the area of employment it is unlawful to discriminate against an individual because he or she is married. The employment provisions cover issues such as:

- advertising

- recruitment

- selection

- promotion

- pregnancy and maternity rights

- training

- sexual harassment

- terms and conditions of employment, retirement, pensions

- redundancy.

The legislation outlaws two types of discrimination: direct and indirect discrimination. It is against the law to treat anyone less favourably than a person of the opposite sex would be treated in the same circumstances. (This would be direct discrimination). It is also unlawful to apply a condition, which, although applied to equally to both sexes, in practice means that one sex is unfairly disadvantaged or advantaged at the expense of the other. (This is an example of indirect discrimination.)

The Race Relations Act 1976 / Race Relations (NI) Order 1997

Background to the legislation

Racism, which has a long history, is the idea that different ethnic groups have particular characteristics and attributes, and that therefore some groups are superior to others. It has often been used to justify the oppression of one ethnic group by another.

One of the earliest examples of racism being used as a justification for oppression was slavery. Ideas about European white racial superiority also played an important role in the colonisation of large parts of the world, as European countries carved out empires for themselves. The biggest of all these empires was the British Empire, which at its largest extent in 1921 covered a quarter of the world's land mass, and contained a quarter of the world's population.

At the end of the Second World War in 1945, the UK, like many other European countries, suffered a labour shortage as they tried to rebuild after the devastation of the war. To fill the gaps in the labour market people from the colonies and ex-colonies were recruited to come and work in the UK. The 1948 British Nationality Act gave British citizenship to all people living in the colonies, and the right of entry and settlement in the UK. Most intended to stay for a short period of time before returning home, but in fact many settled permanently. However, many experienced severe prejudice and discrimination, particularly in employment and housing.

What has been the effect of the discrimination?

Black people and other ethnic minority groups such as travellers (NI Order 1997 cites travellers as a specific minority group) have been unable to participate fully in society. They have been denied access to jobs, housing, education, goods and services. They have been unable to share their cultures for fear of attack or reprisals.

The 1976 Race Relations Act

The 1968 Race Relations Act was repealed by the introduction of the Race Relations Act 1976. This law sought to close several loopholes left by previous legislation. Modelled closely on the Sex Discrimination Act, the Race Relations Act 1976 identifies and outlaws direct and indirect discrimination in the area of race.

The Act makes it unlawful to discriminate against someone on the grounds of their race, colour, and nationality, ethnic or national origins. The Act applies to:

- employment (job advertisements, recruitment, selection, interviewing, and training)

- housing

- education

- other Public Services.

The Commission for Racial Equality was established to oversee the working of the Act. Their function was as follows:

- to work towards the elimination of discrimination

- to promote equality of opportunity and good relations between different racial groups

- to keep under review the workings of the Act, and, if necessary, to draw up proposals to amend it

- to give advice to people with complaints of discrimination and, in some cases, represent complainants in the courts.

Types of discrimination outlawed

Direct discrimination happens when someone is treated worse than others, or segregated from them, because of their colour, race, nationality, ethnic or national origins. Most race complaints are about direct discrimination. Indirect discrimination happens when everyone seems to be treated in the same way, but in practice people from a particular background or ethnic groups are put at a disadvantage. For example, if a law affects one particular ethnic group more than others, without there being a good reason for it, then the law is indirectly discriminatory.

If a person is victimised because they have complained about racial discrimination, or because they have supported another person's complaint, this is also unlawful discrimination.

Race Relations (Amendment) Act 2000

This act was a key part of the Government's drive to implement the Macpherson Report's recommendations. It is also the first significant amendment to the 1976 Race Relations Act. It strengthens the 1976 Race Relations Act in that it gives public authorities a statutory general duty to promote racial equality. The aim of the duty is to make promoting race equality central to the way public authorities work.

> **Key words**
> ---
> Macpherson Report – the report produced as a result of the inquiry into the murder of the black teenager Stephen Lawrence in 1993, for which no one has yet been convicted.

Disability Discrimination Act 1995

Background to the Act

Having a disability affects the person's concept of self; how individuals cope with the experience has been almost totally neglected in most research. Disabled people are a severely disadvantaged minority within British society. Disablement frequently means being unable to take part in social and economic activities that others take for granted, as well as having to endure negative social attitudes. Numerous studies have also shown that in terms of income, employment, housing and access to facilities in the community disabled people are much worse off than their non-disabled counterparts. Disability has two main financial effects: it can result in loss of earned income and in additional expense for equipment etc.

Despite this disabled people are a potentially powerful political force. They have attacked the stereotypical bias in language and have fostered a growing consciousness and identity. Disability pressure groups generally have not been able to exert much positive political change, although some have achieved more successes than others, either because their clients are seen as being more appealing, or because they are more skilled at putting their case.

Existing welfare services have not been developed on the basis of a coherent understanding of the origins and consequences of disability but have emerged in a piecemeal fashion in response to political pressure. Although such services are of enormous benefit to disabled people they are inadequate to secure the full participation of disabled people in all aspects of life.

Disability Discrimination Act 1995

The Disability Discrimination Act recognised that various barriers exist within society that present difficulties for disabled people who are seeking employment and when accessing goods, facilities, services or buildings. In order to address some of these difficulties the legislation, unlike other anti-discrimination legislation, creates a positive duty on employers and service providers to make 'reasonable adjustment' to their policies and premises, where reasonable and appropriate. In addition, unlike other equal opportunities legislation, indirect discrimination is not dealt with explicitly. Instead, it is addressed by both the direct discrimination provisions and the duty to make reasonable adjustments.

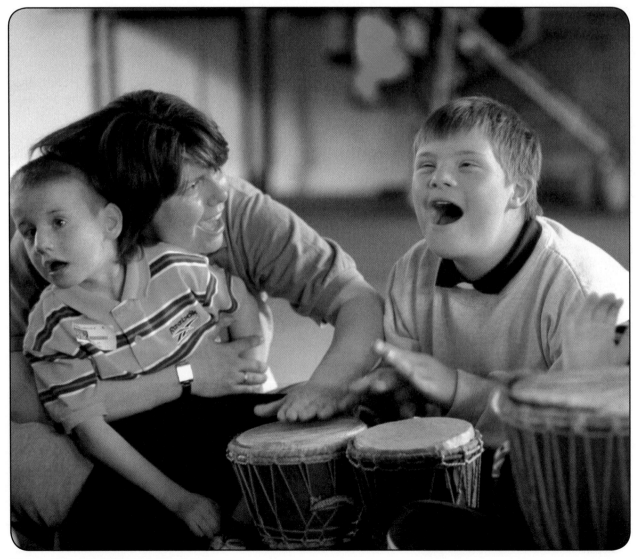

Figure 2.6 Disability adaptations

Disability Discrimination Act 2005

The Disability Discrimination Act was extended to cover education through the Special Needs and Disability Act 2005 (SENDO). This was subsequently amended in 2006 to relate to Further and Higher Education.

Age Discrimination Act 2006

This legislation makes it unlawful to discriminate against a person at work because of their age. The Employment Equality (Age) Regulations 2006 covers:

- recruitment
- terms and conditions of employment
- promotion
- transfers
- discrimination
- training.

Human Rights Act 1998

Although passed in 1998, it was not until Oct 2000 that the UK's Human Rights Act (HRA) came into force. The act applies to all parts of the UK – Scotland, Wales and Northern Ireland (although under the terms of the Good Friday Agreement Northern Ireland was also to have its own Bill of Rights). It entitles anyone who feels their rights have been infringed to seek help from the courts. It covers public, private, voluntary and charitable organisations.

The Act guarantees the following rights:

- the right to life
- the right to freedom from torture and inhuman or degrading treatment or punishment
- the right to freedom from slavery, servitude and forced or compulsory labour
- the right to liberty and security of person
- the right to a fair and public trial within a reasonable time
- the right to freedom from retrospective criminal law and no punishment without law
- the right to respect for private and family life, home and correspondence
- the right to freedom of thought, conscience and religion
- the right to freedom of expression
- the right to freedom of assembly and association
- the right to marry and found a family
- the prohibition of discrimination in the enjoyment of convention rights
- the right to peaceful enjoyment of possessions and protection of property
- the right to access to an education
- the right to free elections
- the right not to be subjected to the death penalty.

Data Protection Act 1998

All information concerning clients and service users is subject to the conditions of the Data Protection Act 1998. The Act covers medical records, social services records, credit information and local authority information. Anyone processing information must comply with the eight principles of good practice, which are that data must be:

- fairly and lawfully processed
- processed for limited purposes
- adequate, relevant and not excessive
- accurate
- not kept longer than necessary
- processed in accordance with the data subject's rights
- kept secure
- not transferred to other countries without adequate protection.

In addition to the legislation outlined on pages 66-69 a number of other laws designed to support and promote the rights of certain vulnerable groups including children, adults and older people, have also been passed.

The Convention on the Rights of the Child 1989

In 1959 the United Nations made a Declaration of the Rights of the Child; this was subsequently amended in 1979 to a Convention the Rights of the Child, which recognises the child as a person worthy of respect and with rights. This was later adopted by the UN General Assembly in 1989 and ratified by the UK government in 1991. Under the Convention children have the following rights:

- the right to life

- the right to adequate standard of living

- the right to education, play, leisure and cultural activities

- the right to protection against all forms of abuse

- the right to a say in matters affecting their lives and opportunities to take part in the activities of their society.

In addition Article 23 emphasises that disabled children also have the right to special care, education and training to help them enjoy a full and decent life.

The Children Act 1989 / The Children (NI) Order 1995

This Act/NI Order supersedes all previous pieces of legislation regarding the safety and protection of children. It is one of the most important pieces of legislation related to the care and protection of children introduced by government over the past 50 years, as it has changed the way society, the state and local authorities perceive their role in protecting vulnerable children.

The act establishes the following principles:

- Children are welfare is paramount

- a child is best looked after within their own homes

- the importance of parental responsibilities – local authorities should work in partnership with parents

- good substitute parenting should be provided where there is family breakdown

- a definition of what a 'child in need' is

- that children have the right to be consulted and listened to when decisions regarding them are being made

- that local authorities must provide a range of services to support children in need

- the provision of a Guardian ad Litem

- the development of a welfare checklist which is used by the courts when deciding a child's best interests.

The Mental Health Act 1983 / Mental Health (NI) Order 1986

This Act focuses on the assessment and treatment of people with a mental disorder. The legislation covers four categories of mental disorder. They are:

- mental impairment

- severe mental impairment

- psychopathic disorder

- mental illness.

Although mental illness was left undefined in the Act the term can broadly be interpreted as meaning:

- persistent interruption of intellectual functioning

- persistent alteration of mood

- delusional tendencies or episodes

- irrational thinking.

Section 2 of the legislation covers admission to hospital for psychiatric assessment for up to 28 days. Compulsory admission for assessment can only take place on the recommendation of two registered medical practitioners. The legislation also allows for compulsory admission for assessment for 72 hours in cases of an emergency. Such an application can be made either by the nearest relative or by an approved social worker and the recommendation of a medical practitioner. The legislation also allows for the provision of a guardian for people over the age of 16.

Mental Capacity Act 2005

This law governs decision making on behalf of adults where they lose mental capacity at some point in their lives or where the condition has been present from birth. It provides a statutory framework to protect and empower vulnerable people who are not able to make their own decisions. It makes it clear who can make decisions, in which situations, and how they should go about this. A code of practice was also developed to underpin the Act.

Nursing and Residential Care Homes Regulations 1984 (amended 2002)

This requires all nursing homes to be registered, as it is an offence to operate without a licence. The Act is accompanied by a code of practice that specifies 14 areas of good practice including inspection, registration, furniture and equipment etc. The Code also promotes the notion that a home should reflect the individual's own environment and therefore in cases of long term stays residents should have the right to bring their own possessions with them.

The Care Standards Act 2000

Care Standards Act 2000 (CSA) provides for the administration of a variety of care institutions, including children's homes, independent hospitals, nursing homes and residential care homes. The CSA, which was enacted in April 2002, replaces the Registered Homes Act 1984 and parts of the Children's Act 1989 that relate to the care

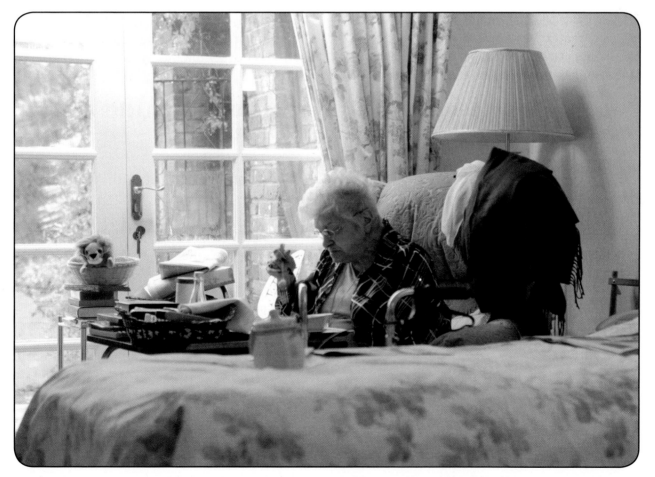

Figure 2.7 A care home must follow strict codes of practice, which are designed to improve residents' quality of life during their stay

or the accommodation of children. The aim of the legislation was to reform the law relating to the inspection and regulation of various care institutions.

The Act also introduced the National Care Standards Commission, which is now responsible for the arrangements for inspection of residential and nursing homes. Underpinning the work of the Commission are the standards published for care homes for older people. The standards cover a number of areas such as choice of home, personal care, social activities, complaints and protection etc. The Act is of particular importance to people requiring specialist care, e.g. service users with dementia.

CODES OF PRACTICE AND CHARTERS

Codes of practice and charters are documents that aim to guide professionals about their professional roles and responsibilities. They lay down standards of practice and therefore serve a role in monitoring and raising professional standards. Codes of Practice guide the professional's behaviour in an everyday context, especially when faced with the constraints placed on them by the bureaucracy of the organisation. They help identify clear boundaries of what is or is not permissible between professionals and users. They are also concerned with how the professional should treat the individual service user rather than with prescribing how resources should be allocated.

There are two main codes of practice that govern the work of health and social care professionals – the General Social Care Council (GSCC) / Northern Ireland Social Care Council Code of Practice and the Nursing Midwifery Council (NMC) Code of Practice.

Research tip

You can download a copy of the GSCC's Code of Practice on their website at www.gscc.org.uk. Visit www.nmc-uk.org to download a copy of the NMC's Code of Practice.

The term Code of Practice is used to cover a broad range of different types of codes of conduct or behaviour. In general codes consist of the following features:

- a statement of the values of the profession

- a statement of commitment to professional integrity

- statements of ethical principles

- general statements of principle.

They range in their size and level of detail and generally do not provide detailed guidance to professionals about how to act in a particular situation.

Codes of practice are necessary for a variety of reasons. Within the health and social care sector many professionals are involved in close, personal work with service users and will use a variety of techniques when working with the services user, which could be open to either neglect or abuse. Also, much of the language used in health and social care is quite technical so a code can help explain simply and clearly the service user's rights. A code of practice will also outline what the practitioner's duty towards the service user is.

ORGANISATIONAL POLICIES AND PROCEDURES

Positive promotion of individual rights

Positive promotion of individual rights occurs when an organisation works in partnership with the individual to ensure that the individual is supported in the care that is being provided. Positive promotion of individual rights covers every aspect of an organisation's activities and is reflected through the policies and practices that the organisation develops.

Affirmative action

Affirmative action or positive action refers to situations when an organisation will actively work to redress a disadvantage. For example, if women aree under represented within the workforce, some organisations will include in their job advertisements that they particularly welcome female applicants. Another example is that a health and social care agency working with a particular minority group may decide to appoint a care worker who comes from that minority background as they will have an understanding of that minority group.

Human rights

The term 'human rights' refers to the rights each individual has with regard to every aspect of life. As previously outlined on page 69, the human rights each individual is entitled to are outlined in the Human Rights Act 1998.

Work practices

Different organisations will vary regarding their own work practices, for example voluntary organisations often operate very differently to in the private or state sectors. Despite these differences, there are accepted rules of good practice for work practices that apply to all organisations:

- regular staff meetings
- induction for all new staff members
- provision of a staff hand book
- induction handbook
- training or mentoring – for example peer observations
- regular audits and monitoring.

Organisations also often formalise their work practices in writing. Equal opportunities statements are statements of intent and include details about what the organisation will do to provide a service free from discrimination and that is accessible to everyone. The content of such statements reflect the principles that underpin equality of opportunity.

Mission statements build on equal opportunities statements but go further in identifying what the service provider hopes to provide in relation to the service. It therefore not only reflects the principle of equality but also deals at length with how the organisation hopes to encourage marginalised groups to participate in the service.

Other statements and policies include:

- Admission Statement
- Induction Policy
- Health and Safety Policy
- Lifting and Handling Policy
- Confidentiality Policy
- Advocacy Policy
- Complaints and Grievance Policy
- Citizen and Patient Charters
- Anti-Harassment, Bullying and Sectarian Statements
- Prevention of Abuse Statements

Staff development and training

Staff development and training have become key areas of activity within most organisations, as it is recognised that the most important asset in making an effective organisation is human resources. Within some health and social care professions it is now mandatory to regularly update skills and knowledge through planned training days that act as refresher courses. Most organisations have their own organisational development plan that outlines how they intend to meet the professional development needs of their staff.

Organisations that carry out regular training with their workforce therefore ensure that staff are aware of key issues affecting the care of service users who access their organisation. Training activities include:

- induction training

- anti-bullying, harassment and sectarian training

- refresher training on legislation

- selection and recruitment training and interview skills

- good practice initiatives, linked with quality assurance

- monitoring of the workforce.

Quality issues

Quality assurance has become a key task for most organisations. It focuses on how an organisation is going to maintain standards and also improve on those standards. Quality assurance begins with policies and procedures developed by the organisation as a benchmark – the minimum standard. As a part of quality assurance, training and professional development are seen not only as an extension of an individual's original training but as a vital means of ensuring effective care and thus maintaining the standards of the organisation. Other important forms of quality assurance include regular inspection and auditing of systems and processes. When quality assurance is effective the service provided becomes more client-orientated, service users are satisfied and happy and resources are used effectively.

Complaints procedures

An important part of exercising rights is being able to complain about a service or the care provided, particularly if it does not meet the service user's requirements. All public and statutory organisations are required to have a complaints procedure. A complaints process is the formal process by which a grievance can be heard and dealt with effectively. A complaints process will normally take place in stages, the first being an informal stage where the person making the complaint will discuss with the organisation the nature of the complaint before proceeding with it further. It is generally in everyone's interests to have complaints dealt with quickly and effectively so if a complaint can be resolved at the informal stage it should be. Complaints procedures are an important way of monitoring the standards provided by the organisation and thus their quality assurance.

Anti-harassment

Harassment means to intentionally hurt or damage and is closely associated to bullying and abuse. Harassment can take many forms, ranging from physical pushing and shoving to verbal abuse. Although most organisations strive to promote a welcoming, happy environment, sometimes employees and service users do face harassment within the organisation. Consequently anti-harassment training has been developed to try and combat the problem and many organisations have developed policies and procedures for dealing with the issue.

Confidentiality

The term confidentiality refers to the security of information about a client or service user. It is one of the central themes of the care value base and involves issues of trust as well as individual rights. However, it is well recognised within the health and social care sector that the issue of confidentiality is a complex one in practice. When is it justified to break a confidence or share information with others? Consequently, most organisations will have a clear policy that will be communicated to the service user regarding the disclosure of information. The issue of confidentiality is further supported by the Data Protection Act 1998, which provides clear guidelines about the use of personal information.

Challenging discrimination

Challenging discrimination can be difficult, particularly if the person challenged is a work colleague or a service user. Finding effective ways of challenging unequal treatment takes time, effort, commitment and a willingness to be equally challenged. Sometimes, because of the risks involved, it is easier to ignore the discrimination and do nothing, but by doing so the individual is supporting discrimination and is equally guilty of it.

Care workers need to develop strategies that enable them to challenge people when their choices or actions infringe the rights of others. Care workers also need to be confident and assertive when putting such strategies in place. Direct challenges take a lot of confidence and some care workers may not feel comfortable doing this on their own. Therefore the support of the organisation and particularly management is essential when effecting real change.

When challenging behaviour it is important to remember that it is the behaviour being challenged, not the person.

EVIDENCE ACTIVITY

P4 – M1 – D1

1. Describe how legislation, codes of practice, rules of conduct, charters and organisations policies are used to promote anti-discriminatory practice. (P4)

2. Explain the influence SENDO or the introduction of Age Discrimination legislation will have on organisational policy with regard to anti-discriminatory practice. (M1)

3. Evaluate how the introduction of SENDO or Age Discrimination legislation could influence organisational and personal practice in relation to anti-discriminatory practice. (D1)

2.4 How anti-discriminatory practice is promoted in health and social care settings

In the previous section national initiatives were highlighted as ways in which organisations can promote good care practice. However, it is also important to examine the role individual care practitioners play in promoting anti-discriminatory practice.

ACTIVE PROMOTION OF ANTI-DISCRIMINATORY PRACTICE

Empowering the client

Empowerment can be used by the professional to promote equality. The focus of empowerment is helping people gain greater control over their lives. Empowerment will not only increase confidence and self esteem but can also help the individual change other aspects of their life. Empowering people can also help tackle inequality, discrimination and oppression.

Partnership

Working in partnership, whether with the individual service user or other professionals involves:

- identifying problems or issues that need to be addressed

- deciding what needs to be done and assigning people to specific tasks

- undertaking the necessary work through a process of collaboration and consultation

- reviewing progress and agreeing any changes that need to be made to the agreed course of action

- evaluating the work done and highlighting strengths and weaknesses and lessons to be learned.

Partnership entails reducing the power differential between professionals and users of services. By putting the service user first the care practitioner demonstrates the importance of respecting the client's culture, their beliefs and the fact that they have rights and choices that need to be reflected in the care provided.

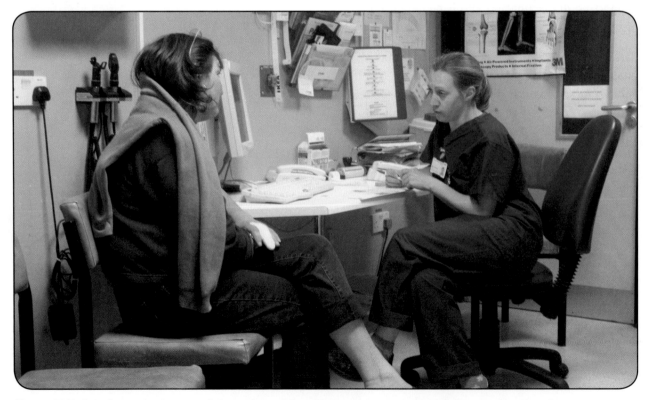

Figure 2.8 It is important to work in partnership with service users and fellow professionals

These key principles can be achieved in a variety of ways:

- appointment of a Key Worker

- development of a care plan for each client, which is reviewed regularly

- monitoring the standards of care through satisfaction questionnaires

- suggestion boxes

- resident's forums

- effective communication with clients and where appropriate the use of advocates and interpreters

- reflective practice

- challenging discriminatory behaviour.

Key words

Key Worker – staff who play a crucial role in the social services, e.g. Nurses, Teachers, social workers, police

Through reflective practice equality can be promoted by encouraging greater sensitivity to issues relating to power or disadvantage. It also enables the practitioner to take account of other factors such as personal, cultural or structural factors, which affect the care provided to clients. For reflective practice to be effective it needs to be critical in the sense that the care practitioner should not take equality for granted or make assumptions that can then reinforce existing patterns of inequality. The starting point for any reflective practice is to ask 'what went well today?', 'what didn't go well today?' and 'what could I have done better?'.

Some practitioners find challenging difficult behaviour extremely difficult to do, but the keys to challenging others' behaviour lies in:

- being tactful and constructive, not critical or punitive

- avoiding 'cornering' people

- choosing an appropriate time and place to address the issue

- being sensitive to the vulnerability, weaknesses or limitations of the challenger

- demonstrating a spirit of good will and compassion rather than taking the moral high ground.

EVIDENCE ACTIVITY

P5 – M2

Nihal has started work as a day care worker in a day centre for adults with physical, sensory and learning disability. He enjoys his work and whenever possible encourages the service users to be as independent as possible. For example, he encourages them to make choices over their lunch menu and to feed themselves. In addition he has obtained permission from the centre manager to start an arts and crafts class on a Wednesday afternoon.

1. Explain how Nihal, through his own practice, is promoting anti-discriminatory practice. (P5)

2. Explain some of the difficulties Nihal may face when implementing anti-discriminatory practice. (M2)

PERSONAL BELIEFS AND VALUES

As a result of socialisation, all individuals have a set of personal beliefs, (that is what they regard as true) and also a set of values that guide their behaviour. Very often the beliefs will influence the ideas. For example an individual might have a belief in God and this may in turn influence their values about the value and importance of human life.

Careful use of language

Although practitioners are more aware of the need to be politically correct when addressing service users, it is worth highlighting that insensitive use of terms and phrases can be discriminatory and can lead to service user oppression. At its worst, the effects of using insensitive language may include a reinforcing of inequality leading to greater social exclusion and marginalisation, and the stigmatisation and devaluing of the service user.

Greater openness

Greater openness can be achieved in a number of ways:

- interactions between staff and service users should be based on openness and honesty

- language (both verbal and written) should be user friendly, for example with minimal use of jargon

- advocates and interpreters should be used as and where appropriate

- decisions should be made jointly or, where this is not possible, fully explained to the service user. This will help avoid conflict and in doing so balance the rights of the service user with those of others.

Use of the law

There are a number of Acts of Parliament that contain provisions for the promotion of equality in one form or another. The law therefore presents an opportunity to develop greater equality and also to challenge discrimination and thus prevent or lessen oppression.

Professionalism

Skilled and trained practitioners should be committed to a set of values that will guide their practice. In addition they should also be committed to high standards of practice that are recognised through professional bodies such as the NMC and GSCC. They should also be accountable for their practice and open to scrutiny.

Committing to the care value base

The care value base is the framework for the social care profession. It identifies the expectations for all individuals who work in health and social care. It defines what quality care looks like and how it can best be achieved. It reflects the basic principles of equality, individual rights and choices.

The care value base is important as it allows carers to check and monitor their own work in relation to the values and standards established. It can help guide a carer's actions and how they behave towards a service user. Service users and their relatives can use it to ensure that they are getting good quality care and it identifies what both the care worker and service user need to do and what is expected. The main elements of the care value base are:

- empowerment

- confidentiality/privacy

- effective communication

- the support of individual rights and choices

- respect for beliefs and identity

- anti-discriminatory practice.

Integrating these principles into practice will ensure that service users are provided with a high level of interpersonal care, that they are empowered and their independence promoted, that they are respected for their individuality, communicated with effectively, given timely and accurate information and that they are not discriminated against.

Implementation of the care value base will provide the opportunity for people to develop to their full potential. On a day to day basis it means understanding assumptions and oppression, prejudice and stereotyping, understanding your own beliefs and valuing the benefits of diversity. In addition it means promoting both rights and responsibilities through developing effective relationships, identifying needs and resources, challenging others when rights are not met and promoting concepts such as confidentiality, choice, dignity, communication, safety and advocacy.

One of the most important concepts in positive care practice is that of confidentiality. This concept reflects the trust and confidence between the service user and the care worker. How the organisation maintains that trust is therefore vital to the relationship between the service user and care worker. Most organisations will have developed clear policy guidelines and procedures for the security of information. However, blurred boundaries and tensions remain, especially on occasions when a confidence has to be broken in the interests of the client and for the safety of others.

Difficulties that may be encountered when implementing anti-discriminatory practice

Although most organisations today have adopted policies and procedures designed to promote equality, diversity and rights, some organisations still directly or indirectly discriminate towards potential service users. There are a number of explanations as to why this might occur.

Organisational culture

Within some organisations the culture is such that it does not lend itself towards promoting equality, diversity and rights for service users. The culture of an organisation may be overtly or covertly sexist, racist etc, and therefore will either not be aware, or choose to ignore, the effects of the culture on both employees and service users.

Physical buildings

The physical buildings themselves may unintentionally prevent some service users from gaining access. This could be because the building cannot accommodate all service users who wish to access the service or because the organisation has not conformed to the regulations laid out in the Disability Discrimination Act 1995, which states that all buildings should be accessible to all disabled people and measures should be taken to ensure this.

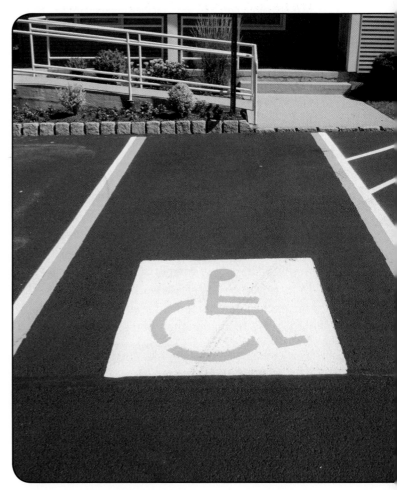

Figure 2.9 Designated parking spaces and ramps make a building more accessible for wheelchair users

Internal conflict

Some organisations encounter difficulties when implementing anti-discriminatory practice if there is a conflict between attempting to promote anti-discriminatory practice and the role (aims and objectives) of the organisation on a day to day basis and the pressures it faces in providing a service. This conflict may be due to the fact that not everyone in the organisation agrees with the idea of equality and promotion of service users' rights. Another reason may be a severe lack of resources (human, financial, physical etc), which may hinder the organisation in implementing effective anti-discriminatory practice.

Individual practitioners

Although all care workers are now required to undertake training, some will slip through the net, or even if they are trained, will not fully understand or agree with the concepts of equality, promoting diversity and service users' rights. If a care worker has developed very entrenched or negative views, either through personal experience or through their socialisation process, it may be very difficult for them to treat each service user equally, especially if they have sexist, racist or homophobic prejudices. Furthermore, the use of professional training and development may be of little use to them as they may choose to ignore the aims of the training or refuse to get involved in group training exercises where they can discuss their feeling and attitudes. In addition, they may feel threatened by the culture the organisation is trying to promote and therefore choose to say nothing but simply comply and pay 'lip service' to it. However, some care workers may have such entrenched and hardened views that it could be impossible to change their perceptions.

The service user

Effective care practice relies on partnership between the organisation, practitioner and service user. Some service users may feel reluctant to complain about a service for fear it may be withdrawn from them. Some service users may not know how to make a complaint about a service. Some service users may not know the difference between an 'effective' service and a 'poor' service. If the organisation has not communicated effectively with the service user and given them information to make choices the service user will be ignorant of what is available to them and therefore will be unable to provide feedback to the organisation.

Loopholes in legislation

Although many organisations conform to legislation, the different requirements of each piece of legislation, which is often extremely complex, make it difficult for some organisations to get it right all the time. Consequently, where loopholes do exist, some organisations will use this as a reason not to promote effective care practice. Some organisations find it difficult to be consistent in applying legislation. This is especially true in small organisations without a personnel officer or human resource officer, where it is left to an administrator who has little training or understanding of equality issues to implement the legislation.

Resources

To effectively promote anti-discriminatory practice resources have to be deployed and used effectively. An organisation will have many resources at its disposal, including human, physical, financial and educational resources. Used effectively and in conjunction with one another the use of resources can greatly promote anti-discriminatory practice – service users are empowered, given choice, independence is promoted, high quality care is given and the individual feels valued. Used ineffectively and wastefully, organisations will have great difficulty in promoting anti-discriminatory practice – individuals may become withdrawn, their physical health may deteriorate, their self esteem affected, and they may feel socially excluded and oppressed.

Good care practice can be effectively promoted within health and social care settings by following some basic principles.

- Promoting all aspects of the care value base.

- Recognising that we live in a society where individuals may face discrimination, inequality and abuse and that there is therefore a need for policies and codes that are designed to protect and safeguard service users.

- Recognising that care workers can hold prejudiced, stereotypical attitudes and values that may affect the quality of care and that regular training and professional development is required to challenge this.

- Identifying that some groups are more vulnerable and need specifically designed policies to protect them.

- Recognising that carers need guidelines to identify the boundaries of their work and protect them from complaints by service users.

- Recognising that care workers and service users need to develop an understanding of the respective boundaries involved in the caring relationship.

The care sector is continually attempting to raise standards and improve provision but this can only be achieved by continual review and evaluation to identify best practice. Best practice acknowledges that there is a distinction between an individual's universal human rights and their rights when receiving services provided by an organisation. Guidance and codes of practice are not always explicit about 'moral' rights (for example treating individuals with equity). An organisation may assume these moral rights are implicit in their policy and procedure and expect care workers to demonstrate this in their practice. There may also be tensions between the rights of the individual and the rights of the organisation (such as allowing individuals to take risks, or balancing health and welfare issues), which the care professional will have to negotiate and make decisions about, not always in favour of the service user.

Key words

Best practice – a working method which is officially accepted as being the best to use in a particular industry. Best practice is usually described formally and in detail

EVIDENCE ACTIVITY

M3 – D2

Ruth works as a practice nurse in a busy GP's surgery. She enjoys her work and is both professional and effective in the care that she delivers. Each Tuesday afternoon she holds a parenting class for young mums who are finding it difficult to cope with the demands of motherhood. Although she enjoys taking the class she doesn't have much sympathy for the mothers and recently told a colleague 'they should have thought about the consequences before they got pregnant'.

1. Analyse how Ruth's personal beliefs and values may influence her practice. (M3)

2. Identify practical ways Ruth could reconcile her own beliefs and values to make her a more effective care worker. (M3)

3. Evaluate these practical strategies in reconciling beliefs and values with anti-discriminatory practice in health and social care. (D2)

Health, Safety and Security in Health and Social Care

unit 3

This unit is about the protection of patients and service users, as well as those who work in health and social care settings. It will explore health, safety and security issues that are important in making sure that services are delivered safely. It will develop your knowledge and understanding of the range of potential hazards in health and social care environments. For example, it will look at the safe handling of food, the principles of manual handling, how to ensure no intruders enter a building and the disposal of waste materials, among other topics.

You will look at the legislation and policies that promote health, safety and security, and their impact on health and social care delivery, as well as at the roles and responsibilities of employers and employees. The risks that are posed by different groups or environments are also explored. For example, the different needs of older people, or those with a loss of hearing or sight, compared with young children; or the difference between an indoor activity and a visit to a local park. You will need to be able to undertake a risk assessment and make recommendations for minimising any identified risks.

The basic principles of emergency first aid are covered, but learners are encouraged to gain a recognised first aid qualification.

Learning outcomes

By the end of this unit you will:

3.1 Understand potential hazards in health and social care — page 85

3.2 Understand how legislation, guidelines, policies and procedures promote health, safety and security — page 99

3.3 Understand roles and responsibilities for health, safety and security in health and social care settings — page 106

3.4 Know how to deal with hazards in a local environment — page 111

So you want to be a...

Deputy Manager, residential care home

My name Paul Butler
Age 27
Income £19,000

If you are organised, flexible and have a real interest in the care of older people, read on.

So, what do you do?

I assist the manager in organising the day-to-day care of the residents and ensuring a high standard of care.

What responsibilities do you have?

I am responsible for the health, safety and security of the residents and the staff. My other responsibilities include managing the staff rotas and identifying their training needs. When the manager is away I stand in for her. Together we regularly review the home's policies and procedures to ensure they are kept up to date. I interview new residents and introduce them to the home.

How did you get the job?

I have a vocational qualification in health care. I worked in a residential home after college and obtained my NVQ Level 2. The units that I had studied in college provided the knowledge I needed for the NVQ. I then got another job as a senior carer and team leader. In that role I was able to complete NVQ Level 3 in social care. After one year's experience I was then in a good position to apply for the deputy manager's job.

How did you find your current job?

I found the job in the local newspaper. I also saw some other positions on national websites.

> ❝ **It is important to have a real interest in older people** ❞

What training have you had?

When I started I spent two weeks shadowing the manager. She made sure that I was confident about all aspects of the home. We have since discussed some courses that I could go on and I will probably start my NVQ Level 4 Registered Manager's Award next year.

What are the hours like?

It is a full-time post and I work 35 hours per week. I have to be flexible about the hours I work to be able to cover for the manager. We take it in turns to be on call in case there are any emergencies.

What skills do you need?

The ability to communicate effectively, manage your time and good interpersonal skills are all necessary. I think it is also important to be a good team worker and have a real interest in older people.

What about the future?

I would like to become a manager of a residential home. I know I am going in the right direction, but need to make sure that I continue to develop my skills. I need to learn more about the financial and business side of running a home.

Grading criteria

The table below shows what you need to do to gain a pass, merit or distinction in this part of the qualification. Make sure you refer back to it when you are completing work so you can judge whether you are meeting the criteria and what you need to do to fill in gaps in your knowledge or experience.

In this unit there are six evidence activities that give you an opportunity to demonstrate your achievement of the grading criteria:

page 88   P1   page 103   P4

page 104   P2   page 110   P5, M2, D2

page 114   P3, M1, D1   page 115   P6, M3

To achieve a pass grade the evidence must show that the learner is able to...	To achieve a merit grade the evidence must show that, in addition to the pass criteria, the learner is able to...	To achieve a distinction grade the evidence must show that, in addition to the pass and merit criteria, the learner is able to...
P1 use work placement experiences to explain a minimum of six potential hazards in a health or social care setting		
P2 describe how key legislation in relation to health, safety and security influences health and social care delivery		
P3 using examples from work experience describe how policies and procedures promote health, safety and security in the health and social care workplace	**M1** explain how legislation, policies and procedures are used to promote the health, safety and security of individuals in the health and social care workplace	**D1** using examples from work experience evaluate the effectiveness of policies and procedures for promoting health, safety and security
P4 examine the roles and responsibilities of key people in the promotion of health, safety and security in a health or social care setting		
P5 carry out a health and safety survey of a local environment used by a specific patient/service user group	**M2** assess the risk associated with the use of the chosen local environment and make recommendations for change	**D2** justify recommendations made for minimising the risks, as appropriate, for the setting and service user groups
P6 demonstrate basic first aid skills	**M3** demonstrate first aid skills on a critically injured individual	

3.1 *Understanding potential hazards in health and social care*

HAZARDS

A hazard is anything that could cause harm. A risk is the chance of being harmed by a hazard. It is important to understand what the potential hazards are in a situation, because in a health and social care setting certain groups of people, such as the sick, elderly or disabled, are particularly vulnerable. Children are also at an increased risk. Some hazards are general to any working environment and others will be specific to working in health and social care. These include hazards that might affect any staff or visitors as well as the clients.

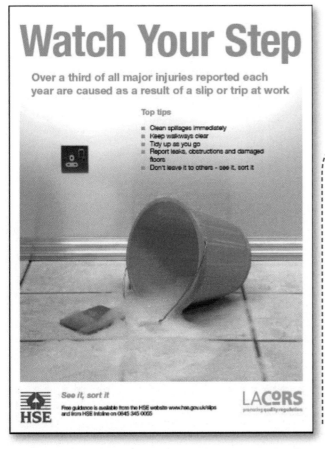

Figure 3.1 A Health and Safety Executive poster warning of potential hazards in the workplace

There are a number of different causes of hazards, including:

- an unsafe working environment
- poor working conditions
- poor staff training
- poor working practices
- wrongly used or badly maintained equipment
- substances, such as chemicals, medicines or food, where safety guidelines are not followed.

> **Think** Can you think of a specific hazard that might result from each of the causes listed above?

WORKING ENVIRONMENT

As someone who works in health and social care, you may visit several different places of work. Some may have similar hazards to each other, but in others the hazards may be different.

Example

Donna is a health care assistant who works with a district nurse. She is based at a health centre, where she works with other members of the primary health care team. In addition to seeing patients at the surgery, she visits other patients in the community. For example, she helps people to wash and dress, dresses wounds and gives injections. Some of her regular patients live in a residential home where there is a special room in which she can perform some procedures. Other patients that she visits live at home and sometimes she finds that the space is very cramped. She drives many miles and often works early in the morning and late at night.

> **Think** How might the hazards that Donna needs to consider differ between the surgery, the residential home and the patient's own home? What hazards might Donna face while out in the community?

CASE STUDY: RESIDENTIAL HOME

Margaret is the manager of a residential home. The home is on a fairly busy road, but it is convenient for the local shops and the residents enjoy going into town to have a coffee and meet friends.

There are 15 members of staff at the home. The staff range in age from 19-year-old students to employees who are over 50. One member of staff is currently off sick with a bad back.

Two years ago a resident slipped while getting out of the bath and fractured her hip.

Margaret has heard that other local homes have been targeted by criminals who raided the residents' rooms while they were having lunch.

Since the accident and the break-ins, Margaret has reviewed the home carefully to see what additional safety features should be installed. She has also set up a programme of staff training and some awareness-raising sessions for the residents.

Some of the staff have complained about the extra time that they have had to spend on training. Margaret has explained how important it is and hopes they will understand that it is for their protection, as well as the residents, that the safety of the workplace is of the highest standard.

QUESTIONS

1. Name some of the hazards for older people in the home.

2. In what ways could these hazards be prevented?

3. Why is staff training important?

4. What responsibilities does Margaret have to the residents?

5. What responsibilities does Margaret have to her staff?

Within an organisation's premises

Hazards may be found either outside or inside premises.

Hazards outdoors

Potential hazards found outdoors include:

- uneven pavements or driveways

- unsafe exits or entrances, for example, obstructed doorways

- lack of parking arrangements

- slippery ground in bad weather

- poor lighting

- steps that may be dangerous, particularly if there is no handrail

- air pollution, particularly on busy roads or near industrial areas.

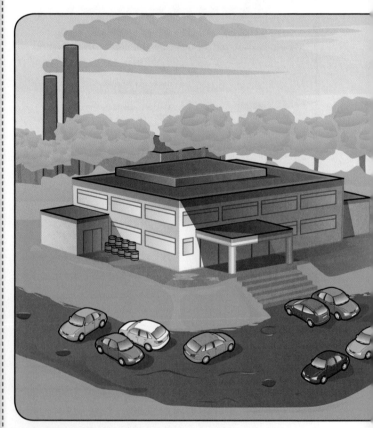

Figure 3.2 Potential outdoor hazards

Think What hazards can you identify outside the premises in Figure 3.2?

Hazards indoors

Indoors, some of the most common hazards are those that cause people to trip, slip or fall. A hazard of this sort may be caused by something that is easily seen, such as a trailing cable, a worn carpet or exposed wiring. It can also be caused by something less obvious, such as a slippery surface. Trips, slips and falls can be caused by a wide range of factors, including:

- rubbish left lying around
- obstructed passageways
- trailing leads
- damaged or torn flooring
- rugs and mats
- changes of slope or level
- poor lighting that hides other hazards
- unsecured windows
- equipment left lying around.

Heating appliances can cause a hazard. Radiators can be very hot and may burn people if they are not protected. Open fires, and gas or electric heaters all have the potential to cause a fire. Very hot water can cause scalds, whether from a badly positioned kettle or from poorly regulated water temperatures.

Some places may be particularly noisy, making it difficult to hear, which may create hazards, for example if you can't hear someone shouting to get your attention.

Children may be at risk from hazards that might not affect adults in the same way.

> **Think** Look at Figure 3.3. What hazards could endanger children?

Figure 3.3 Potential indoor hazards

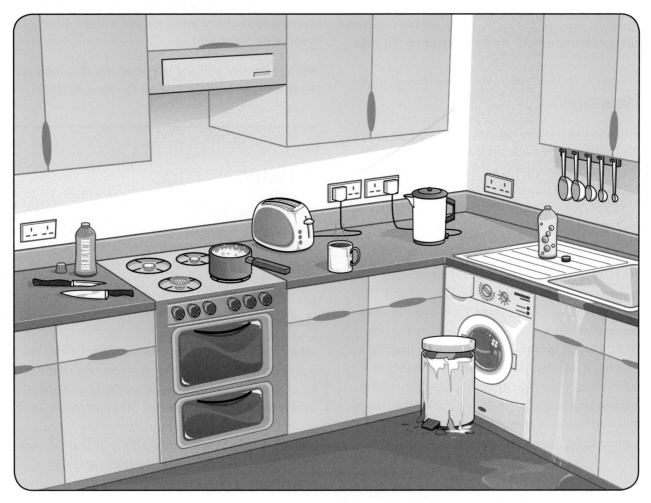

Hazards in the premises of another organisation

In any organisation's premises the staff and service users will get used to the environment. When visiting another organisation's premises it is important to ensure that unexpected hazards do not cause harm. In other premises there are additional issues to be considered:

- accessibility of the premises
- safety of the building
- safety of unfamiliar equipment
- provision of suitable toilet facilities
- safety of transport.

Hazards in the service user's home

If a care worker needs to visit the home of a service user there will be particular issues to consider. There may be obvious hazards that it is not possible to remove, such as rugs, trailing flexes or old equipment. The care worker needs to take precautions and warn the client of the risks.

Example

Mr Khan has lived on his own since his wife died two years ago. His son has become concerned about his father's physical and mental health and has contacted his father's GP. The GP makes a visit with a health care assistant. When they arrive they find that the path is very overgrown and sacks of rubbish in the garden.

Mr Khan is living in very poor conditions. The heating no longer works and he is living and sleeping in one room downstairs in order to keep warm. The house is very dirty and there are piles of rubbish all over the floor. He has injured his leg and has a dressing on the wound that needs to be changed regularly. Mr Khan is very reluctant to change anything. The health care assistant returns the next day to re-dress the leg and to see what she can do to improve the situation.

Think What hazards are found in Mr Khan's house? How should the care worker manage the hazards encountered?

Hazards out in the community

Working in the community involves dealing with several hazards, especially when working alone. All care workers need to be aware of these hazards. Personal safety is important, particularly when visiting areas with high rates of crime or antisocial behaviour.

EVIDENCE ACTIVITY

P1

Use your work placement experiences to explain a minimum of six potential hazards in a health or social care setting.

a) You can do this by drawing a diagram or taking photographs of the premises you worked at on your work placement.

b) Use labels to indicate the positions of at least six hazards, then describe each of the hazards. (P1)

WORKING PRACTICES

As well as identifying the hazards in a working environment that might pose a risk, there are certain working practices that need to be followed to ensure health, safety and security in the workplace.

Activities

Clients may take part in a variety of activities in a health or social care setting, including routine activities, such as cooking or washing, and there may also be opportunities for other activities, such as art or outdoor visits. Any activity may pose a risk to health, safety or security so it is important that a risk assessment is undertaken and all procedures carefully followed.

Procedures

Every worker is responsible for his or her own working practices, but you must also make sure that you follow any systems or procedures in your workplace correctly. Examples of workplace policies and procedures include:

- manual handling techniques
- safety awareness
- providing health and safety information for visitors
- fire drills and training
- first aid
- use and maintenance of equipment
- food hygiene control
- infection control and hand washing
- use and storage of materials
- care of clients' property.

All health and social care organisations will require new staff to have a period of induction. This is for the employee's own safety as well as that of the clients. During the induction period some of the organisation's most important procedures will be explained.

> **Think** How did you prepare to go to your work experience? What information were you given when you arrived?

Clothing

In most situations care workers will be encouraged by their employer to consider what is appropriate to wear while at work. Workplace policies regarding suitable clothing are put in place for health and safety reasons, as well as for the comfort of staff and service users. Uniforms may be used in some workplaces, but in others uniforms

might be seen as a barrier to good communication. For safety reasons or to prevent infection, staff may be required to wear well-supported shoes, ensure that hair is tied up and wear a limited amount of jewellery.

Visitors

Visitors are welcome within care settings, but for the safety of clients and staff it is important to ensure that the organisation knows who is visiting.

> **Example**
>
> Mia is working at a day nursery on a work experience placement. She notices that all the doors have special handles. They are positioned high up, out of the reach of the children. As the children arrive they are checked in very carefully. Once the day has started nobody else is allowed to enter the premises, unless they are let in by a member of staff. Visitors have to sign the visitors' book on entering and leaving. All members of staff must wear identity badges.
>
> One afternoon a man arrives and demands to take his son home. He says he is in too much of a rush to sign in and out. Mia thinks she recognises him as the boy's father.

> **Think** What should Mia do? How should she justify her actions?

Infection control

Clients in care settings are usually particularly vulnerable to infections, which can be spread from one person to another. It is therefore important that measures are taken to ensure that any infections do not spread.

The chance of cross-infection can be minimised by following certain procedures, including the following standard precautions:

- effective hand washing

- wearing gloves when dealing with bodily fluids

- wearing protective clothing

- cleaning equipment effectively

- dealing with waste appropriately

- taking special precautions for certain conditions; for example, cases of food poisoning.

Effective hand washing is one of the most important procedures to get right, for your own safety and that of service users. Alcohol hand rub can also be used when your hands are relatively clean or if you are not near water. There are often dispensers outside hospital wards, which all visitors and staff are requested to use before entering. Staff may have their own container pinned to their uniform, ensuring that they clean their hands between patients.

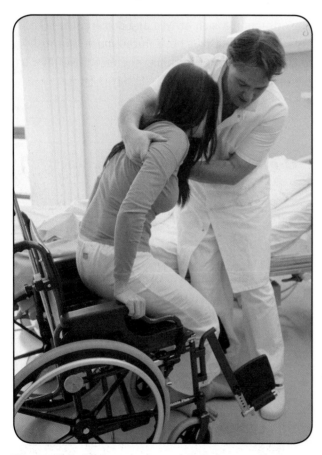

Figure 3.4 Moving a client safely

Storage and use of materials or equipment

Hazards that are associated with materials and equipment include:

- faulty mechanical equipment, for example, brakes on a wheelchair

- damaged or worn out equipment, for example, children's play equipment

- incorrectly labelled substances

- equipment and materials that are badly or incorrectly stored

- property belonging to staff or clients that is not kept securely

- not disposing of waste materials correctly.

There are regulations that cover many of these hazards, which we will look at later in the unit.

Working techniques: manual handling

The safe handling and moving of clients, as well as of materials, is essential to the safety of both clients and care workers. Back injuries can affect anyone, and injuries may be permanent or result in significant periods of time off work. In order to prevent injuries, it is important to understand posture, so that principles of correct moving and handling can be applied in all situations. Many workplaces will have policies that try to avoid the necessity of lifting. Staff may also be required to attend a moving and handling course every year.

> **Think** What are the procedures for moving and lifting in the places you have done work experience?

However, there will be occasions when lifting cannot be avoided. If this is the case, special procedures should be followed to reduce the risk of injury to care workers. This may mean having enough staff in order to be able to lift safely or it could mean that special hoists should be used. Whatever approach is adopted, staff should be trained in the correct procedures.

Working techniques: food hygiene control

> ### CASE STUDY: FOOD POISONING OUTBREAK
>
> An outbreak of food poisoning was reported after a party in a residential home for elderly people in May 1995. The party was attended by 96 residents, staff and guests. Two elderly residents died.
>
> The infection was associated with eating prawns in mayonnaise, vol-au-vents, sausage rolls, corned beef sandwiches and sausages. Two members of staff (who were involved in care of the residents, but not in food preparation) were ill two days before the party. For those who became ill, the onset of illness occurred between 24 and 96 hours after the party. Two members of staff who did not attend the party became ill four and five days after the party; both had looked after residents with symptoms.
>
> The investigation of this outbreak highlighted areas that needed attention. One recommendation was that there should be reminders about basic hygiene precautions to prevent the spread of infection. Secondly, the importance of regular reinforcement in the workplace of formal food-hygiene training for cooks was highlighted. The Food Safety Regulations 1995 came into force soon after this outbreak: their implementation would probably have prevented it.
>
> *[Source: Hansell, Sen, Sufi, McCallum, 1998]*
>
> ### QUESTION
>
> 1. What might have been the reasons for the spread of food poisoning among the residents and staff in this incident?

To help avoid food poisoning it is important to make sure that the food you make for yourself and for other people is safe to eat. The main causes of food poisoning, and its subsequent spread, are:

- cross-contamination and poor personal hygiene
- pests, such as rodents, insects and birds
- ineffective cleaning and disinfection
- food not being kept at the right temperature
- poor labelling of food
- using microwave ovens inappropriately.

> ### Research tip
>
> Visit the website of the Food Standards Agency to find out more about food hygiene control.
> www.food.gov.uk

RISKS

Every day we notice hazards that are all around us. In order to deal with them, we have to make decisions about how likely it is that we will come to harm.

Figure 3.5 We assess risks every day

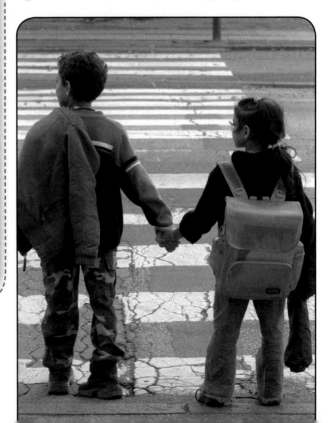

For example, we know that traffic and cars are a hazard, but we assess how much we are at risk or in danger every time we cross a road. The risk is the chance, high or low, that somebody could be harmed by a hazard. Assessing a risk also involves considering how serious the harm could be.

In health and social care settings some clients may be at increased risk because of their age, physical or mental ability, for example. It may not be possible to eliminate all risks, but there is a duty of care which requires that everything possible is done to ensure that clients do not come to harm.

Key words

Risk – the likelihood of a hazard causing harm

Duty of care – a duty to do everything that is reasonably possible to protect others from harm

Possibility of injury and harm to people

The Health and Safety Executive, as part of the Health and Safety Commission, aims to protect people's health and safety by ensuring that risks in the workplace are properly controlled. As part of their work, they have provided the following guidance:

A risk assessment is simply a careful examination of what, in your work, could cause harm to people, so that you can weigh up whether you have taken enough precautions or should do more to prevent harm.

How to assess the risks in your workplace

Follow the five steps:

Step 1: Identify the hazards.

Step 2: Decide who might be harmed and how.

Step 3: Evaluate the risks and decide on precautions.

Step 4: Record your findings and implement them.

Step 5: Review your assessment and update if necessary.

Table 3.1 below shows some of the common hazards, alongside the risks these might cause and what the potential injuries might be.

Table 3.1 Hazards and their consequences

HAZARD	RISK	INJURY
In working environment		
poor external lighting	• unable to see dangers, e.g. broken path	• falls, with injuries such as broken bones
no handrail by steps	• losing balance and falling	• falls, with injuries such as broken bones
floor coverings in poor state	• tripping	• falls, with injuries such as broken bones
rubbish blocking corridors	• losing balance • wheelchairs etc. unable to get through	• falls, with injuries such as broken bones
Working practices		
poor lifting techniques	• client not lifted safely • staff not lifting correctly	• injury to client • injury to staff, especially to backs
inadequate fire training	• staff and clients do not know how to evacuate the building	• burns • smoke inhalation •death
poorly maintained equipment	• equipment may fail	• staff and clients may be injured
cleaning chemicals incorrectly labelled	• chemicals put to wrong use	• clients may be poisoned or injured

Think Can you suggest any other risks that are specific to the client group with which you are working? For example, what are the particular risks in a residential home or in a nursery setting?

Possibility of danger

Some hazards are regarded as posing particularly high and dangerous risks. For example, the danger from fire is always present. All premises must display information about what action should be taken in the event of a fire and must be appropriately equipped with extinguishers and fire blankets. Fire doors should be installed and used correctly, and should not be propped open. All staff should keep up to date with procedures and attend regular training.

It is important to carry out certain activities with particular care in order to avoid increasing the risk of fire. A key risk is cooking, especially, for example, when frying or cooking chips in deep fat.

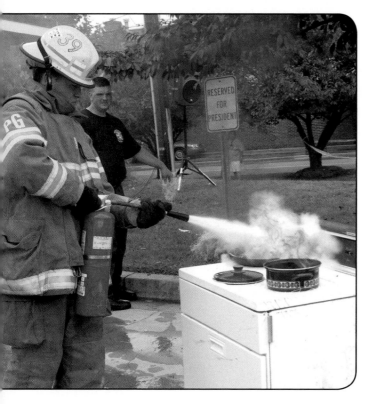

Figure 3.7 Fire safety training

Another key fire risk comes from smoking. New regulations have restricted where individuals may smoke. However, some clients have been lifelong smokers and may find it very difficult to give up. This may mean they will try to conceal their habit.

> **Think** Suggest other risks that might be classified as a danger to staff or clients.

Hazardous waste

Waste can be seen as a possible hazard and the disposal of it may be a risk. This is because some waste is particularly hazardous. It can cause and spread infection and be a risk to clients, staff and the environment. To reduce the risk from disposing of waste, special procedures must be followed when handling different types of waste (see Table 3.2). All waste must be collected and disposed of correctly.

Table 3.2 Dealing with hazardous waste

Type of waste	Risk	Method of risk reduction
Sharps, e.g. needles, syringes	• 'needle stick' injury • infection	• yellow sharps box • must be hard plastic and sealed when full
Clinical waste, e.g. used dressings	• infection	• yellow bags • must be sealed, with special arrangements for collection and incineration
Body fluids, e.g. urine, faeces, blood, vomit	• infection	• wear gloves at all times • clear and flush down toilet area • clean and disinfect area
Soiled linen	• infection	• special laundry bags which disintegrate in the wash

INCIDENTS

From time to time in any organisation an incident may occur that poses a risk to either staff or the clients in a care setting. These can include:

- accidents

- contamination

- chemical spillage

- intruders

- aggressive or dangerous encounters

- lost keys, purses and other personal items

- missing individuals

- individuals locked out

- fires within premises

- bomb scares.

We will look briefly at each of these incidents in the section that follows.

Accidents

Even when things are very well prepared accidents can happen.

CASE STUDY: NURSERY SCHOOL ACCIDENT

Neetha and Kate work as nursery assistants. Neetha has recently left school and this is her first job. She has completed a childcare course at college.

Neetha is working alongside Kate, who is responsible for a group of 3-year-old children. Kate has been working at the nursery for three years and is undertaking a Level 3 NVQ.

Neetha and Kate have planned an outdoor activity. They have set up a 'mini Olympics' course with small obstacles for the children to climb over or squeeze underneath. They have considered the abilities of all the children and believe that the activity should be safe and good fun.

When the activity begins one boy falls over as he is running. He cuts his head and it bleeds. He is very upset and frightened by the sight of the blood. Neetha picks him up and comforts him. She knows that there is a procedure that she must follow in the case of accidents. She takes the child to the first aid room where his injury is treated. She finds a copy of the nursery's procedure and follows it carefully. She finds the form which needs to be completed, and arranges to inform the parents and reassure them that their son is OK. The form requires the following information:

- date, time and place of accident

- person/people involved

- circumstances of the accident

- condition of the injured person

- actions taken following the accident

- any equipment involved in the accident

- any other witnesses to the accident

- who was informed about the accident and when.

QUESTIONS

1. Could anything have been done to avoid the accident?

2. What were Neetha's priorities following the accident?

3. How could she ensure that the other children were safe while she dealt with the injured child?

4. Look at the information required on the report form. Explain why it is necessary to have each piece of information.

Contamination risk

Contamination can be caused by organisms like bacteria, viruses, moulds and mildews. These are often invisible, and some types can travel through the air. Contamination can also be caused by a range of other substances, such as chemicals, animal hair or pollen.

Key words

Organism – any living thing

Bacteria and viruses need nutrients and moisture in order to grow. These conditions can often be found in bathrooms, damp or flooded basements, wet appliances (such as humidifiers and air conditioners) and on some carpets and furniture. Mould or mildew can grow in contaminated central air-handling systems. These systems then distribute the contaminants through the building.

There are a number of health risks associated with contamination:

- Some contaminants, such as pollen, may trigger allergic reactions, including some types of asthma.

- Infectious diseases, such as influenza, measles, tuberculosis and chicken pox, are transmitted by organisms that are carried through the air.

- Some moulds and mildews can release disease-causing toxins.

- Children, elderly people and people with breathing problems, allergies and lung diseases are particularly susceptible to disease-causing organisms in the indoor air.

Legionnaire's disease is a serious illness caused by contamination. This disease gained its name in 1976 when an outbreak of pneumonia occurred among people attending a convention of the American Legion in Philadelphia. Scientists identified the cause as a previously unknown bacterium, which was later named *Legionella*. This contaminant is spread through the air in mist droplets containing the bacteria, which people then inhale. Common sources include domestic hot water systems, showers and water fountains.

Think Why might the residents of a care home be particularly at risk of Legionnaire's disease?

Chemical spillages

Large-scale chemical spillages, which can threaten a large population, tend to receive the most media attention. In fact any chemical spillage can be hazardous. All chemicals are labelled to warn of any hazards that may be connected with them. Before using any substance it is important to check how to use it and to ensure that it is safe to use.

The symbols for dangerous substances are yellow. Figure 3.7 shows some of the common ones.

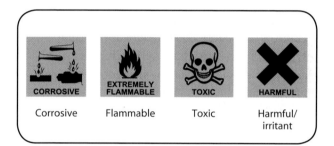

CORROSIVE	EXTREMELY FLAMMABLE	TOXIC	HARMFUL
Corrosive	Flammable	Toxic	Harmful/irritant

Figure 3.7 – Symbols for some common hazardous substances

Many substances that are regarded as hazardous come under special regulations for their control called Control of Substances Hazardous to Health (COSHH). We will look at these regulations in more detail on pages 102 – 103.

If there is a spillage of any substance, including things like adhesives, paints and cleaning fluids, the first thing to do is to check the container to see if there is a hazard symbol. If there is, there will be instructions in the COSHH file about how to clean it up. You must follow the procedures carefully.

Key words

COSHH file – a file kept by health and social care organisations that contains information about hazardous chemicals and their handling. This does not apply just to health and social care organisations.

Intruders

Organisations have a variety of different regulations about how they permit staff and non-staff members to gain access to their premises. Some will have very strict rules, for example:

- issuing all members of staff with badges

- requiring everyone who enters the premises to sign in

- restricting access through locked doors, with only certain staff members having access to keys or code numbers to key pads.

Other organisations, usually smaller ones, rely on more informal methods, such as people recognising each other and being able to identify strangers. The most important rule about access is that only those people who have a right to be on the premises should be there. The more vulnerable a client is, the more danger they are in from intruders. Therefore, the elderly, children and those with special needs are at greatest risk. All staff members need to be prepared to challenge an individual they do not recognise – politely, of course!

Think In what ways could an organisation ensure that its premises are secure from intruders? How could you ensure that someone has the right to be on the premises?

Aggressive and dangerous encounters

Staff working in health care may sometimes find themselves on the receiving end of aggressive behaviour, which may be physical or verbal. The NHS has a policy of 'zero tolerance' on violence towards their staff. However, there are still risks, which may be associated with the mental or emotional condition of the client. Alcohol also plays a large part in causing individuals to behave aggressively.

Key words

Zero tolerance – a policy not to tolerate any instances of undesirable behaviour

CASE STUDY: VIOLENCE AGAINST NHS STAFF IN WALES

Staff working in the NHS in Wales are subjected to an average of 22 cases of violent or aggressive behaviour every day, according to a study. Nurses, midwives and health visitors are most likely to be the victims. A Wales Audit Office study found that violence and aggression towards health service workers cost £6 million a year.

The study looked at figures from 2001 to 2004. Staff working in the mental health, general health and learning disabilities sectors also reported being victims of aggression. The study found one patient threw a fire extinguisher at hospital staff, while another case involved the attempted mugging of a district nurse on a house call. *[Source:* Protecting NHS Trust staff from violence and aggression. *Wales Audit Office, 2005]*

QUESTION

1. In what sorts of situations might there be a greater risk of aggression to care workers?

Example

Ahmed is a nurse. One night he and a female colleague were attacked by a patient who pinned them against a window during a shift:

'He punched me in the face and chest, bloodying my nose and cracking two ribs. My wedding ring got caught and ripped off all the skin on my finger. My colleague had her uniform ripped and ended up with a black eye. We looked like we'd been in a pub brawl'

The 'zero tolerance' approach to violence is the right one.

Lost personal items

In all organisations there is a risk of property being lost. It is sometimes difficult to balance the rights of an individual to privacy and independence with the need to ensure that their property is safe. Each care setting will have its own procedures to manage the care of its property and that of its clients. Examples of these procedures include:

- naming clothes and belongings

- recording possessions on admission, e.g. in a property book

- description of any very valuable belongings

- getting individuals to sign for any valuables they wish to keep to show that they take responsibility for them

- providing keys to rooms, or safes in which to keep property.

If a loss is reported then the organisation's procedures must be followed.

> **Think** What actions might need to be taken if an item is reported as lost?

Missing individuals and individuals locked out

Individuals who go missing from their care setting may be at great risk. People may leave because they are confused, unhappy or because they are very young.

Sometimes individuals or staff may be locked out of a building accidentally. This can be a frightening or frustrating situation for the individual. Most organisations will have procedures in place to ensure that there is someone who can be easily contacted to arrange for the premises to be unlocked.

CASE STUDY: CHILD WANDERS OFF

On Monday 19th June 2006 the following story was reported:

A nursery in Scotland has been criticised after a toddler managed to slip away and walk down a busy street. Damon Wood's mother spotted the two-year-old 60 metres away from the building as she went to pick him up. He was with two strangers.

When she took him back to Seashells Nursery in Eyemouth, Berwickshire, she realised that staff had not noticed he was missing. Following an investigation, the Care Commission has now ordered urgent action to improve security and staffing issues at the nursery.

Three members of staff were given written warnings over the incident, which took place at the end of April, and as a result have resigned from their jobs. The nursery is now temporarily closed due to staff shortages.

Yesterday, the boy's mother, Claire Atkinson, 27, said: "I had dropped him there at 1pm, and when I was driving back at 3.30pm I saw him in the street with a woman and a man. The couple said they had found him wandering."

"Apparently Damon had got out through a main door and a security door which is only meant to be unlocked when you've got through the first one. It must have been because a lot of parents were coming and going at that time of the day that he was able to slip through unnoticed."

[Source: The Scotsman: *Robert Fairburn*]

QUESTION

1. What actions should the nursery have taken if they had noticed Damon missing?

Fires within premises

As discussed earlier, fires are always a risk in any establishment. The procedure if a fire is found should ensure that both the staff and clients are removed from danger as soon as possible. The procedure is likely to be similar to the following:

- raise alarm (individual who finds the fire)

- alert fire service, either by dialling 999 directly or through the switchboard

- move everybody out of danger and ensure they are safe

- individuals leave as quickly as possible without collecting belongings

- if safe to do so, attack fire with correct extinguisher or fire blanket

- assemble at fire assembly point

- check all clients and staff are accounted for

- do not return to the building until told to do so.

Bomb scares

Bomb scares can be threatened by phone, letter or email and should always be taken seriously. The police should be informed and their advice followed. If a bomb scare is reported, the same procedures need to be followed as for a fire alarm, except that clients need to be encouraged to take their own bags with them. When assembling, everybody should keep away from windows and other areas of glass.

ACCIDENTS

As you have seen already, accidents can happen in even the best regulated organisations. These can be due to:

- falls

- hazards in the environment

- poor manual handling

- illness, weaknesses, disability or frailty

- sensory or cognitive impairment.

CASE STUDY: THE GRANGE

Residents of The Grange residential home all have their own rooms. There is a communal area where they have their meals and a separate TV lounge.

Gladys has difficulty walking and needs to use a Zimmer frame. She is very independent and likes to look after her personal needs herself. She comes along to the dining area for her meals; however she sometimes finds it difficult to manoeuvre her frame around obstacles in her way. Brenda is in a wheelchair. She is very heavy and needs help to get out of bed. The staff usually use the portable hoist to lift her. However, the other day she was in a hurry and did not want to wait for the hoist. She persuaded a new member of staff that they could manage without it. Unfortunately Gladys fell onto the floor. She was not badly injured, but bruised her leg. Harry is 98 years old. He hopes to celebrate his 100th birthday in 18 months time. He is very frail and has recently had a bad cold which has left him rather weak and wobbly on his feet. Bill is registered as blind. He started to lose his sight ten years ago and it has become progressively worse. He has been in the residential home for five years. He can find his way around as long as everything stays in the same place. The other day a workman moved his chair from its usual position. Bill nearly fell over it. Margaret may have to move from this home soon. She has become increasingly confused and has started to wander. She has been into other residents' rooms and even tried to get into someone else's bed. She has also wandered out of the home and got lost in the local town. She was brought back by the police after the staff in a cafe became concerned about her behaviour.

QUESTION

1. Identify how each of the residents might be at risk of an accident and why.

3.2 *Understand how legislation, guidelines, policies and procedures promote health, safety and security*

Care settings are governed by a number of different arrangements to ensure the health, safety and security of the staff and the individuals in their care. These fall into three main categories:

- legislation and guidelines

- policies and procedures

- the way in which health and social care services are delivered.

LEGISLATION AND GUIDELINES

The settings in which health and social care is delivered are covered by specific pieces of legislation or laws that set out regulations that must be followed. In addition, there are also guidelines, or codes of practice, which explain, extend or support the regulations. The main purposes of guidelines are to:

- interpret legislation – helping people to understand what the law says

- help people comply with the law

- give technical advice.

All organisations must follow legislation, but following guidance is not compulsory and employers are free to take other actions.

Approved Codes of Practice offer practical examples of good methods of working. They give advice on how to comply with the law by, for example, providing a guide as to what is 'reasonably practicable'. Approved Codes of Practice have a special legal status. If employers are accused of a breach of health and safety law, and it is proved that they have not followed the relevant provisions of the Approved Code of Practice, a court can find them at fault unless they can show that they have complied with the law in some other way.

Health and Safety at Work Act 1974

This Act is the main piece of legislation about safety in the workplace. It applies to all places of work, not just health and care settings. The Act sets out the general duties that employers have towards employees and members of the public. It also outlines the duties that employees have to themselves and to other employees. There are a number of different legal regulations that stem from this Act. The main requirements of the law are as follows:

Employers should:

- provide a safe workplace

- provide health and safety training

- provide information on health and safety

- undertake risk assessments

- set up emergency procedures.

Employees should:

- work with the employer on health and safety issues

- take reasonable care for their own safety and that of others

- look after health and safety equipment.

Both employer and employee are responsible together to safeguard the health and safety of anyone using the premises.

Every workplace that employs five or more people is required to have a written health and safety policy which includes:

- the name of the person responsible for ensuring the policy is acted upon

- a statement of intent to provide a safe workplace

- the names of individuals who are responsible for particular health and safety hazards

- a list of identified health and safety hazards and the procedures to be followed

- procedures for recording accidents at work

- details of how to evacuate the premises.

The Health and Safety at Work Act covers the general principles of safety in the workplace, but there are also many further regulations that apply to specific areas of work. The ones that are most likely to apply in a health and social care setting are:

- Food Safety Act 1990

- Food Safety (General Food Hygiene) Regulations 1995

- Manual Handling Operations Regulations 1992

- Reporting of Injuries, Diseases and Dangerous Occurrences Regulations (RIDDOR) 1995

- Data Protection Act 1998

- Management of Health and Safety at Work Regulations 1999

- Control of Substances Hazardous to Health Regulations (COSHH) 2002

Research tip

The following websites are good sources of information for more detail about these acts.

Health and Safety Executive – www.hse.gov.uk

Food Standards Agency – www.foodstandards.gov.uk

Department of Health – www.dh.gov.uk

Food Safety Act 1990

This is a wide ranging law that affects everyone involved in the production, processing, storage, distribution or sale of food. It is applicable to all food premises. The law aims to ensure that:

- food is what it claims it is, for example, if food is sold as cod it must not in fact be haddock. Food must not contain any foreign objects

- food is not falsely or misleadingly described, for example, making false claims about the food products

- food is safe and fit to eat.

Environmental officers have the power to make checks and to seize foods which are regarded as unfit. They can serve Improvement Notices on owners of businesses that fail to meet the hygiene standards laid down in the regulations. They can close down any premises that are causing an imminent risk to health.

Key words

Improvement Notice - an order to make changes so that standards are met that gives time for the organisation that receives it to make the changes

The Food Safety (General Food Hygiene) Regulations 1995

These regulations are specifically concerned with food hygiene. Here are the ten most important things you need to know about food handling:

1 All food premises must be easy to clean, free from rubbish, well lit, adequately ventilated and protected against all types of infestations.

2 All equipment must be kept clean and in good repair. Equipment made of wood must not be used, for example, chopping boards.

3 Good personal hygiene practices should be observed at all times:

- Always wash your hands after using the toilet, before handling food and between handling raw and cooked food.

- Cuts and boils should be covered with a blue waterproof dressing.

- Food handlers should wear clean, protective clothing, including a suitable hair cover.

4 All food rooms should have a sufficient supply of hot water, liquid soap, and disposable paper towels or a hot air dryer.

5 Food handlers should avoid handling food in such a manner that allows cross-contamination from raw to cooked foods. Separate equipment and work surfaces should be used when handling raw and cooked food. A separate hand basin must also be provided solely for the use of washing hands.

6   Raw and cooked food should always be kept apart so as to avoid cross-contamination.

7   Food must be kept piping hot or cold to prevent the growth of bacteria. Refrigerators should operate at 5°C or colder. Freezers should operate at −18°C or colder.

8   All illnesses should be reported to a supervisor.

9   Smoking is not allowed in food rooms.

10 A large fine may be imposed on any person found guilty of an offence under these regulations. In extreme cases an inspecting officer has the power to close the premises down immediately.

[Source: Walsall Environmental Health and Consumer Services Department]

Manual Handling Operations Regulations 1992

Lifting and handling people is the single highest cause of injuries at work in health and care settings. One in four workers takes time off because of a back injury sustained at work. The legislation aims to minimise risk by requiring that:

- employers avoid all hazardous manual lifting activity where it is practical to do so

- if lifting cannot be avoided, then the risks must be assessed

- appropriate equipment must be available and used correctly

- lifting operations must be planned and supervised by competent people

- employees must follow the procedures.

Remember that this legislation applies to lifting objects as well as people.

> ***Think*** What do you need to consider before undertaking any lifting?

Reporting of Injuries, Diseases and Dangerous Occurrences Regulations (RIDDOR) 1995

It is a legal requirement to report certain accidents and diseases at work. In the UK the Incident Contact Centre collects all of this information so that accidents and injuries can be analysed and causes established. Employers must report:

- deaths

- major injuries

- accidents resulting in more than three days off work

- diseases

- dangerous occurrences.

> **Research tip**
>
> Visit the RIDDOR website to find out more information about reporting accidents.
>
> www.riddor.gov.uk

Reportable major injuries are:

- fractures, other than to fingers, thumbs or toes

- amputation

- dislocation of a shoulder, hip, knee or spine

- loss of sight (temporary or permanent)

- chemical or hot metal burn to the eye or any penetrating injury to the eye

- injury resulting from an electric shock or electrical burn that leads to unconsciousness, requires resuscitation or admittance to hospital for more than 24 hours

- any other injury leading to hypothermia, heat-induced illness or unconsciousness; or requiring resuscitation; or requiring admittance to hospital for more than 24 hours

- unconsciousness caused by asphyxia (suffocation), or exposure to a harmful substance or biological agent

- acute illness requiring medical treatment, or loss of consciousness arising from absorption of any substance by inhalation, ingestion or through the skin

- acute illness requiring medical treatment where there is reason to believe that this resulted from exposure to a biological agent or its toxins, or infected material.

Reportable diseases include:

- certain poisonings

- some skin diseases such as occupational dermatitis, skin cancer, chrome ulcer, oil folliculitis/acne

- lung diseases including occupational asthma, farmer's lung, pneumoconiosis, asbestosis, mesothelioma

- infections such as leptospirosis, hepatitis, tuberculosis, anthrax, legionellosis and tetanus

- other conditions such as occupational cancer, certain musculoskeletal disorders, decompression illness and hand–arm vibration syndrome.

Reportable dangerous occurrences are anything which does not result in a reportable injury but might have done so.

[Source: www.riddor.gov.uk]

Think Look at the list of reportable injuries and diseases above. Why might it be important to know what caused them?

Data Protection Act 1998

The purpose of this Act is to protect the rights of any individual about whom data is obtained, stored, processed or supplied. The Act applies to both computerised and paper records. Data collected must be:

- used only for the specific purposes for which it was collected

- relevant

- accurate

- kept securely

- kept only for an appropriate length of time

- passed on to others only with the consent of the data owner.

Management of Health and Safety at Work Regulations 1999

Often referred to as the Management Regulations, these generally make more explicit what employers are required to do to manage health and safety under the Health and Safety at Work Act. Like the Act, they apply to every work activity. The main requirement they place on employers is to carry out a risk assessment.

Key words

Risk assessment - an evaluation of the health and safety risks that employees are exposed to at work, and of the risks to clients or the public that may be caused by the organisation. The risk assessment should be used to identify measures that need to be taken to address these risks

Control of Substances Hazardous to Health Regulations (COSHH) 2002

These regulations apply to virtually all substances that can be hazardous to health, including substances that are toxic, corrosive or irritants. Any substance that has a warning label on its container is covered by these regulations, including many cleaning materials, disinfectants and bleaches.

Employers are required to take the following steps to protect employees from hazardous substances.

1 Assess the risks – find out what hazardous substances are used in the workplace and the risks that they pose to people's health.

2 Decide what precautions are needed.

3 Prevent or adequately control exposure.

4 Ensure that control measures are used and maintained.

5 If necessary, monitor the exposure of employees.

6 Carry out appropriate health surveillance when employees are exposed.

7 Prepare plans and procedures to deal with accidents, incidents and emergencies.

8 Ensure that employees are properly informed, trained and supervised.

[Source: Health and Safety Executive]

Details of all the hazardous substances used on the premises must be kept in a COSHH file. It should detail:

• where they are kept

• how they are labelled

• what the effects are

• the maximum time that an individual can be safely exposed to the substance

• how to deal with an emergency involving the substance.

Example

Doreen is employed as a cleaner in the Red Bank residential home. She is responsible for cleaning the residents' rooms, the communal areas and the toilets. She has a special trolley on which she carries all her equipment. This includes disinfectant and other cleaning materials. She has been asked to clear up a spillage in the corridor. She does not know what the substance is. There have been some engineers mending some machinery and also some deliveries of new cleaning stock. She realises that there are several possible hazards associated with this accident.

Think What hazards are created by this spill? What actions would you expect Doreen to take to protect herself and others?

EVIDENCE ACTIVITY

P2

Describe how key legislation in relation to health, safety and security influences the delivery of health and social care.

a) Do Internet research to find out further information about the key legislation.

b) Summarise the main points of the key legislation to describe how it influences the delivery of health and social care. You can use printouts of information found on the Internet to provide supporting evidence, but you will also need to provide your own summary. (P2)

POLICIES AND PROCEDURES

In order to ensure the safety of the employees and those in their care, organisations must follow the law. In addition, they will develop their own policies and procedures that meet the legal requirements and apply particularly to their own establishments. These policies and procedures will be reviewed regularly and updated. All members of staff are expected to read and understand them. It is hoped that they will be practical and useful sources of information and reference. The most important policies and procedures are often to be found in a staff handbook. A case study on policies and procedures can be found on page 105.

> **Think** What topics are covered by the policies of the organisation at which you are doing your work placement?

EVIDENCE ACTIVITY

P3 – M1 – D1

1. Use examples from your work experience placements to describe how policies and procedures are used to promote health, safety and security in health and social care workplaces.

a) Collect as many examples as you can from your work placement to show how organisational policies and procedures are used to promote health, safety and security. Make sure you understand what they mean for the staff and the clients.

b) You could use these examples to write a case study about this place of work. (P3)

2. In order to meet the M1 requirement you need to explain rather than describe. This means that you need to give clear reasoning behind your examples. (M1)

3. For D1, you will need to evaluate the effectiveness of the policies and procedures that you describe. (D1)

HEALTH AND SOCIAL CARE DELIVERY

The way in which any care is delivered is governed by the law, the policies and procedures of the organisation, and the working practices that are developed in the light of these influences.

Working practices

Look back at the working practices that were covered on pages 88 to 93. The following important areas were identified:

- manual handling techniques
- safety awareness
- providing health and safety information for visitors
- fire drills and training
- first aid
- use and maintenance of equipment
- food hygiene control
- infection control and hand washing
- care of clients' property.

This unit should have given you an understanding of the legal basis that underpins these practices.

Risk assessment

The results of carrying out a risk assessment will influence the way health and social care is delivered. The Management of Health and Safety at Work Regulations 1999 requires all employers to assess the risks in their workplace. Remember the steps for effective risk assessment:

Step 1: Identify the hazards.

Step 2: Decide who might be harmed and how.

Step 3: Evaluate the risks and decide on precautions.

Step 4: Record your findings and implement them.

Step 5: Review your assessment and update if necessary.

CASE STUDY: POLICIES AND PROCEDURES

BABY UNIT

The two baby units are bright and colourful. The children are able to play and crawl around safely on soft flooring. Play is a very important part of their development and is encouraged in the baby units.

There are both group and individual play activities in which the staff and children participate. The children have plenty of stimulation and interaction with both staff and their peer groups. This includes singing, stories, looking at pictures and staff continually talking to the children. The wide range of equipment helps the children in their physical, intellectual and social development. The children are encouraged to share the equipment and enjoy group games.

All children need comfort, love and attention and that is available at all times, helping their emotional development. Sleep patterns vary from child to child, therefore there is no set sleep time. Children can sleep in their individual cot or, for the older children, on their individual mattress with a sleeping bag. Daily records of the children are kept in the room so that parents can be given an account of the day's activities.

BEHAVIOUR

Good manners are always encouraged. Good communication is important between the home and the nursery. Sometimes, if a child is experiencing a change in the home environment, that may result in changes in their behaviour at the nursery. We will tell you of any problems which may occur with your child at the nursery.

SECURITY

We have an intercom system to ensure that no one can gain access. No child will be handed over to anyone other than the known parent or relative without a written note from that parent being produced.

All our premises and equipment are of the highest standard; our play and learning equipment meets the recognised safety standards.

POLICIES AND PROCEDURES

Our policies and procedures files are available to all parents who wish to review them. They cover areas such as:

child protection	outings
complaints procedures	fire procedures
health and safety	visitors
equal opportunities	staff recruitment

These files are held in the Manager's office and can be seen on request.

MEALS

We have qualified cooks. The weekly menus are designed by them to meet the highest nutritional guidelines. Breakfast is cereal for the younger children and toast for the older children. For lunch the children have a two-course meal in which the emphasis is on fresh food and good nutrition. We use organic meat from a registered butcher. We provide a hot meal (high tea) for children in the afternoon. The daily menu is on our noticeboard.

Figure 3.18 Prospectus for the Start Right Day Nursery

QUESTION

1. What is likely to be covered in the policies and procedures that the prospecus lists?

3.3 Understanding roles and responsibilities for health, safety and security in health and social care settings

The role is what an individual is appointed or expected to do. The responsibilities are what an individual will be answerable for within their role.

ROLES

The different roles of employers and employees mean that they will have different responsibilities for ensuring health, safety and security in the workplace. Table 3.3 is a reminder of the different types of responsibilities that employers and employees might have.

Table 3.3 Responsibilities of employers and employees

Responsibilities of employers	Responsibilities or employer and employee	Responsibilities of employee
undertake planning for a safe and secure environment, including risk assessments	the safety of individuals using the setting	to use the systems and equipment correctly
provide information about health and safety	the safety of the environment	to adhere to policies and procedures
provide training in health and safety		to report any problems, faults or gaps with the equipment or procedures
keep all systems and procedures up to date		

The health and safety requirements that are the responsibility of employees will depend on the limits of their role in the organisation.

Your role may determine what you do in a particular circumstance. There will be some occasions when you can deal with a hazard directly, for example, ensuring that waste is disposed of correctly, removing trip hazards, following the correct procedures if there is a fire, or appropriately challenging visitors. On other occasions, it may be necessary to inform your manager of a hazard so that they can deal with it. This would apply to hazards that are beyond your role or ability to correct, such as faulty equipment, poor flooring or heavy objects causing obstruction.

Example

Jane is undertaking her work experience in a day centre. There are approximately 20 people who attend each day. They do various activities together such as quizzes, bingo or other games before having lunch. It is also an opportunity for individuals to have personal care which they can no longer manage at home. They can have a bath, be given specialist foot care or have their hair washed.

Jane was helping to tidy up at the end of the morning. She noticed that the hairdresser had left the hairdryer plugged in with the lead trailing across the floor. When she entered the bathroom she saw that the sling on the hoist had become loose and unattached.

Think Identify the two hazards that Jane has come across. Which hazard could Jane take responsibility for removing and which should she report to her manager?

RESPONSIBILITIES

We will now look at the responsibilities that need to be assumed to promote a healthy, safe and secure environment. Much of the detail has already been covered, but here is an overview to remind you.

CASE STUDY: RESIDENTIAL SUPPORT WORKER

JOB DESCRIPTION

Senior Residential Support Worker
Directorate of Children's Services, Integrated Services

Reporting to: Residential Home Team Manager

Responsible for: Supervision of Residential Home staff

MAIN PURPOSE OF JOB:

- To assist in the promotion and maintenance of good childcare practice in accordance with departmental policy and practice.

- To support the Management Team of the centre in the creation and maintenance of an environment that has the capacity to respond to the needs of individual young people.

- To act as a source of expertise on childcare methodologies and approaches, giving advice to others as appropriate.

RESPONSIBILITIES, DUTIES AND TASKS:

The Senior Residential Support Worker will:

- assume responsibility for the centre in the absence of managerial staff

- participate in assessing and planning for the needs of young people

- assist in the development of good childcare practice.

- participate in fulfilling the requirements of Care Plans as agreed for residents

- contribute to in-house staff development and training programmes

- undertake the recording of information in line with County guidelines

- maintain such records as may be required, e.g. fire equipment test log, accident book, etc.

- ensure compliance with guidelines for the administration and safe-keeping of drugs and ensure their implementation by all members of staff

- observe the requirements of the Health and Safety at Work Act, including the administration of fire regulations and procedures, and liaison with other parts of the Directorate responsible for keeping the Centre in good repair

- undertake health and safety duties commensurate with the post and/or as detailed in the Directorate's Health and Safety Policy.

NOTES:

- Reasonable adjustments will be considered as required by the Disability Discrimination Act.

- The duties described in this job description must be carried out in a manner which promotes equality of opportunity, dignity and due respect for all employees and service users and is consistent with the Council's Equal Opportunities Policy.

Figure 3.19 Job description for senior residential support worker (source: Worcestershire County Council)

Figure 3.19 is a copy of a job description for a residential support worker. It states the roles and responsibilities of the post.

QUESTIONS

1. What are the main roles that the post holder will be expected to undertake?

2. What are the main responsibilities associated with the job?

3. Identify the responsibilities that are specifically linked with health, safety and security.

Following organisational safety and security procedures

All of an organisation's policies and procedures should be readily available so that staff can easily follow their requirements. Some procedures will need to be followed only occasionally; others will be used every day, and all staff need to be very familiar with them.

> **Think** Look at the safety and security procedures at your workplace. Which ones is it most important that you are very familiar with?

Risk assessment

Risk assessments are vitally important to protect both staff and clients. Before undertaking any task that may present a health or safety hazard, it is important to check whether it has been assessed for risk. It is the employer's responsibility to ensure that risk assessments are undertaken, but the assessment may be delegated to an appropriate member of staff. See page XX to refresh your memory about the steps involved in a risk assessment.

Checking rights of entry and taking appropriate actions

There will be variations in the way access to care establishments is managed. Some premises will have entry that is very strictly controlled while others may rely on a signing-in procedure. Staff need to be aware of the policy of the organisation. However, all organisations expect staff to:

- know the organisation's policy on right of entry
- be aware of everybody who is on the premises
- escort people they do not know rather than giving directions
- report any concerns to the manager immediately.

Identifying and minimising health, safety and security risks

Some risks are accepted as part of a job in the health and social care sector. However, actions need to be taken to ensure that these risks are minimised. People working in an X-ray department have a risk of exposure to radiation. This risk is minimised by wearing protective clothing, such as lead aprons.

> **Think** Give examples of ways in which risks are minimised where you have undertaken your work placement.

Monitoring working practices

Employers are responsible for ensuring that the working practices of employees are monitored. A range of quality assurance measures may be used to do this. The employer may undertake audits or receive feedback from clients about the quality of the care. In addition, all employees have a responsibility to challenge any inappropriate working practices they may see amongst their colleagues.

> **Key words**
>
> Quality assurance – any systematic process of checking to see whether a product or service is meeting specified requirements

> **Example**
>
> Hardeep is working in an after school club. During the afternoon a group of older children are taken to play football in a nearby park. It is the policy of the club that there should always be three members of staff present at any time to ensure the safety of the children. Every afternoon Liz, one of the senior members of staff, goes off to the nearby shop to buy food, leaving Hardeep with only one other member of staff. What should Hardeep do?

Respecting the needs and preferences of individuals

Those working in health and social care settings should respect the rights of the individuals in their care. Enabling and supporting clients to make choices and express their preferences helps them to take control of their situation. It is important that this principle is also applied to allow clients to ensure their own health, safety and security. Therefore, individuals may be encouraged to:

- take responsibility for aspects of their own health and care

- express their own choices

- be shown how to undertake their own risk assessments, if practical

- report anything that might put themselves or others at risk.

Using and storing equipment and materials correctly and safely

There are many regulations that cover the use and storage of equipment and materials. We have looked in detail at some of those regulations, in particular COSHH. Some materials will be supplied with clear instructions about how they should be stored. Some materials, such as foodstuffs, need to be stored at correct temperatures, and so the temperatures of fridges and freezers need to be checked regularly to ensure they are correct. It is the responsibility of the employer and employee to ensure that all instructions for use and storage are carried out correctly.

> *Think* How does your workplace ensure that all foodstuffs are stored safely?

Dealing with spillage of hazardous and non-hazardous materials

Any spillage is a hazard, whatever has been spilled. All employees have an immediate responsibility to ensure that a spillage is cleared up as soon as possible. Wet floors should be dried as far as possible and warning signs put out. A spillage of a hazardous material needs to be dealt with according to the COSHH guidelines. It is the responsibility of the employer to ensure that the guidelines are readily available and that employees follow them.

Disposing of waste immediately and safely

Employers must put procedures in place to deal with waste materials. Employees are responsible for following the procedures and disposing of any waste quickly and safely.

> *Think* What types of waste need to be disposed of in your workplace? How is it done safely?

Implementing correct safety procedures

Employers and employees are both responsible for their own actions in following correct procedures. It is also important that people try to encourage others to adhere to good practice. It is your responsibility to set a good example!

Using correct manual handling procedures and techniques

The Manual Handling Operations Regulations 1992 made employers responsible for avoiding all manual handling where there is a risk of injury. If lifting cannot be avoided, employers are responsible for providing and maintaining appropriate equipment. They must also ensure that staff are adequately trained to use such equipment.

Employees are responsible for ensuring that they take reasonable care of themselves and others who may be affected by their actions when undertaking manual handling. They must always follow the procedures that are set out by their organisation.

Reporting health and safety issues

Employers are required to report health and safety issues to the appropriate authorities. For example, accidents and ill health at work may need to be reported to the Incident Contact Centre, the Health and Safety Executive or the local authority's environmental health department. Employees would normally be expected to report any issues to their line manager for further action.

Completing health, safety and security records

If accidents or injuries occur at work, the details must be recorded. Employers must put in place procedures for recording any accidents. This is a requirement under the RIDDOR regulations and will be checked during any inspection of the organisation. The accident book or report form must comply with the requirements of the Data Protection Act 1998.

Employees are responsible for reporting any accident in which they are involved, either directly or as a witness.

The employee should know where the record book is kept and who is responsible for recording accidents.

> **Think** Find the accident or incident book at your workplace. Who is responsible for completing it? What sort of injuries or incidents have been recorded?

Operating within the limits of your role and responsibilities

It is important that each individual should be very clear as to what their roles and responsibilities are. For this reason, all employees should have a job description which clearly describes the tasks and responsibilities that they are expected to undertake. If an employee is unsure at any point they need to check with their line manager. Most organisations have regular staff appraisals to review how the job is working out and identify any training needs that an individual may have.

EVIDENCE ACTIVITY

P4

Examine the roles and responsibilities of key people in the promotion of health, safety and security in a health or social care setting.

a) Make an organisational chart for the workplace where you carried out your work placement.

b) Identify the key people and what their roles and responsibilities are. You could use this information to write a case study about this organisation. (P4)

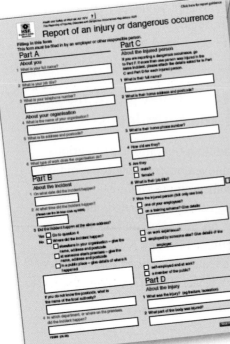

Figure 3.13 Example of an incident reporting form from the Health and Safety Executive

3.4 *Dealing with hazards in a local environment*

As we have already seen, workers in health and social care may encounter hazards for a number of different reasons. They need to know how to deal with them and be prepared to do so. It is important to know how to deal with hazards in the particular local environments in which you are working.

ENVIRONMENTS

Each environment has different hazards which need to be assessed. You are likely to find yourself working in a range of different environments from time to time, including local parks, tourist attractions, shopping malls and play areas.

Local park or children's play area

If you work in a nursery, for example, it is likely that you might take a group of children to a local park or play area. These locations will have a range of specific hazards, which you need to be aware of in order to assess the risk and ensure that you know how to minimise and deal with the hazards.

Hazards in a local park might include grassy areas that have been fouled by dogs, unfenced ponds, busy roads nearby, children's swings and other play equipment, and trees that children might climb. In addition, you need to be aware that there will be other people in the park who you do not know and who may, in some cases, try to approach the children.

> *Think* How would you deal with the risks that might occur on a visit to a local park?

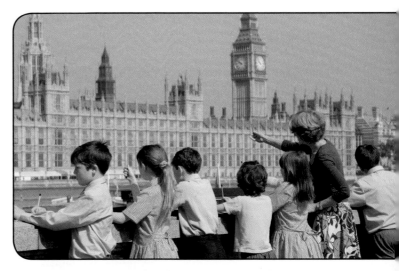

Figure 3.11 *Every environment has hazards*

Tourist attraction or shopping mall

Residential care centres, for example, may take groups of clients to visit a tourist attraction or shopping mall. In these locations, you need to be aware of the specific hazards that may affect the individuals in your care, whether they are older people or people with sensory or cognitive impairment.

> *Think* Choose a local tourist attraction that you know. If you were asked to arrange a visit to this location what information would you need to know, bearing in mind the health and safety aspects you would want to assess for your client group?

PATIENT OR SERVICE USER GROUP

The impact of any hazard may be influenced by the characteristics and needs of the particular patient or service group.

Older people

In Unit 4 you will learn about the effects of the ageing process. As people get older, their physical abilities and functions decline. Older people will have slower physical and mental responses, which means they may be more likely to fall or trip. Table 3.4 outlines the effect of some of these changes.

Table 3.4 Physical implications of ageing on health and safety

Changes due to the ageing process	Possible impact on health and safety
Vision	will not be able to see hazards so easily
Hearing	will not hear danger approaching or warning sounds
Muscles	lack of strength and stamina
Bones	may break more easily, wear and tear on joints may make walking painful
Hearts and lungs	unable to sustain long periods of exercise
Skin	may damage more easily

Example

Jane is planning to take the residents of the care home in which she works to the seaside for the day. All of the residents are in their eighties. They do not have many opportunities to get out so she has booked a minibus for the day. However, when they arrive at the coast she is concerned to find that the car park is a long way from the seafront. They will need to cross several busy roads to get there.

Think What might Jane expect to be the additional problems of taking this group out because of their age? What steps could she take to overcome these problems?

People with sensory or cognitive impairment

Some individuals may have sensory impairment, such as loss of sight or hearing, which is not associated with old age. People who have a cognitive impairment will find it more difficult to think, perceive, reason or remember. These impairments result in the loss of ability to attend to the needs of daily living. Individuals with cognitive impairments may fail to understand the consequences of their actions. For example, individuals with dementia may forget where they are or where they have put things. These needs must be taken into account when analyzing the risk of any hazard.

Children

Children develop very quickly and are usually keen to explore their environment. As their motor skills develop they will tackle more and more challenges. However, their understanding of danger does not necessarily keep pace with their growth. This can lead them into a number of hazardous situations unless their carers understand the risks for them.

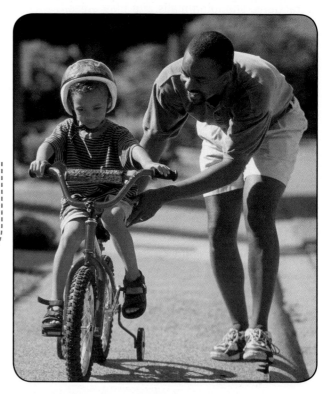

Figure 3.12 Carers need to understand risks to children

Think Identify the motor skills development that is associated with the different stages of childhood, i.e. 18–24 months, 2–5 years, 5–9 years, 10–15 years. What risks might be associated with these different stages of development?

SURVEY OF HEALTH, SAFETY AND SECURITY ISSUES

When undertaking a survey of health, safety and security issues it is important to consider who is involved, what they might be doing and where, considering the staff as well as the clients. As we have already seen, the age, physical or cognitive ability of service users will affect the amount of risk that is involved, so you need to start by identifying who your group of clients is and noting any risks associated with them. Next you will need to consider what activity might take place and whether there any risks involved in the activity. For example, the risk of swimming in the sea might be much higher than going to the park. Next you should consider where: is it somewhere that is well known to the service users or is it a totally new experience? Having identified some of the basic facts it is important to think through the activities that are planned in detail. If appropriate, it may be a good idea to make a preliminary visit to the location as this may make it easier to clearly identify any hazards.

RISKS

The risk is the chance, high or low, that somebody could be harmed by a hazard, together with an indication of how serious the harm could be. For any environment or group of service users, the specific risks need to be known. These could include the possibility of injury or harm, the possibility of infection, or the possibility of danger.

> **Think** Which hazards that might be present in a local park could cause: injury, infection and danger?

RISK ASSESSMENT

Remember the steps to risk assessment.

Step 1: Identify the hazards

First, you need to work out in what ways people could be harmed. If possible, visit the environment beforehand. Walk around to try to identify anything that might cause harm. If you cannot visit, get as much information as possible. Talk to other people who may have visited the environment or somewhere similar. Discuss your visit with others who may be able to think of things you have not thought of that might cause harm. Look back at any accident or incident records to see if anything has happened before.

Step 2: Decide who might be harmed and how

For each hazard you identify, you need to be clear about who might be harmed. Identify the different groups of people who might be at risk, including both different service users and health and social care workers. In each case, identify how they might be harmed. This will help you to identify the best way of managing the risk.

Step 3: Evaluate the risks and decide on precautions

Having identified the hazards, you need to decide what to do about them. The law requires you to do everything 'reasonably practicable' to protect people from harm. If possible the risk should be eliminated. If it cannot be got rid of, then the law requires you to do everything you can to minimise the risks. For example, you can make recommendations of how the activity should be undertaken.

> **Think** Kirsty is planning to take a group of ten children aged 4–5 years old to the local park. Among other things, she has identified that there is a risk of them wandering off and getting into danger. How could she minimise this risk?

Step 4: Record your findings and implement them

Recording what you have planned will help in the future and will ensure that others know what they need to do when the visit takes place.

Step 5: Review your risk assessment and update if necessary

Further recommendations for improvements can be made. Regular updating will ensure that changes in circumstances are allowed for.

EVIDENCE ACTIVITY

P5 – M2 – D2

1. Carry out a health and safety survey of a local environment used by a specific patient or service user group. This can be achieved by surveying a local environment, such as a local park, tourist attraction, shopping centre or children's play area. Your survey should focus on a specific user group, such as older people, those with sensory or cognitive impairment or children. Think about the health, safety and security issues in this environment, which must be a different location from the place where you carried out your work experience. (P5)

2. Assess the risk associated with the chosen local environment and make recommendations for change. Make sure you follow the five steps of risk assessment. (M2)

3. Justify the recommendations that you have made for improvements to minimise the risks, as appropriate, for the setting and service user groups. (D2)

FIRST-AID PROCEDURES

Failure to provide first aid could result in a person's death. Employers are required to make adequate and appropriate first-aid provision for their workforce. All health and social care workers should know what to do in case of emergency and there is no substitute for a recognised training programme and subsequent qualification.

It is important that you only take action that it is safe for you to do. You should not attempt anything outside your skill or responsibility, as this may put you at risk. As part of this unit you are required to know about the following:

- action at an emergency

- emergency first aid

- life-saving procedures

- dealing with injuries, including fractures and sprains

- dealing with bleeding and burns

- asthma attacks

- epilepsy

- diabetes

- bites, stings and allergies.

You will learn about all of these in more detail through a first-aid qualification and your handbook will provide you with the information that you will need.

Research tip

You can look up further details about first aid on the St John's Ambulance website.

www.sja.org.uk

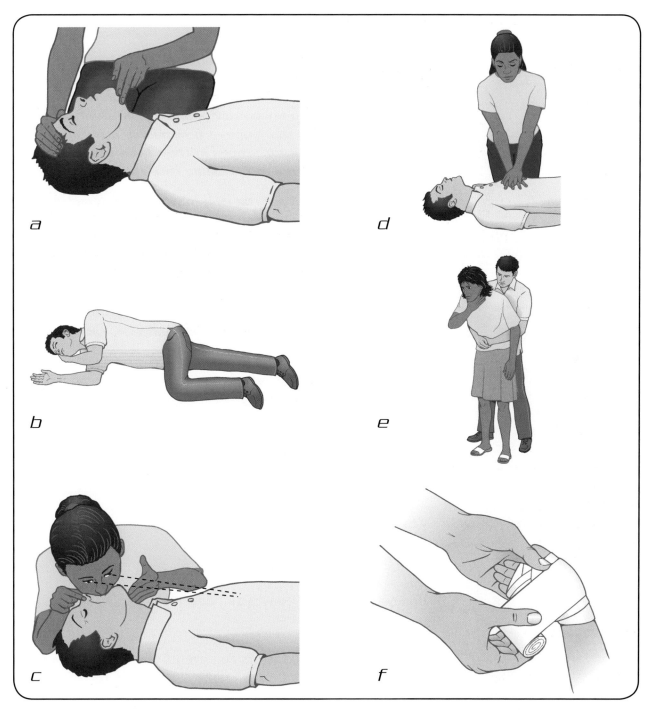

Figure 3.13   a – clearing the airway; b – recovery position; c – giving rescue breathes; d – CPR; e – Heimlich manouevre; f – tying a bandage

EVIDENCE ACTIVITY

P6 – M3

1. You need to be able to demonstrate basic first aid skills. You can do this by obtaining a certificate for a recognised First Aid course. Alternatively, you may be able to choose an appropriate simulated scenario in which to demonstrate your skills. (P6)

2. Demonstrate your first aid skills in a simulated scenario that involves a critically injured individual, for example an individual with more than one serious injury or an individual with life-threatening injuries. (M3)

Development through the Life Stages

If you are going to work in any sector of health or social care, it is important that you understand the needs of the patients or service users you work with. You are likely to encounter people of different ages. Having a good knowledge of how people grow and develop at different stages in their lives will help you understand better the possible care they might need.

Many factors affect the way in which our lives develop. Some of these factors may be present at birth and others will arise during our lives. There may be factors that we have no control over, but there are others over which we can exert some degree of control, such as the amount of exercise we take. There are also events in our lives that can have a big effect, such as starting school, marriage, retirement or serious illnesses.

It is a fact of life that we get older. We cannot stop time or the ageing process. For many people, getting older can be a negative process. However, for others it can be a positive experience. Having an understanding of these different perspectives can help a carer when working with older people.

Learning outcomes

By the end of this unit you will:

4.1 Understand human growth and development through the life stages — page 119

4.2 Understand how life factors and events may influence the development of the individual — page 127

4.3 Understand physical changes and psychological perspectives in relation to ageing — page 144

So, you want to be a...

Health visitor

My name Sushila Mistry
Age 28
Income £31,000

Working closely with a wide range of people in your local community is an important and emotionally rewarding job...

What responsibilities do you have?

I do a lot of work with families - mothers and fathers of young babies. We visit them at home, and we're asked for advice on things like feeding, physical and emotional development, and behaviour management.

We're often the first to spot when things aren't going as they should be. This could be concerns over how the parents are managing their child, or it could be some developmental problem such as a child who seems to be slow to walk or to talk. We might then refer the child on to a physiotherapist or a speech and language therapist. Although we usually work on our own, teamwork is a large part of our job with some families.

How did you get into the job?

I did a vocational qualification in health and social care at college and went on to train as a nurse. I worked in our local hospital for a couple of years, where I realised that helping people be healthy was just as important as helping people who'd become ill! A lot of our work as health visitors' is like that. It's really about health promotion. So I took additional training as a health visitor, as was able to do this part-time over a number of years. Like other nurses I do have to keep my skills up to date through an on-going programme of training

How did you find your current job?

There are some good websites like: http://www.connexionsdirect.com/jobs4u/ and http://www.nhscareers.nhs.uk/, and it's also a good idea to talk to somebody who's doing the job if you want an accurate description of what it's like.

What skills do you need?

Empathising with young parents and understanding the situations they find themselves in is important. Being based in a community setting means you need to be able to communicate with and understand the concerns of people from all different walks of life. The ability to observe a situation and then come up with a solution or way for a parent to address a problem is crucial. You have to remain positive in this job but some things – like child protection issues – can be hard to deal with. So you need to be able to seek and use support from colleagues.

> **"You have to remain positive in the job"**

What about the future?

I'm very happy in present job but might look for a team manager's role later on in my career.

Grading criteria

The table below shows what you need to do to gain a pass, merit or distinction in this part of the qualification. Make sure you refer back to it when you are completing work so you can judge whether you are meeting the criteria and what you need to do to fill in gaps in your knowledge or experience.

In this unit there are 3 evidence activities that give you an opportunity to demonstrate your achievement of the grading criteria:

page 126   P1

page 143   P2, P3, M1, M2, D1

page 149   P4, P5, M3, D2

To achieve a pass grade the evidence must show that the learner is able to...	To achieve a merit grade the evidence must show that, in addition to the pass criteria, the learner is able to...	To achieve a distinction grade the evidence must show that, in addition to the pass and merit criteria, the learner is able to...
P1 describe physical, intellectual, emotional and social development through the life stages		
P2 describe the potential influences of five life factors on the development of individuals	**M1** discuss the nature-nurture debate in relation to individual development	**D1** evaluate the nature-nurture debate in relation to development of the individual
P3 describe the influences of two predictable and two unpredictable major life events on the development of the individual	**M2** explain how major life events can influence the development of the individual	
P4 describe two theories of ageing	**M3** use examples to compare two major theories of ageing	**D2** evaluate the influence of two major theories of ageing on health and social care provision
P5 describe physical and psychological changes due to the ageing process		

4.1 *Understanding human growth and development through the life stages*

LIFE STAGES

You will know people of different ages. We often group people of certain ages together. We do this because the same pattern of growth and development usually happens in everyone's life. We shall learn more about growth and development in this unit. You will find that different text books give different names and age ranges for the life stages. Do not worry about this. For the purpose of this course, Table 4.1 shows the names and age ranges of the different life stages.

Table 4.1 – Life stages

Name of life stage	Age range
Conception	Approximately minus 9 months
Pregnancy	Minus 9 months to birth
Birth and infancy	0–3 years
Childhood	4–9 years
Adolescence	10–18 years
Adulthood	19–65 years
Older adulthood	65 plus
The final stages of life	

Key words

Life stage – an age-related phase of growth and development that a person passes through

Think What are your initial thoughts about these life stages and age ranges? An example might be the lack of an age range for the final stages of life.

Conception

The sperm is the male gamete (sex cell) and the ovum is the female gamete. Conception is the point at which a sperm enters an ovum and fertilises it.

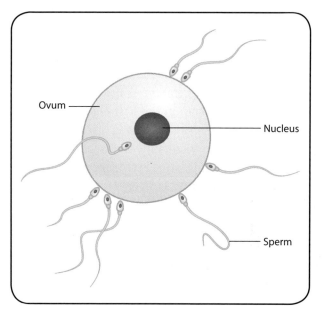

Figure 4.1   Male and female gametes

Look at Figure 4.1. Note the difference in the sizes of the male and female gametes. The female gamete is larger than the male gamete and fewer are produced. The sperm has a tail to help it move. It has an area at the front called an acrosome. This contains enzymes that digest the coating of an ovum. The ovum has a large amount of cytoplasm with many yolk droplets that contain protein and lipids. This provides the embryo with the materials it needs to grow initially.

Pregnancy

There are various definitions of pregnancy:

* the condition of having a developing embryo or foetus in the body

* the process by which a human female carries a live offspring from conception until childbirth.

Think In what other ways could you define pregnancy?

The time between conception and birth is known as the gestation period. This is approximately 40 weeks (280 days), measured from the first day of the mother's last period. For women who become pregnant by a procedure that allows them to know the exact date of conception, such as in vitro fertilisation (IVF) or artificial insemination, then the gestation period is 38 weeks (266 days).

Pregnancy is divided into three stages, called trimesters, each lasting about three months (see Figure 4.2). The term embryo is used to describe the developing human in the first eight weeks of gestation. Foetus is the term used after the eighth week of gestation, when all the systems of the body, such as the digestive system or the nervous system, have formed.

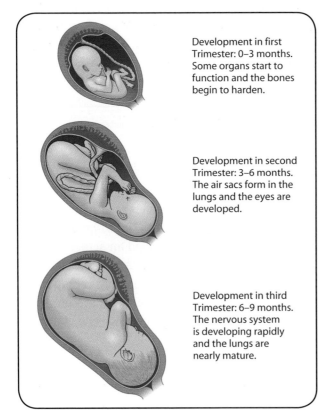

Development in first Trimester: 0–3 months. Some organs start to function and the bones begin to harden.

Development in second Trimester: 3–6 months. The air sacs form in the lungs and the eyes are developed.

Development in third Trimester: 6–9 months. The nervous system is developing rapidly and the lungs are nearly mature.

Figure 4.2 Three stages of pregnancy

We shall see that there are many factors that might affect growth and development during pregnancy.

Think Why might it be difficult to predict a delivery date for some babies?

Birth

Around 38 weeks after fertilisation, the foetus has developed enough for it to survive easily outside its mother's body. Babies are usually born head first, but they can be born bottom first (called breech presentation). Some babies are delivered by caesarean section, if there is a problem with a natural delivery.

The process of giving birth through the vagina to the outside world is called labour. There are three stages of labour.

- Stage 1   The cervix stretches around the baby's head until the opening is about 10 centimetres in diameter. The baby's head can then pass through.

- Stage 2   The baby is expelled. The head usually comes first facing backwards, then the baby rotates so that one shoulder at a time can be delivered.

- Stage 3   The placenta or afterbirth is expelled.

Infancy

Infancy lasts from birth until three years of age. This is a time when there is much growth and development. Table 4.2 gives some examples of the physical developments expected at different ages during infancy. These are just average ages at which infants may be able to do these activities.

Table 4.2   Physical developments during infancy

Age	Examples of physical development
2–3 months	lifting head when lying on front
6 months	sitting up unsupported
9 months	moving independently by rolling or crawling
12 months	walking by holding on to furniture
15 months	walking unaided and crawling upstairs
18 months	running
2 years	walking downstairs
3 years	climbing on play equipment, throwing and catching a ball

Childhood

For the purposes of this course we will say that childhood spans from four to nine years old. This is a time when intellectual, emotional and social developments are particularly prominent. Some of the key features of this life stage are:

- starting school
- being separated from parents or carers
- interacting with other children
- making friends.

Adolescence

Adolescence spans a large age range from 10 to 18 years old. This is a time when there is growth and development in all areas. The main physical changes relate to the secondary sex characteristics, which will be discussed later.

Anyone who has been an adolescent will know what a stormy time this can be. Adolescents are often perceived as moody and unco-operative.

Relationships with friends play a very important part in the lives of adolescents. They probably spend more time with their friends than they do with members of their own families. Stable relationships with friends can play an important part in the transition from family to independent lives.

Adulthood

Adulthood is defined here as 19 to 65 years old. This is a huge age range and people will have very different experiences within this period. You may find some people refer to early and middle adulthood:

- early adulthood: 19–45 years
- middle adulthood: 46–65 years.

Rather than discuss at length here all the possible experiences of adulthood, we shall just look at some of the key features.

Key features of early adulthood

Adulthood starts when the individual has reached physical maturity. Adults may of course gain weight during adulthood, but this may be because of a sedentary life style. Early adulthood is the time when most people will start employment, have a relationship with a partner or get married, and start a family.

Key features of middle adulthood

You may associate middle adulthood with 'mid-life' crises. This is often a period when people take stock of their lives and may feel that they have not achieved all that they might have liked to. Other people, however, may be satisfied with what they have done and achieved. Many people will be at the peak of their careers. Here are some of the key events that generate positive feelings or negative feelings, depending on the person:

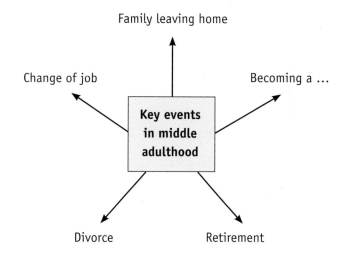

Figure 4.3   Key events that can occur in middle adulthood

> ***Think*** How might positive and negative feelings occur about each of the key events of middle adulthood shown in Figure 4.3?

Older adulthood

When a person is over the age of 65, they are considered to be in older adulthood. Nowadays, with the human lifespan increasing more than ever, many people in this age group do not consider themselves to be old. There are physical changes in the bodies of older people, some which have been occurring gradually over a period of years. You will learn more about these later.

Some older people complain that their short-term memory is not as good as it used to be, but they can usually recall events from way back in the past. I'm sure you know of older people who can recall stories from their younger days. We shall see that how people feel and how they interact with others varies widely at this life stage. Some people are happy and positive in their old age, and others have many causes to feel negative.

The final stages of life

People could in fact die at any of the other life stages. This could be because of:

- serious illness
- accidents
- death during wars
- murder or manslaughter.

For most people, thankfully, the final stages of life will come at the end of older adulthood.

Death and dying are inevitable at the end of the normal life span, yet many people find discussing these topics difficult. Also, the social and biological changes that take place during the last stages of life are important and these are often retained as the most powerful memories of that person by their relatives and friends.

> *Think* You may have experienced the death of someone close to you. What do you remember about that person?

DEFINITIONS

Growth and development

'Growth and development' is often used as a single term and sometimes the two words are used to mean the same thing. However, it is important that we distinguish between them. Growth is an increase in physical size or mass Development is the process of growing to maturity, including changes in complexity, sophistication and use of capabilities

You can see that growth has a fairly precise meaning, whereas development is more difficult to define. When we think of growth, we think of something getting larger. How do we measure whether something is larger? It could be by its size (height or volume) or by its mass.

Human beings start off as a zygote (a fertilised ovum or egg). Initially, the zygote divides in two, then into four, then into eight, with the number of cells doubling with each division. However, we do not end up with just a big ball of the same type of cells. Our cells differentiate into specialised cells, such as muscle cells or nerve cells. These then form organs, such as the heart or liver. This differentiation and the formation of organs is an example of development and it fits with the definition of development that refers to changes in complexity.

> *Think* Consider a baby if it just grew in size and did not develop physically. What would it be like by the age of 10 or even 40? Think now of someone at the beginning of each of the other life stages and imagine what they would be like if they just grew and did not develop.

There are various measures of growth and development. For many years, charts were used to find out if a person's weight and height were within the 'normal' range. Nowadays, a more accurate measurement, called body mass index (BMI), is used. BMI is a calculation that uses a person's height and weight to estimate how much body fat he or she has. Doctors use BMI to determine how appropriate a child's weight is for its height and age.

Developmental norms and milestones

The process of human development follows a predictable pattern and tends to happen within specified time periods. For example, we know that a baby will sit up before it can crawl. Linking this sequence of expected development events to an expected timeframe gives us developmental norms or milestones.

Life course and continuum of life

The life course is the unique pattern of events that a person goes through during their existence. The stages a person goes through during their life, and the order of these, are predetermined and sometimes referred to as the continuum of life. However, everything that happens during the continuum of life will be different for each of us.

Maturation

In 1925, Arnold Gesell was the first person to use the term maturation to describe a genetically programmed sequence of changes in the human body. He suggested that maturation happens regardless of practice or training. For example, during puberty, girls change body shape, grow breasts and start to menstruate. All women will go through the menopause, at which point they stop menstruating. We will all develop wrinkles as we reach later adulthood. It is from this concept of maturation, that we get the idea of a biological clock. We can do nothing about the fact that we all get older. There are many factors that influence how slowly or quickly the clock runs for each individual.

Life expectancy

Life expectancy is the number of years a person might be expected to live for from a given point in time. Life expectancy is increasing all the time. Figure 4.5 shows the life expectancy of males and females at the age of 65. This graph shows that in 1981 a 65-year-old man could expect to live for a further 13 years. This means that his life expectancy would have been 65 + 13 = 78. It also shows that in 1981 a 65-year-old woman could expect to live for a further 17 years. This means that her life expectancy would have been 82 years.

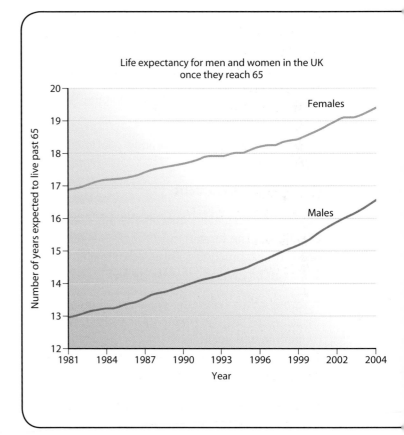

Figure 4.4 Life expectancy at the age of 65 in the UK [Source: Office for National Statistics, 2006. www.statistics.gov.uk]

> ***Think*** What was the life expectancy of a man and of a woman in 2004? Is the gap between the life expectancy for females and males increasing or decreasing?

DEVELOPMENT

Holistic development

Holistic development is development in the widest sense, not just physical or mental alone.

Physical, intellectual, emotional and social development

There are four main areas of development, which can be abbreviated to PIES:

- **P**hysical development – the gradual process of becoming mature biologically
- **I**ntellectual development – developing thinking language skills
- **E**motional development – developing feelings about oneself and others
- **S**ocial development – forming relationships.

Physical development

Physical development involves the differentiation of cells and the formation of the organs of the body. It also involves gaining motor skills. Motor skills can be divided into two areas:

- gross motor skills that use muscles involved in activities such as sitting up, crawling, walking, pulling and pushing
- fine motor skills that involve delicate movement of the fingers, such as using a knife and fork, threading a needle and writing.

The development of motor skills is an area of physical development monitored by health professionals during infancy. Professionals, e.g. physiotherapists, are also involved in helping people regain their gross and fine motor skill ability following an accident, injury or stroke.

Intellectual development

Intellectual development begins when we are born and continues through childhood and into adulthood. During our lifetime we change in the ways we think, in how we communicate, and in how we understand the world around us. If you watch very young babies, you might see them repeating sequences of actions; perhaps flapping their arms to make a mobile move. The baby is learning about cause and effect: that something they do makes something else happen. Older children take this for granted.

Babies also have to learn that things continue to exist when they can no longer see them, which is also something that older children take for granted. A psychologist called Jean Piaget showed young babies a toy, then dropped a cloth over it so it was no longer in view. The babies were able to pull away the cloth, but they didn't do so. Older babies did pull the cloth away because they knew the toy hadn't gone out of existence. They knew that it was still there even though they couldn't see it under the cloth.

> **Think** Babies at a certain age enjoy playing peek-a-boo. What does this tell us about their intellectual development?

Learning to communicate and developing language skills are also part of our intellectual development. Very young babies are already quite skilled communicators: they use looking, smiling and looking away in the same way that we do. They are already communicating before they have any speech or language, and the development of language is usually quite rapid.

During the early part of childhood, thinking can be very 'concrete'. This is a word Piaget used to describe the child's need to use real things as tools in their thinking. For example, in early primary school, children use blocks, other objects or their fingers to count with. By early adolescence, usually by the age of 11 or 12, children develop more 'abstract' thinking.

Psychologists who study intellectual development are most interested in infancy and childhood, as this is the period in which the most rapid changes take place. The examples we have looked at here should show how different young children's thinking is from your own, and how far your own thinking and communication skills have already developed.

> **Think** Can you think of any examples of mistakes in the thinking of younger children that suggest that they don't always think in a logical and 'adult' manner?

Emotional and social development

Like the other areas of development, both emotional development and social development begin at birth and continue all the way through our lives. These two areas are often considered together, as they are usually interlinked. Babies soon recognise those that interact with them. They are happier in the company of those they know than in the company of strangers.

John Bowlby (1870–1937) recognised the importance of early attachments, often known as bonding. Often the baby is given to the mother to hold immediately after birth. This is the beginning of the bonding between a mother and her baby. Bonding does not have to be just with a mother. Strong emotional links may be formed with either parent or main carers.

> **Think** What reasons are there why a baby might not form a bond with its mother?

The popular image of adolescence is that it is a very stormy time – perhaps you or your friends might have opinions on this! Adolescence is a life stage where there are many physical changes happening. It is also a time when we are trying to find a sense of personal identity. Coping with the effects of puberty often triggers concerns about self image and what is 'normal'.

In 1960 Erik Erikson put forward the theory that the main emotional and social challenge of adolescence is in establishing a sense of self, separate from that of your parents. Adolescents, therefore, need to resolve the question, 'Who am I?' They often do this through friendships.

Figure 4.6 shows some of the emotional and social issues adolescents need to cope with.

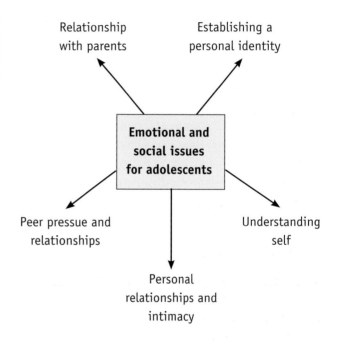

Figure 4.5 *Emotional and social issues facing adolescents*

Friendships become increasingly important during adolescence and these friendships often continue into adulthood. In early adulthood, people begin new roles, as a partner, parent or at work. Each of these new roles in life is likely to affect a person's relationships and their sense of identity. As we move towards middle age, our roles as partners, parents and workers take on a new meaning. We may have a new partner, our children may leave home and we may be promoted at work, or indeed, be passed over for promotion. In older adulthood, the role of parent is often reversed, in that the child may look after their parents. Friendships will remain important for companionship, but older people may have fewer friends of their own age, as they may have died; they may have to adapt to new relationships.

125

CASE STUDY: GED AND MARIA

Ged and Maria are both in their early twenties. They have a son, Pete, who is three years old, and identical twins, Emma and Sarah, who are ten months old. Ged is worried that all the children are not developing as fast as they should be. He thinks that Pete should be talking more, and is worried that he did not walk until he was 18 months old and still takes an afternoon nap. Maris is not concerned. She says that when Pete points to something he wants, she gets it for him, and that she appreciates Pete's afternoon nap, as it allows her to get on with some of the household chores. She reminds Ged he did not walk himself until he was 18 months old. Ged is also concerned about the twins. He is concerned that Emma could sit up before Sarah, but that Emma didn't sit unaided until eight months. He believes that they will not walk until they are 18 months old either.

Maria does not see this as a problem.

QUESTION

1. Why may Pete not talk much?

2. If the developmental norm for sitting up unaided is between 6 and 9 months, does Emma and Sarah's development fall within the norm?

3. Why might Ged expect Emma and Sarah's development to be similar? Suggest a reason why Emma might have sat up earlier than Sarah.

4. The developmental norm for walking unaided is 12–13 months. What do you think about Maria's comments that Ged should not be worried about the children walking until they are 18 months old?

Potential causes and effects of delayed development

There are many reasons why development may be delayed, the details of which we shall learn about later. Figure 4.6 gives an overview of the broad categories of causes of delayed development.

Figure 4.6   Possible causes of delayed development

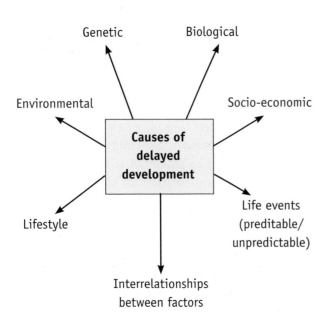

EVIDENCE ACTIVITY

P1

1. Summarise what you have learned so far about physical, intellectual, emotional and social development through the life stages. Make a copy of the table below to help you.

2. Which life stage did you have most difficulty writing about and why? Which area of development did you have most difficulty writing about and why?

3. Write a short paragraph about conception and pregnancy that covers development during this life stage. (P1)

Life stage	Physical development	Intellectual development	Emotional development	Social development
Birth and infancy				
Childhood				
Adolescence				
Adulthood				
Older adulthood				
The final stages of life				

4.2 *Understanding how life factors and events may influence the development of the individual*

THE NATURE-NURTURE DEBATE

It is often possible to tell that people come from the same family. They may look alike, have the same mannerisms, like the same things to eat or, perhaps, have a similar talent, such as playing football or a musical instrument.

> **Think** Think about your own family or another family you know well. What similarities between family members can you see? Group these similarities into the different areas of development – physical, intellectual, emotional or social.

Why do people from the same family have similarities? Is it because they share the same genes or is it because they live in the same environment and share similar experiences? The answer is that it might be because of nature (genes) or nurture (the environment, including experiences), or a combination of both.

> **Key words**
> Nature – those influences on human growth and development that are determined by our genes and we cannot change
> Nurture – those influences on human growth and development that occur during our lifetime, due to our environment (including our experiences)

Key principles

There is a nature-nurture debate because people aren't sure of the relative influence of genes and of the environment or experiences on the way we are and what we do.

Some theorists argue from an extreme nature point of view. They believe that we are genetically or biologically programmed to behave in the

ways that we do and that our environment or experiences play no part in this. For example, they believe that some people are aggressive because 'it is in their genes'. Other theorists argue from an extreme nurture point of view. They believe that our environment and experiences shape our behaviour and that our genes play no role in this. They would believe that people are aggressive because of they way they had been treated in the past or because they live in an environment that is conducive to such behaviour.

You might be wondering whether there is a 'middle ground' approach. Is it possible that both nature and nurture play a part in the way we are and what we do? You will see that for many of our characteristics, this is a possibility. However, there are some of our characteristics that are solely determined by our genes (nature).

Nature: biological programming

Inside the nuclei of all our cells are chromosomes. We have 23 pairs of chromosomes, one of each pair from our mother and one from our father. Each chromosome is composed of several genes, each one of which codes for a particular characteristic, such as eye colour. Deoxyribonucleic acid (DNA) is the chemical that makes up our genes and chromosomes. The relationship between chromosomes, genes and DNA is shown in Figure 4.7.

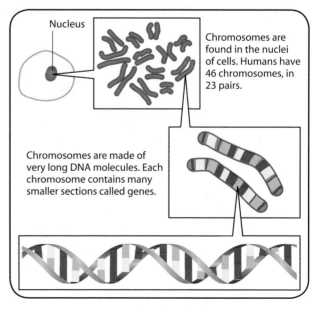

Nucleus

Chromosomes are found in the nuclei of cells. Humans have 46 chromosomes, in 23 pairs.

Chromosomes are made of very long DNA molecules. Each chromosome contains many smaller sections called genes.

Figure 4.7 Relationship between chromosomes, genes and DNA

Characteristics that we cannot change, tend to be determined solely by genes. These include:

• whether we are male or female

• eye colour

• ability to roll the tongue.

You may wonder about the inclusion of whether we are male or female. Someone may have a sex change, which means that their secondary sexual characteristics are changed. However, it is the presence or absence of the Y chromosome in our cells that determines whether we are really male or female, and that cannot ever be changed. You might also wonder about the colour of our eyes. Some people have their irises tinted, but that does not change the underlying colour. The ability to roll the tongue (see Figure 4.9) is possessed by 85 per cent of the population. The other 15 per cent simply cannot do this, no matter how hard they try or how hard they practise. In other words, their experience makes no difference – they cannot learn how to do it.

Nurture: experiences and environment

Nurture may be defined in different ways. We shall look at nurture in terms of the environment and experiences.

Studying nature and nurture

Much of the way we are and what we do is determined by both nature and by nurture. Think about someone who has heart disease. Their father and mother may have died from it, yet their brother does not have heart disease. However, the brother does not smoke, takes lots of exercise and eats healthily, unlike the person who has heart disease. We could then say that the environment and experiences of the brother have had an influence on them not having heart disease. People argue about the relative weightings given to the importance of the nature and nurture components relating to the chances of developing heart disease. This is what the nature-nurture debate is all about.

Identical twin studies

The study of identical twins is very important in determining whether nature or nurture is responsible for determining particular characteristics. Identical twins have identical genes. Therefore, if there are any differences found in their characteristics these must have been due to nurture: their environment or experiences.

Information gathered from twins who have been reared together and from twins who have been reared apart is particularly useful. The example shown in Table 4.3 will help you to understand this. Here the mean difference in height is given for identical twins who were reared apart, for identical twins who were reared together and for non-identical, same-sex twins reared together. The mean difference in mass for the three groups is also given.

Table 4.3 Differences between twins

Mean difference	Identical twins reared apart	Identical twins reared together,	Non-identical, same-sex twins reared together
Height (centimetres)	1.8	1.7	4.4
Mass (kilograms)	4.8	2.0	4.9

Height is more likely to be controlled by nature (genes) because identical twins have little difference in height, whether they are reared together in the same environment or apart. This argument is further supported by the fact that non-identical twins (with different genes) have larger differences in their height even though they are reared together in the same environment.

Mass is more likely to be controlled by nurture (environment and experiences) because identical twins have larger differences in their mass (4.8 kg) when they are reared apart in a different environment compared to identical twins reared together in the same environment (2.0 kg).

CASE STUDY: HENRY AND MARTY

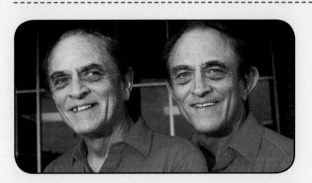

Henry and Marty are 47-year-old identical twins (see Figure 4.8). They were separated from each other shortly after birth, following the death of their mother. Their father decided he could not look after two sons, and so Henry stayed with him, while Marty was raised in a children's home. Years later the twins met up with each other and Marty now lives and works with Henry on Henry's cattle ranch in North America.

As well as looking alike, Henry and Marty have many similar tastes, such as their love of horses, and country and western music. There are some differences between them, however. Henry is right-handed, whereas Marty is left-handed. Also, Henry is about three centimetres taller and half a kilogram heavier than Marty.

QUESTION

1. List the similarities between Henry and Marty. What might be the reasons for these similarities?

2. List the differences between Henry and Marty. What might be the reasons for these differences?

3. Is being right- or left-handed a result of genetic or environmental influence?

LIFE FACTORS

We shall now go on to look at both nature and nurture in more detail to study how different life factors and major life events may influence the development of the individual. It is important that you understand how these may influence the development of individuals. We shall also look at the interrelationships between life factors and major life events.

> **Think** Can you remember what the four main areas of development are?

Life factors may be sub-divided into five categories. These are:

- genetic factors
- biological factors
- environmental factors
- socio-economic factors
- lifestyle factors.

Genetic factors

Genetic predisposition to certain diseases

The occurrence of many common diseases of adult life, such as diabetes, hypertension and schizophrenia, and common congenital malformations (birth defects), e.g. cleft lip, cleft palate and neural tube defects, has a strong genetic element. In these cases, it is thought that a large number of genes each act in a small but significant way to make an individual likely to have the genetic condition.

Scientists have studied identical and non-identical twins to investigate whether people have a genetic predisposition to certain diseases, whether the diseases occur by chance or as a result of something happening in their lives, either environmental or experiences. Identical twins have identical genes and non-identical twins have similar, but not identical, genes. Scientists measure percentage concordance of certain diseases having occurred. If there is 100 per cent concordance, this means if one twin got the disease, then the other would always get it too. If there was 50 per cent concordance, then in half the cases studied, the other twin would get the disease.

Key words

concordance – agreement or similarity between things.

> *Think* What does a concordance of 25 per cent mean? What does a concordance of 0 per cent mean?

Table 4.4 shows that the chance of both identical twins having the same disease or condition is much higher than both non-identical twins having it. We can infer from this that a strong 'non-random' or genetic component is in play.

Table 4.4 – Percentage concordance for some common diseases for identical and non-identical twins

Adult diseases	Twin concordance for some diseases	
	Identical twins	Non-identical twins
Diabetes (mellitus)	50%	10%
Hypertension	30%	10%
Manic depression	80%	10%
Multiple sclerosis	20%	5%
Schizophrenia	40%	10%
Alzheimer's disease	40%	10%

> *Think* Which of the diseases or conditions shown in Table 4.4 has the greatest likelihood of being determined by our genes? Why? What other group of people, who have different genes, might the scientists have included in their studies?

Families with strong links to specific diseases are often very useful to scientists who wish to find out which genes are responsible for determining that predisposition.

Phenylketonuria

Phenylketonuria is an inherited defect, present in individuals who are affected from birth. People who have phenylketonuria have high levels of the amino acid phenylalanine in their blood because they do not possess the enzyme (phenylalanine hydroxylase) needed to break it down. Having too high levels of phenylalanine in the blood will eventually damage the brain.

Phenylketonuria may be treated by putting an individual on a carefully controlled diet that limits the intake of phenylalanine, for example by eliminating meat and dairy products. Early testing is essential because symptoms are not obvious in a newborn baby. Fortunately, screening tests for phenylketonuria are now compulsory for all babies. The dietary treatment must be started soon after birth or some degree of mental retardation may be expected. There is disagreement about how long the diet therapy needs to continue for, but some restriction of dietary phenylalanine is necessary throughout the individual's life. Phenylketonuria affects about one in 11,000 people.

Cystic fibrosis

Cystic fibrosis affects about one in 3,000 births in the UK, currently about 7,500 people have the condition. People who have cystic fibrosis have abnormally large amounts of mucus in the lungs. This causes breathing problems and the inability to clear the airways of fluid, resulting in chest infections because micro-organisms get trapped in the lungs. Daily physiotherapy is needed to clear the lungs of mucus.

Individuals with cystic fibrosis inherit it from their parents, who must both be carriers of the condition. Carriers of cystic fibrosis do not show symptoms as they have one 'normal' copy of the gene which is dominant over their other 'defective' copy of the gene. People who inherit cystic fibrosis have two 'defective' copies of the gene, one inherited from each parent.

Down's syndrome

People with Down's syndrome tend to have similar physical characteristics, such as a rounded face with a flat profile and eyes that tend to slant upwards. Children with Down's syndrome learn new skills more slowly than other children and generally develop at a slower rate, meeting their developmental milestones, such as walking or talking, later. Often a child with Down's Syndrome will not start to use language until the age of two or three. With treatment and support, the average life expectancy of someone with Down's syndrome is about 60 years.

The cells of people with Down's syndrome contain an extra chromosome, 47 instead of the usual 46. Their cells have three copies of chromosome 21, instead of the normal two copies. This triple chromosome condition is called trisomy, and it usually arises because chromosome 21 does not separate properly during the formation of the ovum (egg). The ovum therefore has 24 chromosomes instead of the usual 23. This can happen in any woman, but the chance of this occurring increases with the older woman, and so more Down's syndrome babies are born to older mothers. The relationship between the age of a mother and the risk of her child having Down's syndrome is shown in Table 4.5.

Table 4.5 – The effect of the mother's age on the risk of having a Down's syndrome baby

Age of mother	Risk of Down's syndrome
20–29	1:1500
30–34	1:750
35–39	1:600
40–44	1:300
45+	1:60

Down's syndrome may be detected before the baby is born using a technique called amniocentesis. This involves taking a sample of the amniotic fluid by inserting a long, thin, hollow needle through the wall of the mother's abdomen into the uterus. The amniotic fluid contains cells cast off

from the baby. These cells are cultured and their chromosomes examined.

Of the 600 genetic diseases now known, about a third can be detected in this way. Amniocentesis is not without risks – it may result in a miscarriage. However, it is usually offered to older women because of their increased risk of having a baby with Down's syndrome. Chorionic villus sampling is an alternative method to amniocentesis. It involves taking a small sample of the embryonic tissue from the chorion (developing placenta). It can be performed earlier than amniocentesis, but it carries higher risks of miscarriage.

Sickle-cell anaemia

Sickle-cell anaemia is an inherited genetic condition in which there is an abnormality in the haemoglobin, the oxygen-carrying protein found in red blood cells. It is caused by an alteration in a DNA base that leads to the substitution of one of the amino acids that makes up haemoglobin. This alters the structure of the haemoglobin significantly and makes the red blood cells sickle shaped (see Figure 4.9). These cells then cannot pass easily along the capillaries.

Figure 4.9 Normal and sickle red blood cells

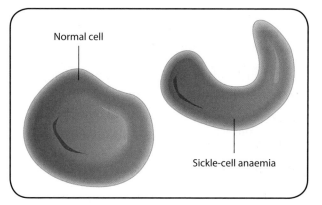

The capillaries of people with sickle-cell anaemia can easily become blocked, preventing oxygen from getting through and causing severe pain and damage to organs. Blockage of a blood vessel causes an attack, known as a crisis. This is most likely to happen when the person is stressed by other illnesses, exhaustion, cold, dehydration and other problems. Organs such as the liver, kidney, lungs, heart and spleen become damaged, causing severe pain. The red blood cells also break up easily, leading to anaemia.

We all have two copies of the haemoglobin gene, one from each parent. Those with sickle-cell anaemia have two genes that create sickle-shaped haemoglobin. Those who have one normal gene and one sickle-cell gene are said to have sickle-cell trait. They are carriers of sickle-cell anaemia and are only at risk of problems under extreme conditions, such as during major surgery.

More than 6000 people in the UK have sickle-cell anaemia. The majority of them are of African or Afro-Caribbean descent. The presence of sickle-cell anaemia in a baby may be tested for during pregnancy, usually using chorionic villus sampling. There is no cure for sickle-cell anaemia, but the frequency and severity of crises and their complications can be reduced by prompt recognition and treatment. Bone marrow transplants have been used in some cases.

Biological factors

Biological factors are defined here as those that affect the foetus in the uterus. Many of these may be caused by the lifestyle of the mother, such as whether she smokes or drinks too much.

Foetal alcohol syndrome

The consumption of alcohol during pregnancy can have devastating effects on the brain of a developing foetus. The alcohol can cross the placenta and may stunt foetal growth or weight and cause permanent damage to the central nervous system. It may also cause the child to have distinctive facial features.

Figure 4.10 A baby with foetal alcohol syndrome

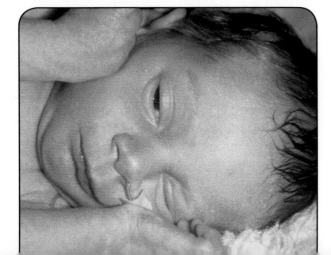

Infections during pregnancy

Infections are a normal part of life. Many infections present no danger to the unborn baby.

Coughs, colds and flu should not cause any harm to the unborn baby. Urinary tract infections should also cause no problems, as long as they are treated early. Vaginal infections, e.g. thrush, caused by the yeast *Candida albicans* are more common in the early months of pregnancy. More serious sexually transmitted diseases, e.g. chlamydia and gonorrhoea infections can be passed to the baby during delivery, causing eye infections. Chickenpox is a viral infection, but is not often contracted as many people have the antibodies against it in their blood. Pregnant women can ask their doctor to test for the presence of these antibodies if they think they may have come into contact with the virus.

Some viruses can cause miscarriage or birth defects in a baby. One of the most significant is rubella (German measles). Birth defects occur in about half of all women who get rubella in the first month of pregnancy. The rate of birth defects drops to 20 per cent in the second month and 10 per cent in the third month. The birth defects caused by rubella include:

- eye defects, such as cataracts, glaucoma and blindness

- deafness

- heart defects

- mental retardation.

The risk of rubella causing birth defects drops dramatically after the first three months of pregnancy. After the twentieth week of pregnancy, there are rarely any complications caused by rubella. Fortunately, rubella is rare today. Many babies are vaccinated against rubella and teenage girls are tested to see if they have antibodies against rubella and, if not, they are vaccinated. Since 1969 almost all teenage girls have been given the rubella vaccine if they had not been vaccinated as babies.

> **Think** Why is it that only teenage girls are tested and vaccinated?

Environmental factors

Water and sanitation

The World Health Organization (WHO) states that drinking water quality is an issue of concern for human health in developing and developed countries worldwide. The risks arise from:

- infectious agents

- toxic chemicals

- radiological hazards.

The levels of contaminants in the UK's drinking water are seldom high enough to cause acute or immediate health effects. Examples of acute health effects include nausea, lung irritation, skin rashes, vomiting, dizziness, and even death.

Most UK water quality standards are based on World Health Organization guidelines. The standards generally include wide safety margins and cover:

- bacteria

- chemicals, such as nitrate and pesticides

- metals, such as lead

- the way that water looks and tastes.

Today most of our drinking water is made safe by the use of chlorine. This is an essential part of the purification process used by water companies to supply our homes and ensure that discharges of waste water to rivers and seas are safe.

CASE STUDY: CHOLERA

In 1854, in the Soho district of London, 600 people died from cholera in just 10 days. At that time there was no known cure for cholera and people started to panic. They believed that 'vapours' were coming from corpses buried in a nearby cemetery, some of whom had died from cholera a century before.

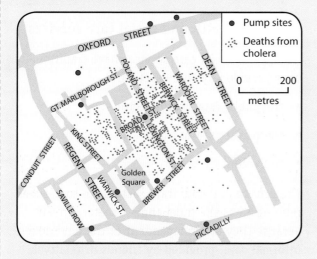

Figure 4.11 Location of the water pumps and the homes of the people who had died from cholera

John Snow, a physician, knew that they would have to identify the source of the disease in order to stop the disease from spreading. He believed that the cause of the cholera was drinking water. At that time, people got their drinking water from pumps in the streets. Snow produced a map showing the location of the pumps and the homes of the people who had died from cholera.

Snow concluded that the pump that was the source of the problem was the one in Broad Street. Can you think how he proved this? He removed the handle of the pump and the number of cases of cholera decreased significantly. Although this does not prove conclusively that the pump contained infected water, it strongly supported the hypothesis that the disease was transmitted by something carried in drinking water and that the infected water came from that pump.

Pollution

The two major forms of pollution are air and water pollution. Air pollution is a cause of health problems worldwide. Urban and rural outdoor environments contain toxicants and irritants that reduce the quality of life and cause disease. The main causes of air pollution are:

- **Smoke** – contains tiny particles of carbon and tar that come from burning coal either in power stations or in the home. The tarry drops contain a chemical that may cause cancer.

- **Sulphur dioxide and nitrogen oxides** – coal and oil contain sulphur, and when these fuels are burned, they release sulphur dioxide into the air. The sulphur dioxide dissolves in rainwater and forms an acid, which creates 'acid rain'. Nitrogen oxides form nitric acid, another form of acid rain. Acid rain can irritate the lungs and skin.

- **Smog** – a thin fog that occurs in cities in certain climate conditions, usually created from a mixture of smoke and fog. Smog is irritating to the eyes and lungs.

- **Carbon monoxide** – is produced when fuels do not burn completely in the engines of cars. It is also present in cigarette smoke. When inhaled, carbon monoxide combines with the haemoglobin in the blood to form carboxyhaemoglobin. This makes the blood less able to carry oxygen.

- **Chlorofluorocarbons** – are used as refrigerants and as propellants in aerosol sprays. They react with the ozone in the atmosphere that protects us from the sun's harmful ultraviolet rays. A reduction in the ozone layer means that we may be more at risk from skin cancer.

> **Think** What is air pollution like where you live? Do you feel that you have suffered from any of the effects of the pollution?

Access to leisure and recreational facilities

Leisure and recreation facilities are provided by city and town councils. Here are some extracts from the websites of two councils in the UK.

Example

Exeter City has a comprehensive selection of sports and leisure facilities. Facilities are provided for use by the public and by clubs including sports centres, running tracks, indoor bowling greens, a petanque terrain, a golf course and a driving range, swimming pools, sports pitches and an artificial turf pitch.

Manchester Leisure is responsible for the city's parks, for sports development and the Parkside Training Centre. In partnership with the City Council, Serco Leisure Manchester manages twelve of the city's indoor facilities.

Manchester has over forty allotments city wide. There are over sixty innovative safe, and exciting play areas spread throughout the city. For older residents and visitors, Manchester Leisure has a comprehensive programme of activities and events.

Leisure facilities are beneficial for the physical development of people at every life stage. They provide opportunities for people to keep fit and help to prevent cardiovascular diseases. They also help people's emotional and social development. Think how much better you feel after exercise or just relaxing in the fresh air. They also provide the opportunity to meet new people or catch up with friends who share the same interests.

Access to health and social care services

Health and social care services have traditionally been provided by three sectors:

- the public (statutory) sector

- the private sector

- the voluntary sector.

The private and voluntary sectors are sometimes referred to as the independent sector. This is because they are independent of the government. Informal care, provided by friends or relatives, is also important to the provision of care. Figure 4.12 summarises the types of care providers. The care system in the UK is what is known as a 'mixed economy of care' because of the different methods of funding that support each of the different care sectors.

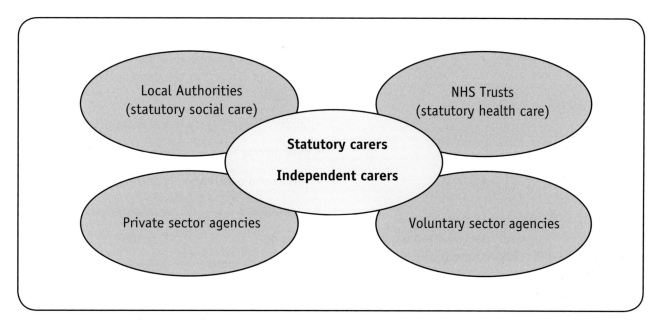

Figure 4.12 Different types of care providers

Think What does the organisation of different types of care providers tell us about the role of the informal carers?

Barriers to accessing health and social care services

Factors that hinder the access of some service users to obtaining health and social care are called barriers to access. Such barriers may result from the way in which a care organisation operates. However, barriers to access can also be the result of factors that are out of the control of a care organisation, such as service users living in a remote part of the country. Figure 4.13 shows some of these barriers.

Example

Mark is a wheelchair user. He has a full-time job. He has recently moved to a new area and wants to make an appointment with a dentist, but doesn't want to take time off work. He lives three miles away from the nearest dental surgery, which has steps at the entrance, and no other means of entry. He contacted the surgery and was told that there were only places for private patients left.

Think What barriers to access has Mark encountered? How might each of these barriers be overcome?

Figure 4.13 Barriers to accessing health and social care services

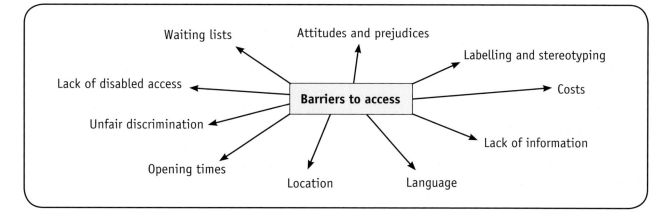

Access to employment and income

Access to employment and income depends on many factors. Some of the most common are:

- qualifications

- language and communication

- emotional

- geographical and physical.

In addition, some people might experience discrimination. The main bases of discrimination are gender, disability and ethnicity. We shall look at discrimination in more detail later in the unit.

Qualifications

The charts in Figure 4.14 show the effect of different types of qualifications on percentage employment rates and gross weekly earnings. These show that there is a clear relationship between higher qualifications and higher earnings. The increased weekly earnings for those possessing a degree are particularly high. The average gross weekly income of full-time employees in the UK with a degree was £632 in spring 2003. This was more than double the weekly income of £298 for those with no qualifications. The likelihood of being employed is also higher for those with higher qualifications.

Figure 4.14 Impact of qualifications on employment and earnings [Source: Office for National Statistics, www.statistics.gov.uk]

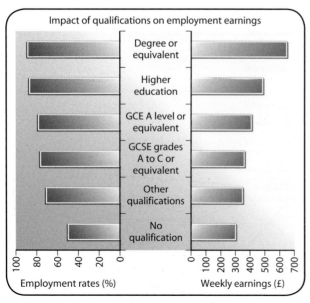

Socio-economic factors

All of the following socio-economic factors can have an impact on the development of an individual:

- family
- peer groups
- values and attitudes
- expenditure
- housing
- culture and belief
- discrimination
- bullying.
- community
- social class
- income
- employment status
- media
- gender
- education

Socio-economic factors stem from the others around us (the social part) and the amount of money we have (the economic part). We shall see that socio-economic factors have a major bearing on all aspects of our development, physical, intellectual, emotional and social, and in all our life stages.

Social class

The main elements that define an individual's social class are their job and their skills. Over the years, there have been changes in the detail of how social class is defined.

> **Think** Why has it been necessary to make changes to how social class is defined?

In 1921 the Registrar General set up a classification of society into five social classes. This classification was modified in 1971 as the status attached to certain jobs had changed.

At the beginning of this century, the classification was further updated to reflect the innovations associated with technological developments and the increased educational attainment of those entering the labour market. The Office for National Statistics' socio-economic classification is now used for all official statistics and surveys. There are eight classes, with the first one being subdivided. This classification is shown in Table 7.1 on page 233.

There are many examples of the link between social class and health. Douglas Black published a report in 1980 called Inequalities in Health. One of the startling discoveries was that 'in 1971 the death rate for adult men in social class V (unskilled workers) was nearly twice that of adult men in social class I (professional workers) even when account has been taken of the different age structure of the two classes'. Donald Acheson published a report in 1998 that traced the roots of ill health to 'such determinants as income, education, housing, pollution, nutrition and employment'.

Figure 4.15 shows the relationship between social class and long-term illness and disability that restricts daily activities. You can see that, among those in employment, people in routine occupations had the worst self-reported health. The percentage of people in this category who also rated their health as 'not good' was more than double that of people in higher managerial and professional occupations.

We shall now look at other factors that affect our development. Many of these are interrelated with social class.

Income, expenditure and employment status

We have seen that social class is determined mainly by the type of job someone has. The income we receive depends on the job we do, but is it always the case that income reflects the class of the occupation? For example, it is quite possible that a teacher in group 2 of the National Statistics socio-economic classification would earn less than a self-employed builder in group 4.

> **Think** Can you think of any other examples where someone in a lower occupation group might earn more than someone in a higher occupation group?

If someone has a higher income, you might imagine that they have more money to spend. However, this might not always be the case. Think of a man who has left his wife and family and now has a new partner and family. He will have a high expenditure because he has two families to support.

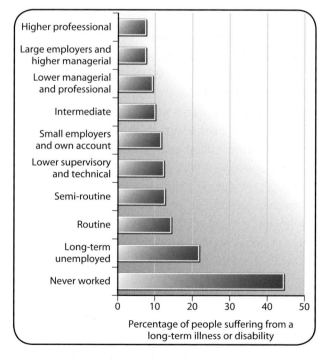

Figure 4.15 Age-standardised rates of long-term illness or disability that restricts daily activities [Source: 2001 Census of England and Wales. Office for National Statistics. www.statistics.gov.uk]

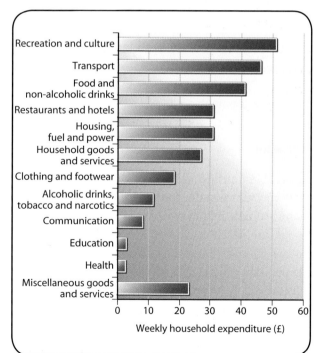

Figure 4.16 Weekly household expenditure, Wales, 2001/2 [Source: Office for National Statistics. 2001/2. www.statistics.gov.uk]

What do people actually spend their money on? Figure 4.17 shows the weekly household expenditure in 2001/2002 in Wales. You can see that the largest item of average weekly household expenditure in Wales was recreation and culture (£51) followed by transport (£46) then food and non-alcoholic drinks (£41).

> **Think** Which areas of an individual's development will benefit from a high proportion of money being spent on recreation and culture?

Unemployment in the UK fell from a peak of three million in 1993 (just under 11 per cent of the working age population) to 1.5 million (around 5 per cent) in 2001. Since then there has been a further and more gradual decline. Long-term unemployment can have detrimental effects on all areas of development. It will mean less money and thus reduced household expenditure. If expenditure is not reduced, then there may be increased financial debt. Less money could lead to buying cheaper, less nutritious food. This could impact on health, for example increasing levels of obesity. It could mean less money to spend on recreation and leisure, but it could also mean more time to take forms of exercise, like walking, that do not cost money. Being unemployed can mean less social contact, with less opportunity to participate in shared activities with others. This may have a detrimental effect on emotional and social development.

Housing

Affordable housing was one of the aims of the modern welfare state, founded in 1945. There are many studies linking poor housing conditions to premature death or chronic illness. For example, houses that are damp may cause asthma and make people likely to get infections. Cramped conditions may adversely affect a person's emotional development as they have no time to themselves. Living in such close proximity to others may result in more disagreements. However, it could be said that members of a family may benefit from being together more. What do you think?

Education

The level of education of individuals can affect the type of job they get and the amount of money they have to spend. Knowledge about issues such as eating healthily, the importance of exercise and the problems caused by smoking, all of which can result from education, can benefit a person's physical development.

The more education a person has, either formally or informally, benefits their intellectual development. Older people who keep their minds active, for example by doing crosswords, are likely to improve their memories. Education can make a person more confident, leading to higher self-esteem. People meet other like-minded people when they attend evening classes, thus broadening their social development.

> **Think** Can you think of any ways in which education may adversely affect a person's development?

Family, community, peer groups, media, values and attitudes

Our development is affected greatly by those around us. Our first socialisation is with our family. Secondary socialisation takes place with people in the community outside the family, such as friends, teachers and workmates. Our friends are part of our peer group, a group of people who share certain common characteristics, such as age. Peer groups have a very important influence on development during childhood and adolescence, more than parents or immediate family. An adolescent's social attitudes and values, their ways of behaving and sense of self-worth are significantly affected by the expectations their peer group have. Albert Bandura stressed the importance of peer pressure and role models on shaping behaviour.

The media can also affect our views, through advertising, documentaries and even TV soaps. Storylines in programmes such as Coronation Street and EastEnders show how many socio-economic factors affect the lives of the characters.

Discrimination, culture and beliefs, gender and bullying

People living in the UK are entitled to enjoy life free from discrimination on the grounds of race (culture and beliefs), gender, sexual orientation, disability and age, and there is legislation in place to support this. Discrimination occurs when a person or group of people is treated differently to others. Prejudice is the main cause of discrimination. This is a dislike towards another person or group of people, usually based on inaccurate information or unreasonable judgements.

Racism is the belief that one ethnic group is superior to another. In the UK it mainly affects the emotional development of members of black and minority ethnic groups. Gender discrimination arises if a woman receives lower pay for doing the same or equivalent job as a man. Bullying can have a very detrimental effect on a person's emotional development. It can take many forms from physical to mental. It can also differ in its severity.

> **Think** Look back at a time when people were not nice to you. Did you think of it as bullying? What did you do about it? Did anyone help you?

Lifestyle factors

Lifestyle factors are those over which we have some degree of control. By adopting a 'good' lifestyle people can increase their chances of being healthy and living longer. A healthy lifestyle impacts positively on emotional and social development. Learning about healthy lifestyles also has a positive effect on intellectual development.

CASE STUDY: SOCIO-ECONOMIC INFLUENCES

Richard and Ian are both 20 years old. They both play football for the same local team. That is where the similarity ends. Richard's father left home when he was very young and, following this, his mother became an alcoholic. They lived in a very small flat near the industrial estate. Richard is an only child and was bullied at school because his clothes were old and dirty. His school years were very unhappy and he did not gain many qualifications. He tried to make friends, but it was always with people who got into trouble for misbehaving. He never had enough to eat because his mother was unable to find a job. Richard now has a low-paid job as a cleaner, but he hopes to go to college to train as a mechanic.

Ian's life has been easier. His father is a doctor, originally from India, and his mother is a teacher. They live in a detached house with a large garden on the edge of the town. He has two brothers and one sister. They have always enjoyed doing things as a family. Richard did well at school and is now at university, studying engineering. He was popular at school and had many friends. He hopes to work abroad when he finishes university.

QUESTION

1. What socio-economic factors have affected Richard and Ian?

2. For each of the socio-economic factors you have identified, decide how it has affected Richard and Ian's physical, intellectual, emotional and social development.

3. Which of the socio-economic factors has had the most influence on the difference between Richard and Ian's emotional development?

Nutrition and dietary choices

There are particular aspects of nutrition and diet that are important for certain areas of personal development. You have already seen, for example, that the lack of a particular enzyme to break down one amino acid in food results in phenylketoneuria, a condition that can result in brain damage.

The food we eat provides our bodies with the energy to carry out chemical reactions that enable us to move, and for cells to build and repair themselves. Our diets need to be balanced. They should contain the correct proportions of carbohydrates, fats and proteins, as well as vitamins, minerals and fibre. The proportion that we need of these different types of food changes depending on which life stage we are in. Some examples of the effect of nutrition and diet include:

- poor maternal nutrition is linked to low birth weight in babies

- adequate levels of vitamins, particularly folic acid, are important in the diet of pregnant woman for normal embryonic development

- calcium and vitamin D are important for the healthy growth of bones

- diets that contain plenty of fibre are linked to reduced incidence of cancer, diabetes and cardiovascular disease

- high salt intake can lead to high blood pressure

- additional iron helps avoid anaemia due to menstruation.

> **Think** Which life stages and which area of development do each of these statements apply to?

Exercise

Exercise is good for you because it increases stamina and muscle strength, and has a positive effect on physical growth and development. Any form of exercise that raises the heart rate by at least one-third of its normal value is beneficial for the cardiovascular system and reduces the chance of developing heart disease. The type of exercise people do as they get older changes. Brisk walking is a very good form of exercise, particularly for older people who are unable to take part in sports.

Exercise may also affect other areas of development positively:

- intellectually: stimulates thinking and encourages planning skills

- emotionally: increases confidence and self-esteem

- socially: provides a way of meeting others and develops co-operation and team work.

> **Think** What specific examples can you think of for each of the benefits listed?

Stress

Stress is the inability to cope with everyday life. When people are stressed adrenaline is released in their bodies at an inappropriate time. Adrenaline is the 'fight or flight' hormone which, among other things, makes the heart beat faster so that we can exercise. Stress can affect the way in which we relate to other people. It can also make us feel ill and make our immune system less effective, making us more likely to catch illnesses, such as colds and flu. Some might argue that stress is always bad, but others would say that stress is a normal part of living and that we should only be concerned when it becomes excessive. Some people work better when they are under a little bit of stress.

> **Think** Think of a time when you felt under stress. What did you feel like? What caused you to feel the way you did? What did you do to make the symptoms of stress easier?

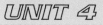

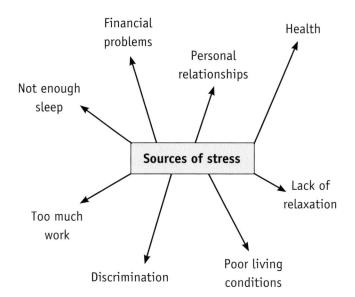

Figure 4.17 Some sources of stress

> ***Think*** Whichs area of development are affected by each of the sources of stress?

Substance abuse

The Mental Health Foundation defines substance abuse as '*the continual misuse of any mind altering substance which severely interferes with an individual's physical and mental health, social situation and responsibilities.*' We will consider three common instances of substance abuse: smoking, alcohol and drugs.

Smoking

Many lung diseases are linked to smoking, including lung cancer, bronchitis and emphysema. The tar in tobacco can cause cancer, and the hot gases in the smoke destroy the cilia (hairs) on the cells that line the respiratory passages. This means that dust particles and bacteria, which are normally trapped and removed, find their way into the lungs.

Smoking rates have declined across all age groups in the last 50 years, with the largest decrease amongst people aged 50 and over. People in their early twenties have the highest rates compared with other age groups.

Alcohol

Alcohol is misused when a person consumes excessive amounts or becomes dependent on it. There are many health risks associated with drinking more than the recommended maximum amount of alcohol: 14 units for a woman per week and 21 units for a man per week.

There is a culture of 'binge' drinking among some teenagers and young people, which involves drinking excessive amounts of alcohol, especially at weekends. Alcohol consumption for teenage boys has declined slightly since 2000, whereas the alcohol consumption of teenage girls is still increasing.

Drugs

The most commonly misused illegal drugs are:

- amphetamines (commonly known as 'speed' or 'whizz')

- cocaine (commonly known as 'crack')

- MDMA (commonly known as 'ecstasy')

All of these drugs are class A drugs, although if amphetamines are taken by mouth, instead of being injected, they are deemed to be a class B drug. Illegal drugs in the UK are classified into three groups, A, B and C. Class A drugs are treated by the law as the most dangerous. Table 4.7 shows the penalties under the Misuse of Drugs Act for possessing and supplying drugs.

Table 4.6 – Maximum penalties under the Misuse of Drugs Act

Drug class	Possession	Supply
Class A	7 years + fine	Life + fine
Class B	5 years + fine	14 years + fine
Class C	2 years + fine	14 years + fine

Drug misuse leads to potentially fatal physical illnesses. There is also a danger of infection caused by sharing hypodermic needles. It also leads to psychological and social problems. In some cases, people turn to crime to pay for their drug habits.

MAJOR LIFE EVENTS

Major life events fall into two categories: predictable and unpredictable. However, what may be predictable for some people might be unpredictable for others. The following classification takes the most common view.

Predictable life events include:

- starting school or nursey

- employment

- leaving home

- marriage

- parenthood

- retirement

- ageing.

Unpredictable life events include:

- birth of a sibling

- moving house

- redundancy

- serious injury

- divorce

- bereavement

- abuse.

> **Think** What areas of development might be adversely affected by the birth of a new sibling? In what ways might the birth of a new sibling have a positive effect on the social development of an older sibling?

Rather than look at each of the life events in turn, we will consider a series of case studies that illustrate the combined effects of different life events.

CASE STUDY: GURDEEP AND IMOGEN

Gurdeep and Imogen are both 26 years old. They have a five-year-old daughter, who has just started school, and a two-month-old son. Both parents have a healthy lifestyle. They eat sensibly, go to the gym twice a week and used to cycle most weekends before the children were born. Three years ago, Gurdeep was knocked off his bike by a car and broke his leg badly in several places. He was off work for six months, but has now returned to work full time. He has worked hard to get fit again, with Imogen's support, but he knows that he might not be able to ride a bike again. Gurdeep's grandmother lives nearby. She is 76 years old and she also has a healthy lifestyle. Although her arthritis gets worse as she gets older, she tries to be as active as she can. She swims once a week and walks to the local shops to buy fresh vegetables most days. She cares for her husband who has had a series of heart attacks since he retired ten years ago. She is worried that her husband might die soon, just like her brother who died last year. She is glad that Gurdeep and Imogen lead a healthy lifestyle as she blames her husband's heart attacks on the fact that he smoked.

QUESTIONS

1. What are the predictable and unpredictable events illustrated in this case study?

2. Describe and explain how each of the unpredictable events could have both a positive and negative impact on a person's emotional development.

3. Exercise is a lifestyle factor that is usually beneficial for all areas of development, yet in Gurdeep's case it could be argued that it had a negative effect as he was injured while excercising. What are the positive and negative effects of the other lifestyle factors in this case study?

CASE STUDY: JOE AND TRACEY

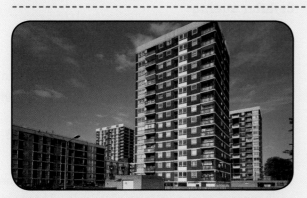

Joe is 14 years old. He lives with his mother, Tracey, in a block of flats on the outskirts of a large city. Joe's parents are divorced. Joe is glad because his father was abusing him and threatened to cause him serious injury if he told anyone. Joe knew that most people don't leave home until their late teens or early twenties. However, he was so unhappy that he wanted to run away there and then.

Joe and Tracey have just moved into a block of flats and do not know anyone well. Joe hangs around with some unemployed youths who are older than him and who drink alcohol and take drugs. Joe sometimes plays truant from school to spend more time with them and Tracey is worried that he will end up just like them. Tracey works as a cleaner in Joe's school and has asked the head teacher if there is anything the school can do to help.

To leave home when you are a young adult is considered to be a predictable event. In this case study, the fact that Joe was considering leaving home earlier was an unpredictable event. It was a consequence of being abused by his father. Abuse can affect a person's emotional development, through the unhappiness that it causes. It may also affect a person's social development as someone who has been abused may find it difficult to form relationships in the future.

Another unpredictable event in this case study is moving house. This could affect a person's emotional development in both a positive and negative way. Joe and Tracey do not know anyone in their new area well. This could mean that they do not interact easily with other people. Joe's social relationship with the unemployed youths, could have a negative effect on his physical development if he starts to take drugs. It will not help his intellectual development if he plays truant from school as it will decrease his chances of gaining qualifications. This will have a knock-on effect on his chances of getting a fulfilling, well-paid job. Many of the life factors and life events that affect people are interrelated and hard to separate.

EVIDENCE ACTIVITY

P2 – P3 – M1 – M2 – D1

Create a PowerPoint presentation about a person you know well, that explores the influence of life factors and events on that individual.

1. Describe the potential influences of five life factors on their development. Explore one life factor from each of the groups covered in this unit: genetic, biological, environmental, socio-economic and lifestyle. (P2)

2. For each of the factors, identify whether it is a 'nature' or 'nurture' factor. Include some slides in your presentation that discuss the nature-nurture debate in relation to the individual you have chosen. (M1)

3. Consider the relative importance of each of the factors on the individual. Write a conclusion about whether nature or nurture has had the most influence on their development. (D1)

4. Describe the influences of two predictable and two unpredictable major life events on the development of the individual. (P3)

5. Explain how these major life events may have influenced the development of the individual. (M2)

4.3 *Understanding physical changes and psychological perspectives in relation to ageing*

THEORIES OF AGEING

Ageing does not begin at a particular age. People age throughout their lives, and so it is not only those in older adulthood or the final stages of life who experience ageing. People do not age in a fixed way as they are constantly changing in individual and different ways. Many of these changes are in response to external events. For example, an arthritic joint in later life might be the result of a much earlier sports injury, rather than the natural ageing process.

> **Think** Can you think of two people who are the same age, but who don't look the same age? Can you suggest an explanation for this?

For most people, death occurs because the body wears out rather than because of accidents and disease. Some current theories of ageing support the view that life expectancy in developed countries is unlikely to increase much beyond the present level. For example, some suggest that certain human cells are programmed for only a limited number of divisions. Other scientists believe that in the not too distant future people might expect live to the age of 200.

Theories of ageing fall into two main categories:

- biological theories, for example cellular ageing and evolutionary ageing
- psychosocial theories, for example activity theory and disengagement theory.

There are a huge number of different theories of ageing, probably over 300. Most of the theories are not exclusive, but overlap, so it is possible to believe in more than one.

Biological theories of ageing

Cellular ageing

Some of our cells are frequently renewed, such as skin cells; others, including nerve cells, are long lived. This means that the concept of an 'old' human cell does not always correlate with the age of the cell. In a matter of days a short-lived cell shows the same signs of ageing as will ultimately appear in a long-lived cell years later.

Irrespective of the type of cell, there are a number of changes that characterise older cells. These are:

- the appearance of a protein, lipofuscin, which slows down cellular processes
- an increase in a cell organelles called lysosomes, which contain enzymes that break down the cells
- an increased number of abnormal chromosomes, because of damaged DNA.

These changes contribute to cell death.

Many beauty products would lead us to believe that we can slow down the ageing of the skin. You might find it interesting to investigate this further. One of the reasons that it is important to eat healthy food, including lots of fruit and vegetables, is that these contain antioxidants that protect our cells against oxidants that can damage our DNA. There are also claims that red wine, drunk in moderation, has beneficial effects on the ageing of skin, although many disagree with this. Health and social care providers can ensure that service users look after their skin properly and are given plenty of fresh fruit and vegetables.

> **Think** What advice would you give to a service user who did not want to eat fruit and vegetables? If you were manager of a residential home for older people, how would you go about educating your staff on the importance of good care for the physical development of the service users?

Evolutionary theory of ageing

Humans are one of the few species that live long enough to show signs of ageing. Some of the changes that we display when we age are not particularly pleasant, such as decreased mobility or poorer eyesight.

We might ask why natural selection has not resulted in a greater proportion of the population being free from the changes that ageing causes, if they are not to our advantage. The theory of evolution predicts that individuals who are less well adapted would leave fewer surviving offspring. However, the unpleasant changes that ageing causes occur after we have passed on our genes to our children. In terms of continuing our species, it does not matter what happens after we have had children, so evolution does not slow down the ageing process. For women, giving birth and feeding babies involves considerable physiological stress, and giving birth can result in death. By preventing further reproduction, menopause removes the associated risks.

In summary, there are no known advantages of ageing. It is not an adaptive process that has evolved by natural selection. However, without menopause, the last born babies would not have their mothers around for long. Menopause also allows women a time when they can offer their caring skills to close relatives. Health and social care provision should recognise this important role that older people have in life. It is important that a service user should have as much access as possible to other members of their family and that they should be respected for their experience and wisdom.

> **Think** How would you respond to a service user who says, 'I don't matter anymore. I can live on through my children'?

Psychosocial theories of ageing

Here we shall look briefly at two theories: the activity theory and the disengagement theory. There are also many other theories, including the life-course theory, put forward by Eric Erikson.

This views ageing as a process, where at each life stage the person faces a crisis or dilemma that must be resolved to move on to the next stage. Another theory is the continuity theory, which states that older adults try to use strategies that allow them to adapt to their ageing, by considering past experiences in setting goals for the future. We shall see that this has some similarities with the activity theory.

Activity theory of ageing

This theory was first put forward by Havinghurst in 1963. It argues that older people need to be kept active and integrated into society so that society as a whole functions well. The theory emphasises the importance of ongoing social activity. It also suggests that a person's self-concept is related to the roles held by that person, so after retiring it is important for people to have other roles, such as volunteer and community roles. This is a positive view of ageing that argues that well being in old age is achieved by older people refusing to accept the limitations imposed upon them.

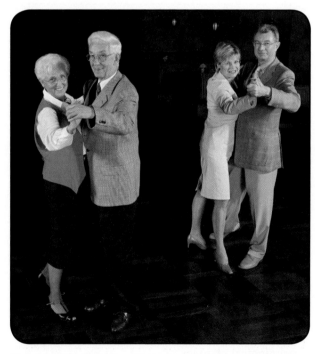

Figure 4.18 Social activity helps older people stay part of the community

> **Think** Which areas of development of these older people shown in Figure 4.19 are being affected by walking?

Others argue that the activity theory is unrealistic for older people, because the structure of society prevents many older people from maintaining any major activity in later life, making them dependent. Many health-care settings, however, encourage the activity theory by providing activities such as bingo, communal singing and excursions.

Disengagement theory

The disengagement theory was put forward by Cumming and Henry in 1961 and suggests that older people voluntarily withdraw from society in preparation for death, and that this is necessary for society to continue to function. In some ways, the theory is positive, in that it sees old age as a time of serene preparation for death, with the older person adjusting to the losses of old age. The older person contentedly pursues solitary, passive activities. Many people think that this is an outdated theory. However, it could be argued that many older people do not want to be forced into social activities and should be allowed the option of disengagement.

> **Think** Imagine you are a care worker in a residential home for older people. Another care worker tries to persuade a reluctant service user to take part in a bingo session. What explanation would you give to that care worker, for why the service user should be exempt from participating?

PUBERTY AND THE MENOPAUSE

Hormonal control

Before considering physical and psychological changes in the body, we will look at hormonal control, which has a particularly important role in the changes that occur during puberty and the menopause. They impact on both physical and psychological changes.

Puberty

The male and female sex organs are known as the primary sex characteristics. During early adolescence changes happen to boys and girls that lead to sexual maturity. These changes are controlled by hormones, and the time when they happen is called puberty. Puberty involves two key developments: the production of sex cells in boys and the adaptation of the bodies of both sexes to allow reproduction to take place. These events are triggered by hormones released by the pituitary gland called follicle-stimulating hormone (FSH) and luteinising hormone (LH).

You may have heard of these hormones in connection with the menstrual cycle, but they also play a part in the development of male secondary characteristics. In males, FSH stimulates sperm production. LH controls the secretion of the male sex hormone testosterone from the testes. Testosterone controls the development of the male secondary sexual characteristics. In females, FSH and LH control the release of a female sex hormone called oestrogen from the ovaries. Oestrogen produces the female secondary sex characteristics.

Table 4.7 – Male and female secondary sex characteristics

Male	Female
sperm production starts	menstruation starts
growth and development of male sexual organs	growth and development of female sexual organs
increase in body mass, especially chest and shoulders	increase in body mass, development of rounder shape (hips)
growth of body hair under the arms, in the pubic area and on the face	growth of body hair under the arms and in the pubic area
voice breaks	breasts develop

> **Think** Which secondary characteristics are common to both male and female? Which are peculiar to each sex?

The menopause

The word menopause literally means 'the end of menstruation'. It is a natural part of the ageing process. Every woman who has periods will go through the menopause, usually between the ages of 42 and 58. The menopause occurs when a woman's reproductive cycle stops. This period is marked by decreased levels of oestrogen and progesterone, and increased levels of FSH and LH. The changing hormone levels are responsible for the symptoms associated with menopause; for example, the 'hot flushes' that many women experience. The fall in oestrogen levels in particular can have long-term health effects e.g. osteoporosis, heart disease and increased blood pressure.

Some women receive hormone replacement therapy (HRT). Oestrogen is not usually taken alone as it increases the risk of cancer in the lining of the uterus. A combination of oestrogen and progesterone is taken, although this causes bleeding every month.

PHYSICAL CHANGES

There are many age-associated physical changes in the body. The ones we shall consider here are in the:

- cardiovascular system: atherosclerosis and coronary heart disease

- respiratory system: asthma, emphysema, chronic obstructive pulmonary disease

- nervous system: degeneration of sense organs, motor neurone disease and cognitive changes

- musculo-skeletal system: muscle thinning, arthritis and decline in mobility

- skin: loss of elasticity.

Cardiovascular system

The cardiovascular system consists of the heart and blood vessels. Cardiovascular ageing is a continuous and irreversible process. Heart disease is the most common cause of death in elderly people. The coronary arteries on the outside of the heart can narrow due to atherosclerosis, the building up of fatty plaques in the lining of the arteries (see Figure 4.19).

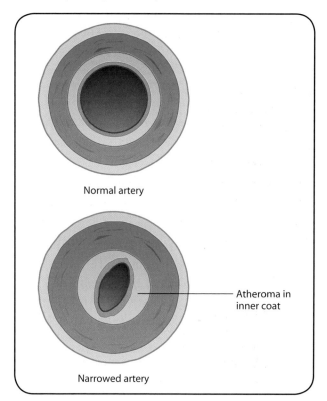

Normal artery

Atheroma in inner coat

Narrowed artery

Figure 4.19 Comparison of a normal artery and one with atherosclerosis

You can see that the space inside the artery, the lumen, is reduced in size where there are atheroma present. You may also notice that the inner surface is rough. This may cause the body to think it is damaged, leading to the formation of blood clots which will block the flow of blood. If this happens in the coronary arteries supplying the heart muscle with blood, then a heart attack will occur as the muscle cells cannot function without food and oxygen.

Think What advice about lifestyle would you give to someone who has heart disease?

Respiratory system

The respiratory system includes the lungs and airways. As people get older their vital capacity decreases. This is the maximum amount of air you can breathe out following a large breath in. This is because the diaphragm muscles and intercostal muscles (between the ribs) become less strong. Asthma is caused by a narrowing of the airways, often aggravated by air pollution, and can be present in any life stage. The occurrence of asthma in people over 65 is increasing, often affecting former smokers. Chronic obstructive pulmonary disease (COPD) includes chronic bronchitis and emphysema, and has recently been defined as non-reversible lung function impairment. The World Health Organization estimates that COPD is the fourth leading cause of death worldwide. The main cause is smoking and the UK is now experiencing a growth in this, as a generation that had a high rate of smoking reach old age.

A person with emphysema will have decreased gas exchange in their alveoli (air sacs). Figure 4.2 shows the effects of emphysema on the alveoli. You can see how the walls of the alveolus of someone with emphysema have been broken down. This means that less gas exchange will occur.

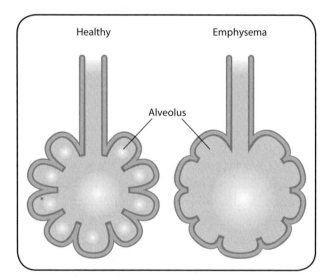

Figure 4.20 Effects of emphysema on the alveoli

> ***Think*** How will a decreased amount of oxygen entering the blood affect a person's ability to exercise?

Nervous system

Many older people experience memory loss. Neurones (nerve cells) are not able to replicate, so cannot be replaced if they die. The brain contains billions of cells, so even though estimated cell loss is about 100,000 neurones a day in adult life, it is a very small proportion of the total. A person with Parkinson's Disease has a high loss of neurones in a particular area of the brain, resulting in shaking, loss of fine motor skills and loss of precision in walking. Symptoms may be controlled to some extent with drugs.

Our sense organs deteriorate as we get older and some changes may occur in middle adulthood, e.g. it becomes much more difficult to read small print. This is because the ciliary muscles that control the shape of the lens in the eye do not work as well. This can be corrected with spectacles. Some people develop cataracts, which is a clouding of the cornea that may be corrected with an operation. Hearing may deteriorate, especially at high frequencies – hearing aids can help this.

Motor neurone disease can affect any adult, but significantly increases in people over 65. It affects the nerve cells in the brain and spinal cord which control our ability to walk and talk. Degeneration of these motor neurones leads to weakness and wasting of muscles, often initially in the arms or legs. Some people develop weakness and wasting in the muscles of the face and throat, causing problems with speech, chewing and swallowing.

Musculo-skeletal system

Creaking joints, aching bones and stiff muscles often affect older people. This may result in a loss of mobility. There is evidence that people lose up to 30 per cent of muscle fibres between the ages of 30 and 80, and there is often a loss of motor neurones at the same time. Studies suggest that both types of cells die if they are not used, so exercise can help to reduce this loss.

Age-associated changes in the bones can pose a serious threat to health, especially in women. Osteoporosis occurs when the level of bone mass falls below a critical point, resulting in an increased risk of fractures. The use of HRT can decrease the risk of osteoporosis occurring.

CASE STUDY: AGNES AND MARION

Agnes is 86 years old and lives in a one-bedroom bungalow in a complex for older people. She cannot walk far, although she goes out occasionally in the minibus. Her hands tremble and she sometimes spills things. This is a source of great embarrassment for her so she avoids seeing people.

Most of all she complains of tiredness. She makes herself do household chores, but it always takes it out of her. Agnes has felt under a lot of stress for a long time. Most of this was due to an unhappy marriage. Following the death of her husband, she had to work night shifts in a factory to make ends meet.

Agnes' friend Marion is 89 years old and in good health. She owns her own house and does all her own shopping, cooking and cleaning. She still walks a lot with friends and swims once a week. Her hearing is not good and she has a hearing aid. She had bad eyesight, but since her cataract operation her confidence in using her computer has been restored. Her only complaint at the moment is itchy skin, but she says she is lucky that this is all that bothers her.

For her, health is about being able to carry on with her usual activities. She attributes her own good health to her upbringing. She was a schoolteacher and enjoyed working with children. She never married and says that she would probably have been too independent. She clearly takes charge of her life.

Agnes has a negative perspective on retirement. Marion, on the other hand, has a positive outlook on her retirement.

Skin

The condition of someone's skin is one of the ways that we can tell their age. Collagen in the skin loses its elasticity as we age. The appearance of ageing skin has become associated with unattractiveness by some people. This can have harmful effects on their sense of well-being.

PSYCHOLOGICAL CHANGES

The psychological changes that happen as people age can affect their confidence and self-esteem. There are both positive and negative perspectives on the changes that occur.

Table 4.8 – Perspectives on changes due to ageing

Positive perspectives	Negative perspectives
effects of retirement	effects of retirement
role changes	role changes
learning for pleasure	loss of partner and peers
leisure pursuits	financial concerns
culture variations	ageism

EVIDENCE ACTIVITY

P4 – P5 – M3 – D2

Use the case study about Agnes and Marion to help you complete the following activities.

1. Choose two theories of ageing. Use five key ideas of each theory to write a description of the theory. (P4)

2. Describe the physical and psychological changes that have occurred to Agnes and to Marion due to the ageing process. (P5)

3. Compare the two theories you have chosen by explaining how well each of them relates to the case of Agnes and of Marion. (M3)

4. You have been asked to recommend care services for both Agnes and Marion. What services would you recommend for each of them? Explain your choices, based on the theory of ageing that best applies to each of them. (D2)

Fundamentals of Anatomy and Physiology for Health and Social Care

unit 5

If you are going to work in any sector of health or social care, it is important that you understand the fundamental aspects of the anatomy and physiology of human body systems. You are likely to encounter people with health problems, so having a good knowledge of the structure of the body and how it works will help you better understand the care they might need.

The human body consists of cells, tissues and organs, and is made up of several different systems. It is important that you develop a detailed knowledge of these and how they are involved in energy metabolism. To ensure the maintenance of good health, the body systems need to be controlled and work together efficiently. You will find out how to take measurements that give indicators of how well the body systems are working and to investigate normal responses to routine variations in body functioning.

Learning outcomes

By the end of this unit you will:

5.1 Understand the organisation of the human body — page 153

5.2 Understand the functioning of the body systems associated with energy metabolism — page 162

5.3 Understand how homeostatic mechanisms operate in the maintenance of an internal environment — page 179

5.4 Be able to interpret data obtained from monitoring routine variations in the functioning of healthy body systems — page 189

So, you want to be a...

Nurse

My name Simon Petrov

Age 24

Income £ 19,000

If you are a patient and caring individual who wants a job that directly improves the day-to-day lives of others, nursing is the job for you...

What job do you do?

I'm a nurse. I've only recently qualified and I'm working in my local hospital.

Have you always wanted to be a nurse?

I wasn't very sure what I wanted to do when I was at school, but I'd always enjoyed looking after people and helped to look after my grandma when she became ill. It was one of the personal advisers from Connexions who asked me to think about nursing.

What qualification did you need?

I didn't enjoy school very much but I went on to college and I did a BTEC in Health and Social Care as it appeared to be more practical than a lot of my GCSE subjects. From there I did a diploma in nursing at university. There's a diploma and a degree course; I decided to do the diploma.

What was your training like?

It was three years, full-time, and it was done partly through lectures and partly on placement in local hospitals and health centres. It's about 50:50, theory and practice. A good mix really. And I got an NHS bursary while I was training. That helped me financially.

I think all the training courses in nursing have a Common Foundation Programme in the first year. That introduces us to the basic principles of nursing,

> **❝ I'd always enjoyed looking after people ❞**

and then you specialise for the rest of the course in one of four areas: adult nursing (that's what I did), children's nursing, mental health of learning disabilities.

Did you have to know a lot about biology?

It helps! It wasn't my favourite subject at school but it's a lot easier to learn when you're using the knowledge to help people become well. It's more important in some areas of nursing than others I suppose.

Why did you choose to do adult nursing?

There is a huge range of work in adult nursing, and I wanted to keep my options open. For example, you can work in a specialist area such as accident and emergency, care of the elderly, cancer care, women's health, practice nursing, etc. You can also work in different settings, for example in a hospital, in the community or in the armed services; you might be able to work abroad, and you can even work on cruise ships!

Where can you get more advice on careers in nursing?

The NHS has a really good website and anyone interested in working in the NHS can find out about jobs there. It gives you great career information, and there are lots and lots of jobs advertise there. That's where I found my job. Just go to: www.nhscareers.nhs.uk

Grading criteria

The table below shows what you need to do to gain a pass, merit or distinction in this part of the qualification. Make sure you refer back to it when you are completing work so you can judge whether you are meeting the criteria and what you need to do to fill in gaps in your knowledge or experience.

In this unit there are 3 evidence activities that give you an opportunity to demonstrate your achievement of the grading criteria:

page 179   P4, M1, D1

page 189   P5, M2, D2

page 193   P6, M3

Please note that there are no evidence activities for P1, P2 and P3. The systems, structures and functions referred to in these pass grades are all clearly detailed in the text and therefore a reading and understanding of the unit will provide adequate opportunity to practice your achivement.

To achieve a pass grade the evidence must show that the learner is able to...	To achieve a merit grade the evidence must show that, in addition to the pass criteria, the learner is able to...	To achieve a distinction grade the evidence must show that, in addition to the pass and merit criteria, the learner is able to...
P1 describe the functions of the main cell components		
P2 describe the structure of the main tissues of the body and their role in the functioning of two named body organs		
P3 describe the gross structure and main functions of all major body systems		
P4 describe the role of energy in the body and the physiology of three named body systems in relation to energy metabolism	M1 explain the physiology of three named body systems in relation to energy metabolism	D1 use examples to explain how body systems interrelate to each other
P5 describe the concept of homeostasis and the homeostatic mechanisms that regulate heart rate, breathing rate, body temperature and blood glucose levels	M2 explain the probable homeostatic responses to changes in the internal environment during exercise	D2 explain the importance of homeostasis in maintaining the healthy functioning of the body
P6 measure body temperature, heart rate and breathing rate before and after a standard period of exercise, interpret the data and comment on its validity	M3 analyse data obtained to show how homeostatic mechanisms control the internal environment during exercise	

5.1 *Organisation of the human body – overview*

INTRODUCTION

If you ask most people how the body is organised, they will probably say things like, 'we have a heart and lungs and a digestive system ...' Indeed, they may give you a long list of the different parts of the body, but they may not know how these relate to each other. Most people have a rough idea of how their bodies function, but if you are going to work in the health and social care sector you should have a clear understanding of the structure of the body and how it works. Anatomy refers to the structure of the body and physiology refers to how the structures work. To clearly understand how the body functions, we need to know how the different structures are organised to work together. It is important to have an overview of the organisation of the human body before we learn any detail.

OVERVIEW OF CELLS, TISSUES, ORGANS, SYSTEMS

All living organisms are made of small units called **cells**. These may be seen fairly easily using a light microscope. You will learn the names and functions of the different parts of cells.

There are some very small, microscopic organisms which consist of only one cell. They are able to carry out all the processes necessary for them to survive. Most living organisms, like us, are multicellular. However, in order for us to survive, our cells must be grouped together and work closely with each other. There must also be mechanisms for cells to communicate with each other. **Tissues** are groups of similar cells with similar functions. **Organs** consist of several different tissues grouped together to make a special structure which has a specific function. **Systems** are special groups of organs whose functions are closely related.

One of the simplest tissues is **epithelial tissue**. This consists of a sheet of cells which fit neatly together. This type of tissue forms the lining in many parts of our body. One of its main functions is to protect the structures beneath it. (Later we shall see that there are many different types of epithelial tissue.) Another very common tissue is **non-striated** or **smooth muscle**, which is found surrounding internal organs such as the alimentary canal or blood vessels where movement is required.

Tissues may be combined together to form organs – structures that have a specific job to do. The diagram below shows how epithelial tissue and non-striated/smooth muscle tissues combine to form part of the wall of the gut.

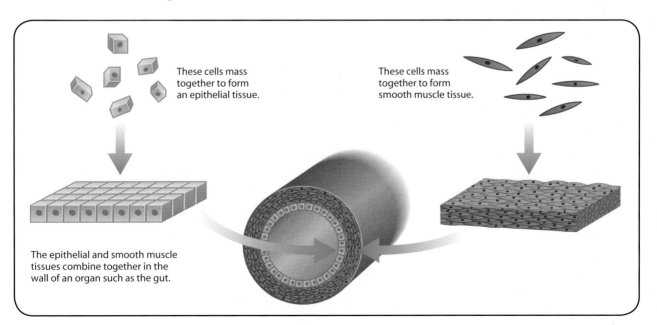

These cells mass together to form an epithelial tissue.

These cells mass together to form smooth muscle tissue.

The epithelial and smooth muscle tissues combine together in the wall of an organ such as the gut.

Figure 5.1 How cells form tissues and organs

In the body certain jobs are carried out by several organs working together. An example is the **digestive system**, which consists of the stomach and intestines, along with the oesophagus, liver, pancreas and gall bladder. The job of the digestive system is to digest and absorb food.

You have now been introduced to cells, tissues, organs and systems. We have seen how these link to each other. We shall now look at them in more detail.

> **Think** Define a tissue and an organ. Give an example of an organ and the different tissues it consists of.

CELLS

An overview of cells was given in the previous section. We saw that they could be grouped together to make tissues, that different tissues could be found in organs and that different organs could work together in a system. We shall now look at cells and their component structures, which are called **organelles**.

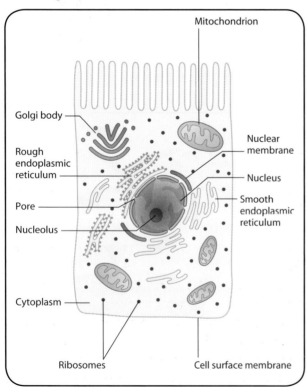

Figure 5.2 *The ultrastructure of a typical human cell*

Figure 5.2 shows the ultrastructure (or detailed structure) of a typical animal cell, and the organelles that can be seen with a very powerful microscope, called an electron microscope.

Cell (surface) membrane

There are many membranes in a cell. The one that concerns us here is the **cell (surface) membrane** that surrounds the cell. There are also membranes surrounding the organelles and a network of them throughout the cell itself.

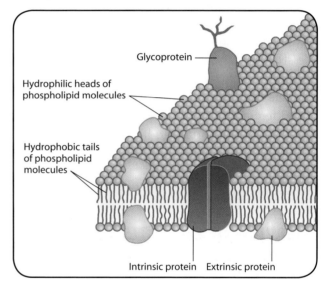

Figure 5.3 *A cell (surface) membrane*

All these structures are important for the different functions of the cell (surface) membrane. The table below shows the main functions of the cell (surface) membrane and the structures that are associated with these functions.

Table 5.1 *Functions of the cell membrane*

Function of cell (surface) membrane	Membrane structure that carries out this function
holds together the cell's contents	phospholipids
controls what enters and leaves the cell	phospholipids, intrinsic proteins
contains receptors for hormones and other substances	glycoproteins

Cytoplasm

Cytoplasm means 'cell fluid'. It contains many different organelles that can only be clearly distinguished with an electron microscope. The exception to this is the largest organelle – the nucleus.

Nucleus

The **nucleus** is usually spherical and bounded by a double membrane with many pores. The nucleus is where DNA, arranged in chromosomes, is found. DNA is responsible for cell division and protein synthesis.

Key words

DNA – chemical containing the genetic code
chromosome – thread shaped body consisting of DNA

Mitochondria

Mitochondria is plural, the singular is mitochondrion. Mitochondria are the powerhouse of the cell. Here, in a series of biochemical reactions called respiration, energy is released from glucose.

Key words

respiration – the series of chemical reactions that releases energy from food materials (glucose)

Endoplasmic reticulum

This is a series of interconnected flattened sacs or tubes which spread throughout the cell. **Endoplasmic reticulum** is concerned with the manufacture and transport of materials. Figure 5.4 shows two types of endoplasmic reticulum.

- **Rough endoplasmic reticulum (RER)** has small structures called ribosomes on the surface of some of its membranes. It is involved in transporting proteins made by the ribosomes to other parts of the cell, or out of the cell if the protein is a hormone or an enzyme involved in digestion.

- **Smooth endoplasmic reticulum (SER)** does not have ribosomes on its surface. It is involved in the manufacture and transport of lipids (fats) and steroids.

By looking at the type and amount of endoplasmic reticulum we can get an idea of the function of the cells.

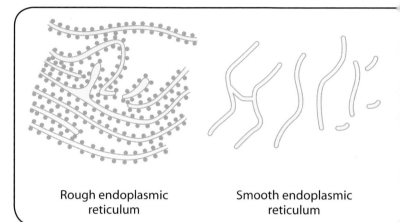

Rough endoplasmic reticulum   Smooth endoplasmic reticulum

Figure 5.4 Rough and smooth endoplasmic reticulum

Think Look back at Figure 5.2 and identify the RER and the SER. How would you expect the proportions of the RER and the SER to change if the cell was involved in the production of a protein such as insulin?

Golgi apparatus

The **Golgi apparatus**, sometimes known as the Golgi body, is made up of a series of flattened sacs stacked on top of each other. They are named after Camillo Golgi who first observed them about 100 years ago, but they have only been seen clearly since the advent of the electron microscope. They link with, but are not joined to, the RER where protein is made. It is thought that in the Golgi apparatus the protein is joined with sugars to make glycoproteins. An example of a glycoprotein is mucus, which is used in lubrication. The membrane of the Golgi apparatus can close off to form a small sac called a vesicle. Vesicles then break off from the Golgi apparatus and move through the cell, where they fuse with the cell

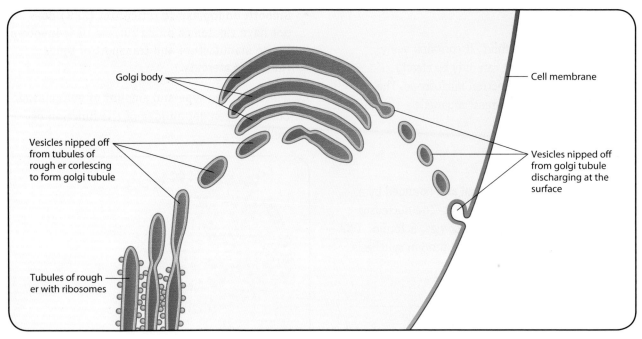

Figure 5.5 Golgi apparatus

surface membrane and release their glycoprotein contents. Figure 5.5 shows the Golgi apparatus and how it works.

Lysosomes

Vesicles can also form from the rough endoplasmic reticulum. Some of these vesicles contain enzymes to destroy worn out organelles. These particular vesicles are called **lysosomes**. Their enzymes have to be kept separate from the rest of the cell otherwise the cell would self-destruct. Lysosomes are also used by white blood cells called phagocytes. They are used to destroy foreign material such as bacteria.

> ***Think*** Why is it important that the contents of a lysosome is kept separate from the rest of a cell?

TISSUES

Having looked inside cells, we shall move up a level and look at tissues, then organs and finally systems. For your assessment, you need to be able to be able to describe the structure of the main tissues of the body and their role in the functioning of two named body organs. You also

need to be able to describe the gross structure and main functions of all major body systems.

Epithelial tissues

Epithelial tissue provides protective covering for surfaces inside and outside the body. There are two main types of epithelial tissues (see page 153): **simple** and **compound (stratified)**. Simple epithelial tissue is only one cell thick, whereas compound epithelial tissue consists of two or more layers of cells. We shall look at the structure of the different types of simple and compound epithelial tissue, where they might be found and their role. The best way to show the structure of a tissue is to draw it.

Simple epithelial tissues

- **Squamous epithelium**, sometimes known as pavement epithelium, consists of flat, thin cells. It forms the lining of blood vessels and the air sacs in the lungs. Gases can be exchanged rapidly because of the thinness of the cells.

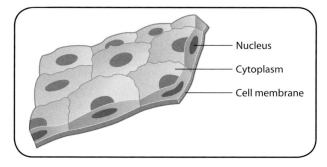

Figure 5.6a Squamous epithelium

- **Cuboidal epithelium** consists of cube-shaped cells and is found in the kidneys and ovaries. It is involved in absorbing and releasing substances.

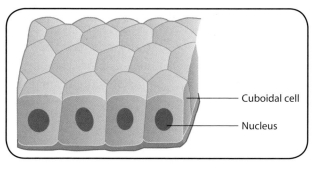

Figure 5.6b Cuboidal epithelium

- **Columnar epithelium** consists of tall column-like cells and lines the whole of the digestive tract. As well as protecting the lining of the gut, it contains cells that produce mucus to aid the passage of food.

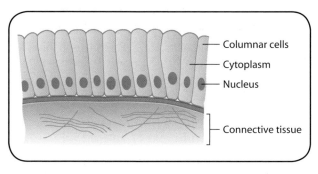

Figure 5.6c Columnar epithelium

- **Ciliated epithelium** consists of tall column-like cells which have hair-like structures called cilia. It is found in the respiratory passages of the lungs and in the fallopian tubes of the female reproductive system. The cilia helps move dust and bacteria, trapped in mucus from the respiratory passages, and ova (eggs) in the fallopian tubes.

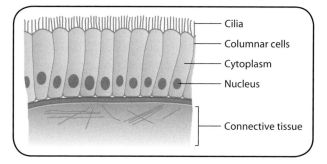

Figure 5.6d Ciliared epithelium

Compound epithelial tissues

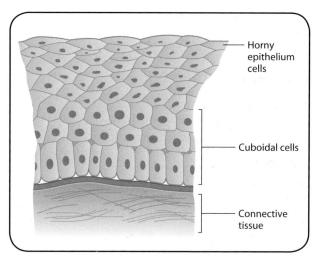

Figure 5.7 Compound epithelial tissue

Simple compound or **stratified epithelium** is found where body linings have to withstand wear and tear. If the top layer contains a tough, resistant protein called keratin the epithelium is referred to as keratinised compound epithelium. Our skin contains **keratinised** compound epithelium, but the linings of the mouth, anus and vagina contain non-keratinised compound epithelium.

> ***Think*** Create a table to show the different types of epithelium and where each is found in the body.

Connective tissue

Unlike epithelial tissue, **connective tissue** typically has cells scattered throughout a material called the extra-cellular matrix. The function of connective tissue is to protect, support and bind other tissues.

Areolar tissue

Areolar tissue consists of a thin gel supporting a network of fine, white fibres made of collagen. These give strength to tissues like blood vessels, neurones and muscle fibres. Areolar tissue in the skin also contains elastic fibres.

Adipose tissue

Adipose tissue consists of fat cells and has three main functions: storage, insulation and protection. It is found all over the body, in areas such as the hips and buttocks, and around various organs, such as the kidneys, heart and liver.

Bone tissue

Bone tissue consists of fibrous material, which gives it its strength, and calcium salts, such as calcium phosphate, which gives bone its rigidity.

Blood

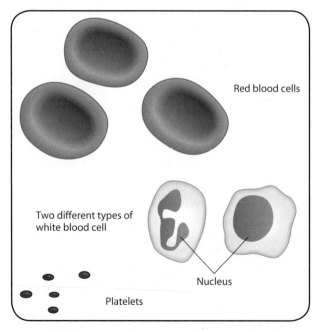

Figure 5.8 Blood cells – red, white and platelets.

Interestingly, **blood** is considered to be a type of connective tissue, although it has a different function compared to other connective tissues. It does, however, like other connective tissues, have a liquid extra-cellular matrix called plasma. Red blood cells (erythrocytes), white blood cells (leucocytes) and platelets are suspended in the plasma. The table shows the functions of the different components of blood.

Table 5.2 Blood components

Component	Function
Red blood cells (erythrocytes)	Transport oxygen round the body
White blood cells (leucocytes) • phagocytes (P) • lymphocytes (L)	(P) Surround and destroy foreign material such as bacteria (L) Produce antibodies that destroy foreign material such as bacteria
Platelets	Clots blood when the body is damaged
Plasma	Transports material such as food, carbon dioxide and hormones

Cartilage

Cartilage tissue is strong but flexible and is found in joints and as rings of cartilage holding open the trachea.

Muscle tissues

Humans have three different types of muscles, which are known by various names. Figure 5.9 shows the various names for each of the different types of muscle.

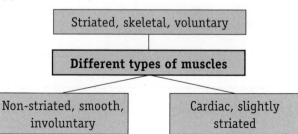

Figure 5.9

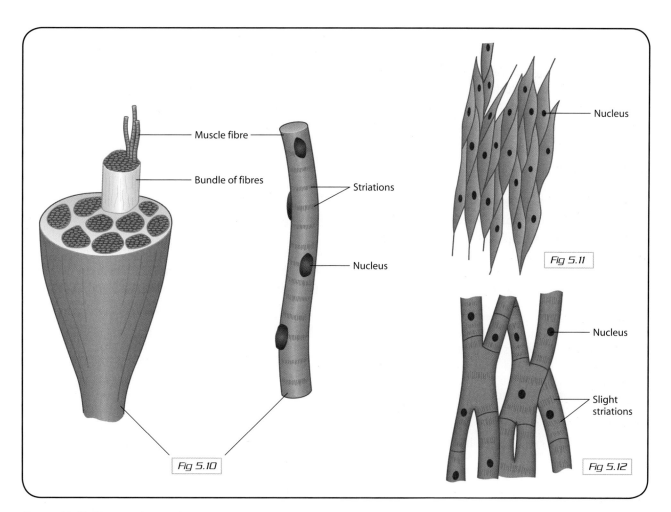

Figure 5.10 Striated muscle
Figure 5.11 Non-striated muscle nucleus
Figure 5.12 Cardiac muscle

Striated muscle

Striated muscle gets its name from its appearance. You can see its striped appearance in figure 5.10, which shows the arrangement of bundles and fibres in striated muscle.

Striated muscle is often referred to as 'skeletal muscle' because it is attached to the skeleton. These muscles contract and relax to make our skeleton move. Striated muscle is also known as voluntary muscle because we can control its actions.

Non-striated muscle

Non-striated muscle also gets its name from its appearance. You can see from the diagram that it has no stripes. This is why it is often referred to as smooth muscle.

You can see that non-striated muscle is composed of spindle-shaped cells arranged in bundles. These muscles contract rhythmically and do not tire easily. They are found in the alimentary canal (gut), the walls of blood vessels and in the tubes leading to and from the bladder (ureter and urethra, respectively). They are sometimes referred to as involuntary muscles, as we have no control of their contractions.

Cardiac muscle

Cardiac muscle is found only in the walls of the heart. It is capable of rhythmical contraction and relaxation over a very long period – a lifetime, in fact! You can see from Figure 5.12 that it has slight striations.

Nervous tissue

There are many types of nervous tissue including the tissue inside the brain and spinal cord, as well as the peripheral nerves. The two types you need to know about are neurones and neuroglia.

Neurones

A **neurone** is a single nerve cell. They carry information from one part of the body to another in the form of nerve impulses. There are several types of neurone:

- sensory neurones – going from receptors to the spinal cord

- motor neurones – going from the spinal cord and brain to effectors such as muscles and glands.

- relay neurones – found within the spinal cord itself

A motor neurone can be seen in the diagram below.

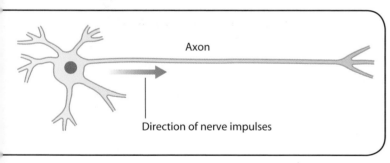

Axon

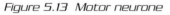

Direction of nerve impulses

Figure 5.13 Motor neurone

> **Think** Where have the impulses come from? Where are the impulses going to? Describe how the shape of the neurone makes it particularly suitable for its function.

Neuroglia

Neuroglia are also known as 'glia' or 'glial cells'. They are non-neuronal cells that provide support and nutrition in nervous tissue. They also destroy harmful foreign material and remove dead neurones. It is believed that there are ten times as many neuroglia in the brain as neurones.

SYSTEMS AND THEIR ORGANS

We shall deal with organs and systems together. For your assessment, you need to have an overview of the structure and function of the main systems in the body, including the locations of various organs. We shall cover the organs you need to know as we look at each system in turn. The exception to this is the skin. The skin is classified as an organ and does not belong to any system.

The systems you need to know about, including the location of their associated organs, are:

- cardiovascular system – heart

- respiratory system – lungs

- digestive system – stomach, liver, pancreas, duodenum, ileum, colon

- renal system – kidneys, bladder

- nervous system – brain

- endocrine system

- reproductive systems – testes (male), ovaries and uterus (female)

- lymphatic system

- musculo-skeletal system

- immune system.

The structure of three systems and the location of the organs are shown in figures 5.14, 5.15 and 5.16, with other body systems illustrated throughout the unit. The main function of each system detailed above is then given in table 5.3.

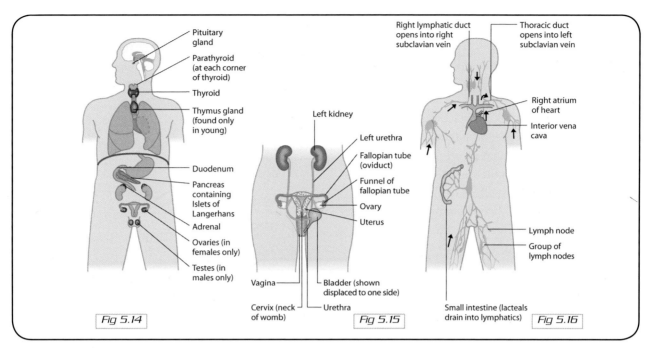

Fig 5.14
Fig 5.15
Fig 5.16

Figure 5.14 Endocrine system

Figure 5.15 Female reproductive system

Figure 5.16 Lymphatic and immune system

Summary of the main body systems and their functions

Table 5.3 gives a summary of the main body systems and their functions.

Think For each of the body systems, write an additional sentence that gives more detail about its function.

Table 5.3 Body systems and their functions

Body system	Main functions
Cardiovascular	transports materials around the body
Respiratory	takes in oxygen and gets rid of carbon dioxide
Digestive	digests and absorbs food
Renal	excretes waste products such as urea
Nervous	conducts messages from one part of the body to another via electrical impulses
Endocrine	secretes hormones that conduct messages from one part of the body to another via the blood
Reproductive	ensures the continuation of the species
Lymphatic	pathway that returns some tissue fluid from the cells back to the blood and helps in fighting against disease-causing organisms
Musculo-skeletal	enables movement
Immune	protects the body against disease-causing organisms

5.2 The role of energy in the body

WHY DO WE NEED ENERGY?

Most of the processes taking place inside our cells need energy in order to happen. When large molecules are formed, such as proteins from amino acids or glycogen from glucose, they need energy; when muscles cells contract or neurones conduct electrical impulses, they need energy; to maintain our body temperature, we need energy. So, you can see we need a lot of energy.

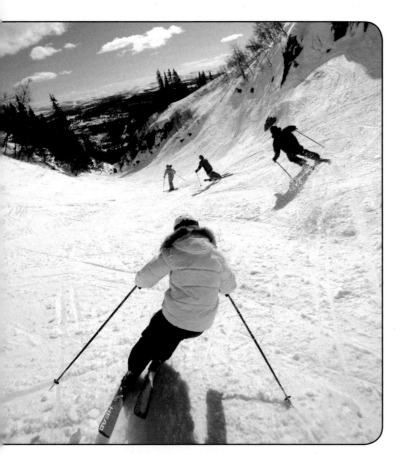

Figure 5.17 Being active in a cold environment requires a lot of energy

HOW MUCH ENERGY DO WE NEED?

Energy is measured in kilojoules (kJ). You may also see energy measured in kilocalories. (1 kilocalorie = 4.2 kilojoules)

The table shows the daily energy requirements of different types of people.

Table 5.4

Age/sex/occupation of person	Daily energy requirement (kJ)
Newborn baby	2,000
Child aged 2	5,000
Child aged 6	7,500
Girl aged 12-14	9,000
Boy aged 12-14	11,000
Girl aged 15-17	9,000
Boy aged 15-17	12,000
Female office worker	9,500
Male office worker	10,500
Woman breast-feeding	11,300
Pregnant woman	10,000
Heavy manual worker	15,000

Think Explain why a heavy manual worker has the highest daily energy requirement. Explain why a woman who is breast-feeding has a higher energy requirement than either a female officer worker or a pregnant woman.

WHERE DOES OUR ENERGY COME FROM?

Our energy comes from the food we eat. However, we might say that our energy and all the energy used by all organisms on Earth comes from the sun. However, we don't use the energy from the sun directly. We need plants to do that for us.

Plants are able to absorb sunlight and use the light energy to make food molecules from carbon dioxide and water, in a process called 'photosynthesis'. When we eat plants, we digest the complex food molecules back into simpler ones. We then change the energy contained in these simple food molecules, such as glucose, into a more useable form in a process called 'respiration'. Respiration is essentially the reverse of photosynthesis.

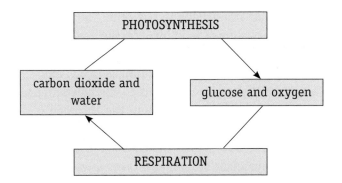

Figure 5.18 Respiration and photosynthesis

Think What are the main uses of energy in the body? Digestion and respiration are both associated with energy in the body. Explain the different roles they play.

ENERGY LAWS, FORMS OF ENERGY AND ENERGY METABOLISM

Energy cannot be created or destroyed – this is the **law of conservation of energy**. What it can do, however, is be transformed from one form into another. Some of the different forms of energy found in the body are:

- chemical
- heat
- electrical
- sound
- light.

Look at how the different forms relate to where energy comes from.

- The sun provides light energy, which is stored as chemical energy in the bonds of food molecules, such as glucose.

- The chemical energy in glucose is transferred to more accessible chemical molecules, ATP (or adenosine triphosphate), during respiration. ATP is a relatively small molecule that can diffuse around the cell quickly.

- Some of the chemical energy is also transferred into heat energy during respiration.

Splitting ATP provides readily available energy in small, useable amounts for the wide variety of energy-requiring reactions that occurs in the body. The chemical energy from the bonds of ATP is transferred into other forms of chemical energy, electrical energy and into sound energy. We need chemical energy for some other reactions, electrical energy for nerve impulses, and sound energy for our voices.

Energy metabolism refers to a cells capacity to acquire, store and use energy. The word 'metabolism' comes from a Greek word meaning change. The term can be applied to all the chemical processes that occur within cells. The reactions are arranged in intricately branched pathways called metabolic pathways, along which compounds are transformed in a series of steps. Some chemical reactions release energy which is used directly in other reactions that require energy. In other cases, energy is stored temporarily until it is required; this is the role played by ATP. Storing energy in the bonds of ATP is rather like keeping your money in an accessible bank account until it is needed.

There are two types of metabolic pathways:

- **Catabolic pathways** break down large molecules into smaller, simpler ones. Examples of this are proteins being broken down to amino acids or glycogen being broken down to glucose in digestion. Another example is respiration. Catabolic reactions release energy.

- **Anabolic pathways** build up large molecules from smaller, simpler ones. Examples of this are amino acids being joined together to form proteins or glucose molecules being joined to form glycogen. Another example is photosynthesis. They are the reverse of the catabolic reactions in that anabolic reactions require energy.

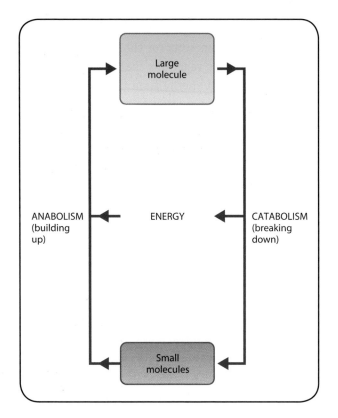

Figure 5.19 Relationship between catabolic and anabolic pathways.

COLLABORATION BETWEEN BODY SYSTEMS TO PROVIDE US WITH ENERGY

Here we shall take an overview of the role the cardiovascular, respiratory and digestive systems play in providing us with energy. The next section will explain how they do this is more detail. However, it is important to see the big picture, as this is what you will need to achieve a pass. The detail of each system is required for a merit. To achieve a distinction, you will also need to use examples to explain how these body systems relate to each other. You will begin to see this here as we take a holistic view of how the systems work together in relation to energy metabolism.

We need food to provide energy and oxygen in order to release that energy efficiently. Energy is released from food in the process of respiration. Respiration takes place inside our cells. We need to

get the food and oxygen to our cells. The digestive system breaks down food into simpler molecules, like glucose, which can be absorbed into the blood stream. The respiratory system takes in air, and oxygen diffuses from our lungs to the bloodstream. The cardiovascular system moves the absorbed food and oxygen to our cells where the energy is released into a form that the cells can use easily. The cardiovascular system also takes away the waste products of respiration – carbon dioxide and water – from the cells. The carbon dioxide is then diffused from the blood back into the lungs where it is exhaled.

> **Think** Summarise the role of each system in a table. Imagine you are a molecule of oxygen. Describe your route from the air to a cell in your body. What abbreviation represents the name of the chemical that is the cell's usable form of energy? (Hint: it is made in respiration)

THE CARDIOVASCULAR SYSTEM AND ENERGY METABOLISM

The cardiovascular system consists of the heart and blood vessels. Its workings are a vast topic. Here, we shall concentrate on the heart and blood vessels in relation to providing the materials for energy metabolism to the cells of the body. You need to know about:

- the heart:
  - structure
  - cardiac cycle
  - heart rate
  - stroke volume
  - blood pressure.

- blood vessels:
  - arteries
  - arterioles
  - capillaries
  - venules
  - veins
  - pulmonary and systemic circulation
  - structure and functions of blood.

The heart

The heart is the organ that moves blood round the body. It consists of a complex four-chambered muscular bag. It is a cone-shaped organ about the size of a clenched fist and it is found in the chest, located just beneath the sternum (breast bone). The apex is directed downwards, slightly to the left and ventrally towards the chest wall.

The structure of the heart

We have seen that the wall of the heart consists of cardiac muscle tissues. The atria have relatively thin walls and function as collection chambers for blood returning to the heart, pumping blood only a short distance to the ventricles. The ventricles have thicker walls, especially the left ventricle, which pumps blood round the whole of the body. The cardiac muscle is supplied with glucose and oxygen for its energy requirements by the coronary arteries. If these get blocked then a heart attack may occur. An external view of the heart is shown in the diagram below.

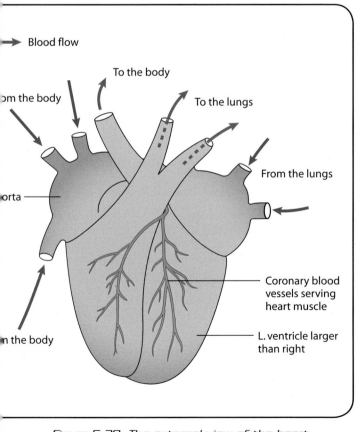

Figure 5.20 The external view of the heart

The following diagram shows a detailed view of the heart. The heart is divided by a septum (a partition), into right and left sides. Between the atrium and ventricle on each side is an opening, guarded by the tricuspid valve on the right and the bicuspid valve on the left side of the heart. When the valves are closed they seal off the atria from the ventricles. These valves only allow blood to flow downwards from the atria to the ventricles. Note that there are inelastic tendons called 'chordae tendineae' to prevent the flaps of the valves being forced back too far.

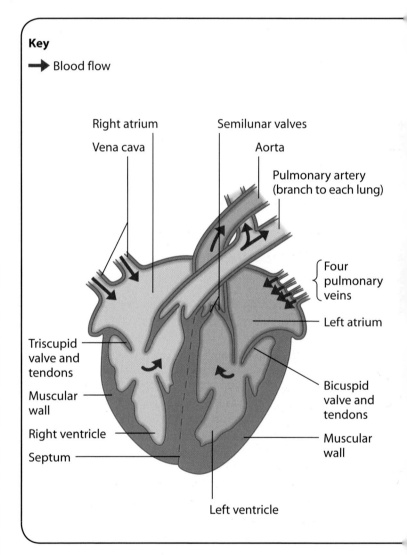

Figure 5.21 A detailed view of the heart

There are another two sets of valves, both called semilunar valves, between the right ventricle and the pulmonary artery, and between the left ventricle and the aorta. These stop the blood flowing back into the heart from these vessels.

The heart cycle

The sequence of events during each heartbeat is referred to as the **heart cycle**. The cycle has two main phases: systole and diastole. Systole is the phase of the cycle where the heart contracts. There are two contractions, the atrial contraction and the main ventricular contraction. Diastole is the phase where the heart is relaxed and is filling with blood.

A full cycle lasts about 0.8 seconds when a person is at rest, with systole and diastole lasting about the same length of time. During the first 0.1 second of systole, the atria contract, forcing the blood into the ventricles. Then, in a powerful contraction, the ventricles pump blood in the arteries during 0.3 second. For 0.4 second, the atria are relaxed and filling with blood returning from the veins. Throughout diastole, the ventricles are also filling and the atrial systolic contraction just finishes this off. These events are summarised as follows:

- While the heart is at rest, blood flows from the veins into the atria and on into the ventricles.

- The atria then contract, forcing more blood into the ventricles.

- Overfilling of the ventricles causes the tricuspid and bicuspid valves to close. This causes the first heart sound, 'lub'. The atria relax and the blood flow from the veins resumes.

- The distended ventricles contract and blood is forced into the arteries. The ventricles relax and the drop in pressure allows the tricuspid and bicuspid valves to open. Blood flows passively from the atria into the ventricles.

- The arteries are now filled with blood and the semilunar valves close with a snap, 'dupp' – the second heart sound. The arteries contract, forcing the blood onwards.

Here we have only referred to the left side of the heart. Note that the events occur simultaneously in both sides of the heart. Oxygenated blood moves through the left side of the heart and deoxygenated blood moves from the right side of the heart; the heart has a double circulation.

Cardiac output, heart rate and stroke volume

Heart rate or pulse rate refers to the number of heart beats per minute. You can count your own heart rate by counting the pulsations of arteries in your wrist or neck. During each heart cycle, the ventricular contractions during systole are of such a force that the elastic arteries stretch from the pressure. For a person at rest the pulse is about 75 beats per minute, although people who are fit often have lower resting pulses than those who are less fit.

The volume of blood that the left ventricle pumps into the aorta each minute is called the 'cardiac output'. This volume depends on two factors:

- the **heart rate** (pulse rate)

- the **stroke volume** – the amount of blood pumped out at each contraction.

The cardiac output is equal to the stroke volume multiplied by the heart rate per minute. The cardiac output is roughly equal to the amount of blood we have in our bodies. This means the total volume of blood in our body passes through the heart each minute.

Example

An average stroke volume is about 0.075 dm³ (or litres). Someone with a heart rate of 70 beats per minute will have the following cardiac output:

70 × 0.075 = heart beats/min × average stroke volume
= 5.25 dm³ (litres) per minute.

This means that the total amount of blood leaving the heart each minute is 5.25 dm³.

Think You need to understand the relationship between cardiac output, stroke volume and heart rate. What would the effect on the cardiac output be if either the stroke volume or the heart rate changed?

Blood pressure

The pressure of the blood can be measured with a sphygmomanometer, which presses on the artery in the upper arm. It records the pressure of the blood as the heart contracts and relaxes. Normal pressures are about 120 (systole) and 70-80 mmHg (diastole). Over time the blood vessel walls can become less elastic, raising the blood pressure.

Blood vessels

Blood is carried in three main types of blood vessels, which are shown in the diagram below. There are two other types of blood vessels you need to know about. These are arterioles (little arteries) and venules (little veins). Remember that the general function of blood vessels is to carry material to and from the cells where respiration occurs.

Figure 5.22 An artery, a vein and a capillary.

Arteries

Arteries always carry blood away from the heart. They usually carry oxygenated blood (except the pulmonary artery which carries blood to the lungs). They have an outer coat of fibrous and connective tissue, mainly for protection. Inside this they have a thick layer of circular muscle fibres in the wall. This muscular layer exerts a steady pressure on the blood. When an artery is cut, the muscular wall remains active, so that blood continues to flow in spurts, coinciding with the pumping of the heart and the contractions and relaxation of the muscles of the artery walls. The lumen is lined by epithelium composed of a single layer of cells – the endothelium. This is very smooth and offers very little resistance to the flow of blood.

Unfortunately, later in life adhesions such as atheroma (fatty deposits) can form here. This condition is known as atherosclerosis and causes narrowing of the arteries.

Veins

Veins carry blood back to the heart from the tissues. They usually carry deoxygenated blood (except the pulmonary vein which carries blood back to the heart from the lungs). Veins have much thinner and less elastic layers and are more likely to collapse than arteries.

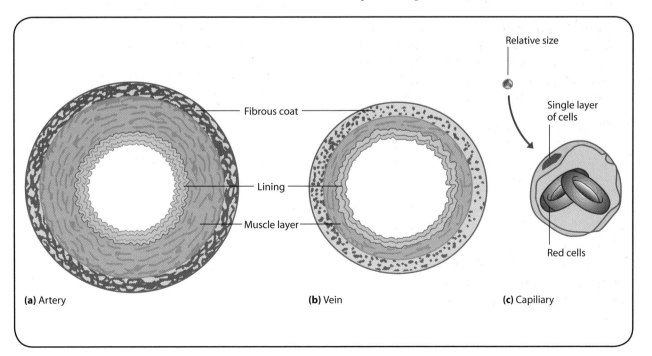

(a) Artery   (b) Vein   (c) Capiliary

The lumen in veins is larger than that in arteries. Also the blood travelling in them is at a lower pressure than the blood in arteries. When blood in veins travels against gravity (for example up the legs), there are valves to stop the blood flowing backwards. Sometimes these valves do not work properly, causing varicose veins, which show through the skin as a series of knots running up the vein. If they become particularly painful, surgery may be necessary.

Blood is able to flow up our legs towards the heart thanks to muscles in our legs contracting. For example, when we walk the muscles become shorter and fatter and squeeze the veins. This has the effect of moving the blood upwards.

Capillaries

Capillaries are tiny vessels found in all body tissues where material needs to be exchanged with the cells. Remember, cells need glucose and oxygen for respiration, and carbon dioxide and other waste materials need to be removed. Capillaries have thin walls which consist of endothelium alone, one cell thick. This provides a short diffusion pathway. The walls are permeable and material can pass through them so that water and dissolved substances can be exchanged between the capillaries and the cells. See Figure 5.23.

A fluid called **tissue fluid** (or **lymph**) surrounds the cells and this helps to transport substances to and from the cells. The tissue fluid drains into vessels called 'lymphatics' and this is an alternative way for certain materials to be returned to the heart.

Arterioles and venules

There are two other blood vessels you need to know about. The largest arteries divide again and again. The smallest branches, the **arterioles**, further divide into capillaries. The capillaries which emerge from the tissues unite to form **venules**, which in turn give rise to veins.

Double circulation

Humans, like all vertebrates, have a double circulation - the pulmonary circulation and the systemic circulation. This means that blood passes through the heart twice, once through the right-hand side as deoxygenated blood and a second time through the left-hand side as oxygenated blood. The blood in the pulmonary circulation goes to the lungs to pick up oxygen. It is then returned to the heart to be pumped through the systemic circulation to the rest of the body. Figure 5.24 shows the circulatory system in more detail.

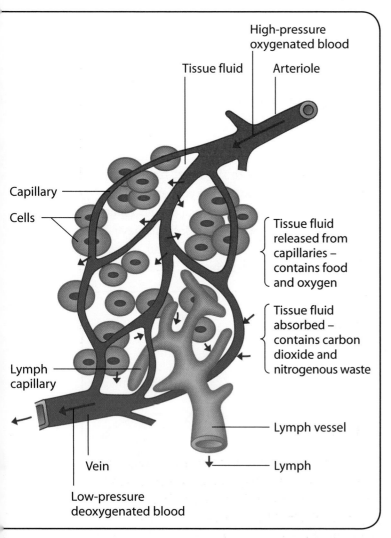

Figure 5.23 Pathways between cells and capillaries

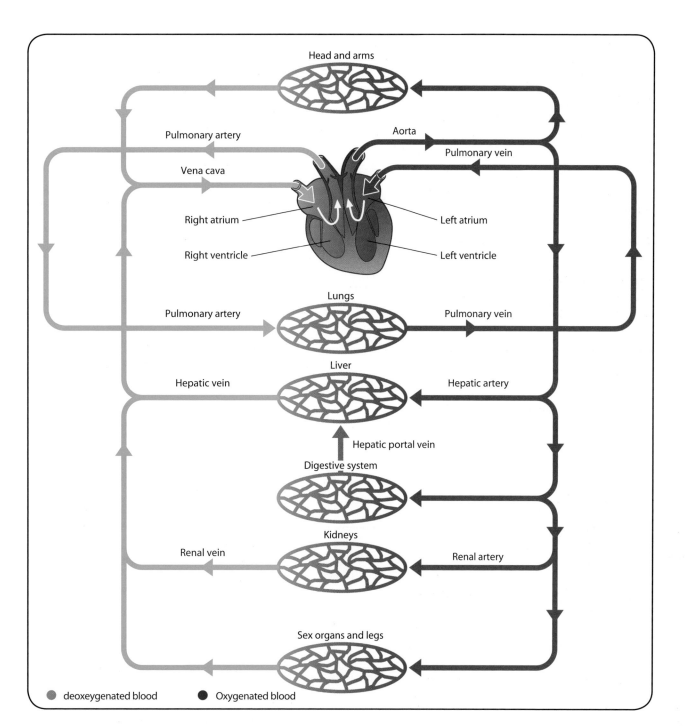

Figure 5.24 The circulatory system

Think Use Figure 5.24 to identify the pulmonary circuit and the systemic circuits.

Structure and functions of blood

We have already discussed the structure and functions of the different components of blood (see page 158). Here we shall look and see which parts of blood are specifically involved in energy metabolism.

Red blood cells

Red blood cells carry oxygen from the lungs to cells in our tissues. They contain haemoglobin which can combine with oxygen to form oxyhaemoglobin. This happens in the lungs where the concentration of oxygen is high. In the tissues the concentration of oxygen is lower, so oxyhaemoglobin breaks down, releasing oxygen.

Plasma

Respiration requires food as well as oxygen. Digested food such as glucose is transported in plasma. In the tissues, it diffuses from the capillaries into the cells at the arteriole end of the capillary. Carbon dioxide, a waste product of respiration, diffuses from the cells back into the capillaries, at the venule end of the capillary. Look back at Figure 5.23 which shows the pathway between cells and capillaries to see this.

THE RESPIRATORY SYSTEM AND ENERGY METABOLISM

The function of the respiratory system is to provide oxygen for efficient respiration and to take away carbon dioxide, a waste product. The respiratory system works in two ways:

- **ventilation** – breathing air in and out of the lungs

- **gaseous exchange** – the exchange of gases between the lungs and the blood.

Our lungs are deep inside the thorax (chest cavity) and it is important that they are well ventilated. The lungs are delicate structures and, together with the heart, they are protected by the rib cage. The ribs can be moved by intercostal muscles and the bottom of the thorax can be moved by the muscular diaphragm. Air flow is tidal, air entering and leaving along the same route. It enters the nostrils and mouth and passes down the **trachea**. It enter sthe lungs via the two **bronchis** which subdivide into many **bronchioles** (sometimes called the bronchial tree), ending up in air-sacs called **alveoli**.

THE STRUCTURE OF THE RESPIRATORY SYSTEM

The structure of the respiratory system is shown in Figure 5.25 below.

> **Think** One way to learn the structure is to imagine a molecule of oxygen travelling from the outside world in to the blood. How would you describe the journey it would take?

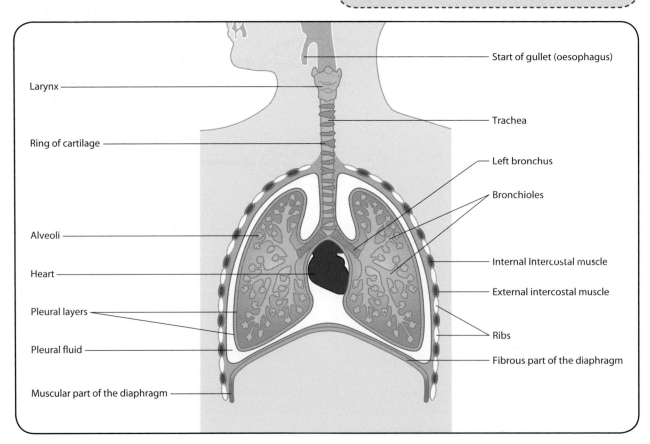

Larynx

Ring of cartilage

Alveoli

Heart

Pleural layers

Pleural fluid

Muscular part of the diaphragm

Start of gullet (oesophagus)

Trachea

Left bronchus

Bronchioles

Internal Intercostal muscle

External intercostal muscle

Ribs

Fibrous part of the diaphragm

Figure 5.25 Diagram of the structure of the respiratory system

Within the nasal (nose) channels, mucus is secreted by goblet cells in the ciliated epithelium. This mucus traps dust particles and bacteria and the cilia move them to the nose where they can be removed when the nose is 'blown', or to the back of the mouth where they are swallowed. The mucus also serves to moisten the incoming air, which is warmed by superficial blood vessels.

The air then passes through the pharynx (throat) and past the epiglottis, a flap of cartilage which prevents food entering the trachea. The larynx or voice box, at the top of the trachea, is a box-like cartilaginous structure with a number of ligaments, known as the vocal cords, stretched across it. Vibration of these cords, when air is expired, produces sound. The trachea is lined with cilia and has rings of cartilage to prevent it collapsing when there is reduced air pressure.

The trachea divides into two bronchi; each of which then branches several times into smaller and smaller bronchioles, and the supporting cartilage ceases to be necessary. Eventually, at the end of each branch is an air-sac or alveolus. There are over 350 million alveoli in each human lung; these form a total respiratory surface of about 90m^2.

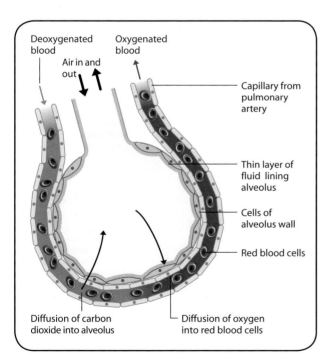

Figure 5.26 A single alveolus

Labels on figure:
- Deoxygenated blood
- Oxygenated blood
- Air in and out
- Capillary from pulmonary artery
- Thin layer of fluid lining alveolus
- Cells of alveolus wall
- Red blood cells
- Diffusion of carbon dioxide into alveolus
- Diffusion of oxygen into red blood cells

> **Think** Why is it important to have blood capillaries in such close proximity to the alveoli? What is moving from the cells to the alveoli in the lungs? Why is this different to other tissues?

Figure 5.26 shows gas exchange in an alveolus. Oxygen moves into the red cells from the alveolus and carbon dioxide moves back into the alveolus from the plasma. Movement in each direction is because of the diffusion gradient of the gases, the concentration of oxygen being higher in the alveoli and of carbon dioxide being higher in the plasma.

The capillaries are very narrow and the red blood cells are squeezed as they pass through. This not only slows down the passage of blood, allowing more time for diffusion, but also results in a larger surface area of the red blood cell touching the endothelium, thus facilitating the diffusion of oxygen.

The oxygen in the inspired air (air that has been inhaled) dissolves in the moisture of the alveolar epithelium and diffuses across this and the endothelium of the capillary into the red blood cells. We have already learned that inside the red blood cell, the oxygen combines with the respiratory pigment haemoglobin to form oxyhaemoglobin. Carbon dioxide diffuses from the blood into the alveolus, to leave the lungs in the expired air.

> **Think** Why does carbon dioxide diffuse from the blood into the alveolus? What would happen to the diffusion if the concentration of carbon dioxide in the lungs increased to a higher level?

MECHANISM OF VENTILATION

Humans ventilate their lungs by breathing: the alternate inhalation and exhalation of air. Ventilation maintains a maximal oxygen concentration and minimal carbon dioxide concentration within the alveoli. The actual mechanism is negative pressure breathing, which works like a suction pump.

Air moves into the lungs in the following way:

- The **intercostal muscles** contract, raising the ribcage, which is pivoted on the vertebral column. At the same time, circular muscle fibres in the **diaphragm** contract, causing it to flatten. In this way, the volume of the chest cavity is increased.

- The chest is a closed cavity and so an increase in volume will produce a fall in pressure. As a result the lungs, which are naturally elastic and at rest compressed, expand.

- Lung expansion is assisted by the pull of the pleural membranes – the outer membrane is attached to the chest wall and the inner membrane to the lungs. The two adhere to each other because of the fluid film between them. As the outer membrane is pulled out with the expanding chest wall, it pulls the inner membrane and the lungs with it.

- Expansion of the lungs reduces pressure within. The lungs are open to the air (via the bronchi and trachea), which rushes in to equalise the pressure.

Exhalation is largely a passive process. Intercostal muscles and diaphragm muscles relax and the rib cage falls, compressing the lungs and pushing air out. Voluntary contraction of the abdominal muscles causes more air to be expelled. Figure 5.27 gives a summary of ventilation (inhalation and exhalation).

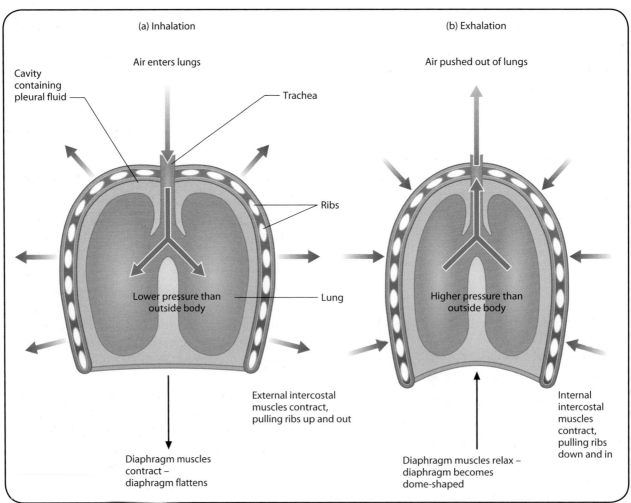

Figure 5.27 A summary of ventilation

THE DIGESTIVE SYSTEM AND ENERGY METABOLISM

The function of the digestive system is to break down complex food into a simpler, soluble form. This is necessary for the absorption of the food through the gut wall into the body itself.

Most of the complex material in food consists of carbohydrates, fats and proteins, which are too large to pass through membranes and enter cells. Also, the material in the food may not be in the form that the body requires. Carbohydrates are broken down to simple sugars, fats are broken down to fatty acids and glycerol and proteins are broken down to amino acids. The digestion of these macromolecules is catalysed by enzymes. We will learn more detail about this shortly.

The digestive system consists of the **alimentary canal** and various organs associated with it, which secrete digestive juices containing enzymes into it. The wall of the alimentary canal is made up of distinct layers. Next to the lumen (cavity) is a mucous membrane called the mucosa. Outside this is a layer of connective tissue, followed by a layer of muscular tissue. The outermost layer is a sheath of connective tissue attached to the membrane.

The accessory organs associated with the alimentary canal are three pairs of **salivary glands**, the **pancreas**, and the **liver** (with its associated storage organ, the gall bladder). We will now follow the movement of food through the canal, seeing what happens to it at the various stages.

Ingestion

Pieces of food are bitten off by the incisor teeth and reduced to small particles by the grinding of the molars and the action of the tongue against the hard palate. See Figure 5.28.

The small particles are mixed with saliva, a watery mucous solution produced by the salivary glands. There are three pairs of salivary glands, which secrete saliva in response to the sight, smell or even thought of food. Saliva has two functions: digestion and lubrication.

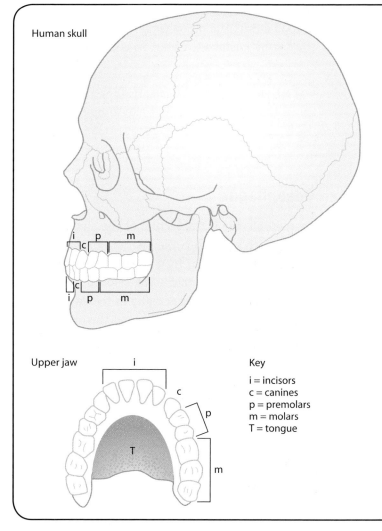

Figure 5.28 Ingestion

We secrete more than one litre of saliva into the mouth every day. It contains the glycoprotein mucin, which protects the soft lining of the mouth from damage as well as lubricating the food to make it easier to swallow. Saliva also contains buffers which help to neutralise the acid produced from food and kill bacteria. These processes also help to prevent tooth decay. Most importantly, saliva contains the enzyme **salivary amylase**, a digestive enzyme which begins the breakdown of starch to the disaccharide, maltose.

The tongue is used not only to taste food, but to help shape the food into a ball, called a bolus, ready for swallowing. The back of the mouth is called the pharynx and it leads to both the oesophagus and the trachea or windpipe. When we swallow, the top of the wind pipe is closed off by a cartilaginous flap called the epiglottis.

The swallowing mechanism ensures that the bolus of food enters the oesophagus. If it enters the trachea by mistake, we start to choke.

> **Think** In a table summarise the roles of the various parts of the mouth in digestion.

Oesophagus

The oesophagus is the section of the alimentary canal which leads from the pharynx to the stomach. The bolus of food is squeezed towards the stomach by peristalsis. The smooth muscle of the alimentary canal is actually in two layers, one running in a circular direction and the outer one running in a longitudinal direction.

When the circular muscles in one region contract, they make the alimentary canal narrow in that region. A contraction in one region of the alimentary canal is followed by another contraction just below it, so that a wave of contractions passes along the canal, pushing food in front of it.

Peristalsis ensures that food travels in one direction, from the pharynx to the stomach. This will still occur when we are horizontal or even upside down, proving that the movement of food down to the stomach does not rely on gravity. Note that the muscle contractions require energy.

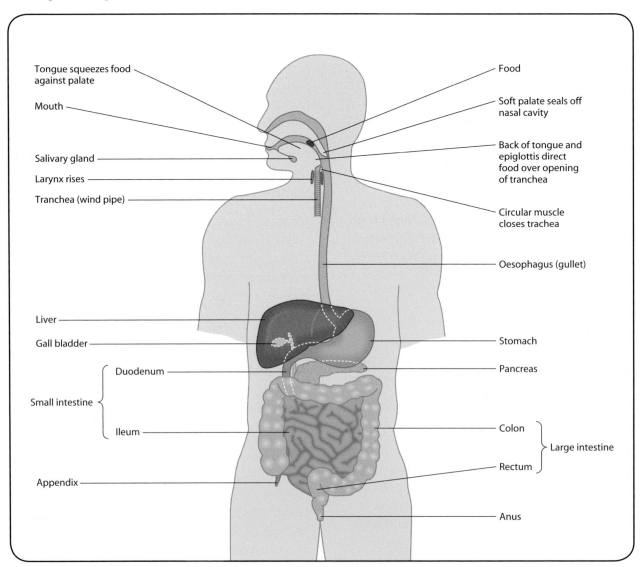

Tongue squeezes food against palate

Mouth

Salivary gland

Larynx rises

Tranchea (wind pipe)

Liver

Gall bladder

Duodenum

Small intestine

Ileum

Appendix

Food

Soft palate seals off nasal cavity

Back of tongue and epiglottis direct food over opening of tranchea

Circular muscle closes trachea

Oesophagus (gullet)

Stomach

Pancreas

Colon

Large intestine

Rectum

Anus

Figure 5.29 The digestive system

Stomach

You can see the stomach in this diagram of the entire alimentary canal.

The stomach is located on the left side of the body, just below the diaphragm (see figure 5.29). It is able to stretch to store a whole meal, and therefore we do not have to eat constantly. There are sphincters (rings of circular muscle) both at its entrance (cardiac sphincter) and at its exit (pyloric sphincter), which regulate the amount of food entering and leaving, respectively.

The epithelium that lines the stomach secretes a fluid called gastric juice. This is very acidic and helps kill any bacteria present. It also contains the enzyme pepsin which breaks down proteins into smaller chains of **amino acids** called **peptides**. It is not able to break down proteins to individual amino acids because it only breaks the bonds between certain amino acids.

What stops the pepsin and the acid in gastric juice digesting the wall of the stomach itself? Pepsin is released in an inactive form, pepsinogen, which needs hydrochloric acid to change it into pepsin. As pepsinogen and acid are released from different cells they do not come into contact with each other until they are in the lumen of the stomach. There is a coating of mucus, secreted by epithelial cells, which forms on the inside of the stomach wall. The inside of the wall is constantly having its cells regenerated, but if this regeneration is not fast enough, and pepsin and acid attack it, an ulcer will occur.

The smooth muscles in the stomach wall churn the food regularly. If they operate on an empty stomach we can sometimes hear the rumbling. The food and gastric juice eventually become a nutrient broth known as acid chyme. At the bottom end of the stomach, the pyloric sphincter helps regulate the passage of chyme from the stomach into the small intestine. It takes from two to six hours for a meal to empty completely from the stomach.

> **Think** How is the stomach adapted to perform its functions? Write a short summary in your own words

Small intestine

This is where most digestion takes place. Up until now there has been only limited digestion of carbohydrates in the mouth, and the start of protein digestion in the stomach. The small intestine can be up to six metres in length. (It is called the 'small' intestine because of its small diameter compared to the large intestine.) It is not only responsible for a large part of digestion, but also for the absorption of the digested food into the blood or lymph.

The first 25 centimetres of the small intestine is called the duodenum and it is here that the secretions from the pancreas, liver, and gall bladder enter. The larger part of the small intestine is called the ileum. Here digestion is completed and the digested food is absorbed into the blood and lymph.

Several other organs contribute to digestion in the small intestine and they are shown in the Figure 5.30.

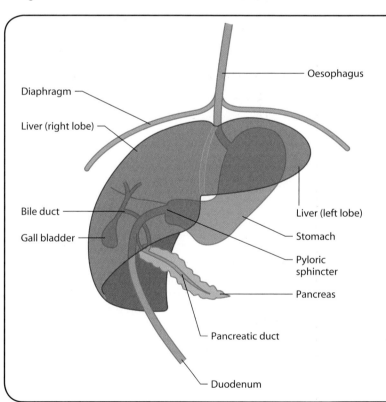

Figure 5.30 Diagram to show relationship between the stomach, liver and pancreas

175

The pancreas secretes pancreatic juice into the duodenum, which contains various enzymes (we will look at these later) as well as an alkaline solution that neutralises the acid from the stomach.

The liver performs a wide variety of functions, one of which is the production of bile, which is stored in the gall bladder until it is needed. Bile aids the digestion of lipids (fats) by emulsifying them to increase their surface area for enzyme digestion. Bile also contains pigments which are the by-products of red blood cell destruction in the liver. These bile pigments are eliminated from the body with the faeces.

Carbohydrates

Salivary amylase starts the digestion of carbohydrates in the mouth and this is continued in the duodenum by pancreatic amylase. Both enzymes digest starch into maltose, a disaccharide. Digestion of maltose is completed by the enzyme maltase, which is secreted from the walls of the ileum. Other sugars such as lactose and sucrose are also broken down to glucose, by the enzymes lactase and sucrase respectively.

Proteins

Digestion is initiated in the stomach by the enzyme pepsin, but protease enzymes in the duodenum continue the digestion to peptide and amino acids. Digestion is completed to amino acids in the ileum by other proteases.

Lipids (fats)

Nearly all of the fat in a meal reaches the small intestine completely undigested. Bile breaks down the fat into smaller droplets, a process called emulsification. This increases the surface area to help digestion by lipase, the enzyme that hydrolyses lipids into fatty acids and glycerol.

SUMMARY OF FOOD DIGESTION

During their passage through the alimentary canal, complex food molecules are completely digested into simpler ones, small enough to be absorbed through the ileum wall into the body itself. A summary of food digestion is given in Table 5.5.

Table 5.5 Food digestion

Part of the digestive system	Carbohydrates	Proteins	Lipids
Mouth	Starch to maltose by salivary amylase		
Stomach		Protein to peptides by pepsin	
Duodenum	Starch to maltose by pancreatic amylase	Protein to peptides by proteases Some peptides to amino acids by proteases	Fat globules to emulsified fat by bile Lipids (fats) to fatty acids and glycerol by lipases
Ileum	Disaccharides such as maltose to glucose by maltase	Peptides to amino acids by proteases	Lipids (fats) to fatty acids and glycerol by lipases

ABSORPTION IN THE SMALL INTESTINE

To enter the body, digested food must leave the lumen of the alimentary canal by crossing the lining of the digestive tract. This happens in the ileum.

The mucosa of the ileum is folded into fine, finger-like projections into the lumen. Each projection is called a **villus** (plural is villi) – see Figure 5.31.

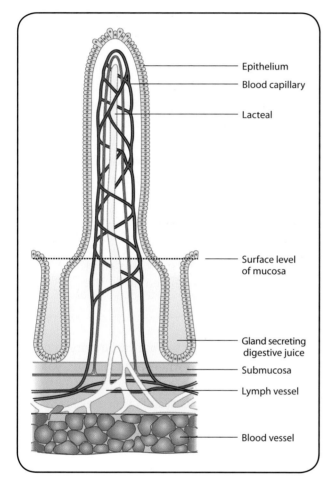

Epithelium
Blood capillary
Lacteal
Surface level of mucosa
Gland secreting digestive juice
Submucosa
Lymph vessel
Blood vessel

Figure 5.31 A single villus

The epithelial cells of the villi possess **microvilli**. The villi and the microvilli increase the surface area through which absorption can take place. Each villus contains a network of blood capillaries. Most digested food in the lumen enters these capillaries by diffusion or by active transport. However, fatty acids and glycerol enter a tube in the middle of the villus called a **lacteal**. The lacteals form part of the body's lymphatic system, which transports lymph. This lymph drains back into the blood system eventually.

The blood vessels from the ileum join up to form the hepatic portal vein, which leads to the liver. This processes the digested food further. Excess glucose is stored as glycogen. Excess amino acids are converted to urea by a process called **deamination**. Urea is excreted from the body by the kidneys.

> **Think** In which ways is the structure of the ileum well adapted to the absorption of digested food?

ROLE OF DIGESTED FOOD IN THE BODY

The role of digested food is summarised in the table below:

Table 5.6 Role of digested food

Digested food	Role in the body
Glucose	first source of energy – used in respiration
Amino acids	build up to form proteins – used for building up and repairing tissues
Fatty acids and glycerol	used as a secondary energy source – build up into lipids for insulation and phospholipids for cell membranes

THE LARGE INTESTINE

The role of the large intestine is to eliminate waste. By the time the contents of the gut have reached the end of the small intestine, most of the digested food has been absorbed. The waste material consists mainly of cellulose (fibrous plant material) and other indigestible material. It also contains water, bacteria and cells lost from the lining of the gut. The first part of the large intestine is the colon and it is here that most of the remaining water is reabsorbed into body. This leaves a semi-solid paste called **faeces**. This is stored in the rectum until it is egested from the body through the anus.

HOW THE BODY SYSTEMS WORK TOGETHER IN ENERGY METABOLISM

We have looked at the cardiovascular, respiratory and digestive systems in detail. We shall now see how they interrelate to each other in energy metabolism. We shall see that other systems, such as the nervous system and endocrine system, have a part to play as well.

There is an overview of the role of the cardiovascular, respiratory and digestive systems on pages 160 and 161. Have another look at this before reading on.

CARDIOVASCULAR, RESPIRATORY AND DIGESTIVE SYSTEMS ROLE IN ENERGY METABOLISM

We have learned that respiration is the process that releases energy from food inside our cells. We have also learned that oxygen is needed to make this process efficient. Think for a minute how the cardiovascular, respiratory and digestive systems work together to make this happen.

- the digestive system breaks down the food so that it may be absorbed into the blood

- then the cardiovascular system carries the digested food from the ileum to all our cells.

At the same time:

- the respiratory system brings in oxygen into the blood through ventilation and then diffusion

- then the cardiovascular system carries the oxygen from the blood capillaries surrounding the lungs to the cells.

> *Think* Rewrite the four bullet points above in your own words, expanding each one to give more detail. Then, think about how carbon dioxide, a waste product of respiration, gets from the cells back into the atmosphere. Write your own bullet points to describe this.

OTHER SYSTEMS INVOLVED IN ENERGY METABOLISM

Let us think a bit more about how oxygen gets from the air to our cells and the part that other body systems play.

Overview the nervous system's role

You will find out more about the role of the nervous system when we discuss homeostasis on page 179, but here we shall give an overview.

The nervous system plays a part in the ventilation of the lungs. We have learned that, in order to breathe in, our diaphragm and intercostal muscles must contract. The stimulus for this contraction comes from the nervous system. Likewise, the stimulus for them to relax, so we can breathe out, also comes from the nervous system.

> *Think* How is the nervous system involved in breathing in and breathing out? Produce a table to show this (hint: consider what is happening to the different muscles).

Consider what happens to your respiratory and cardiovascular systems when you exercise: you breathe faster and deeper, and your heart beats faster. It is the nervous system that makes this happen and we shall learn more about this on pages 182 and 183.

Overview of the endocrine system's role

Many hormones are involved in energy metabolism. The one you are probably most familiar with is adrenaline, which is secreted from the adrenal glands. Adrenaline is released into the blood at times of 'fight or flight' – when we are stressed or when we exercise. It stimulates the heart to beat faster, and faster and deeper breathing. This, of course, brings more oxygen to the cells for respiration.

There are two hormones secreted by the pancreas that are involved in energy metabolism. Insulin stimulates excess glucose in the blood to be stored as glycogen. Glucagon stimulates stored energy to be broken down to glucose when the body requires more energy.

Recent studies have pointed to the adipose tissue (see page 158) as a highly active endocrine organ secreting a range of hormones that take part in energy metabolism. An example of this is leptin, which regulates appetite and energy balance.

EVIDENCE ACTIVITY

P4 – M1 – D1

For P4 you need to describe the role of energy in the body and the physiology of three named body systems in relation to energy metabolism. To gain M1, in addition, you need to explain the physiology of three named body systems in relation to energy metabolism. To gain D1 you also need to explain how body systems interrelate with each other.

To achieve this, consider which three systems you are going to discuss. The key systems described here are the cardiovascular, respiratory and digestive systems, and so it seems sensible to choose these systems. Note the key difference between the pass criteria and the merit criteria – you have to explain as well as describe for a merit. It would seem sensible to explain how each system relates to energy metabolism as you describe it, rather than doing the explanations all at the end after the descriptions. For a distinction, you also need to consider how these systems relate to each other and also consider what role additional systems play.

Here is one way in which you might gather evidence for the latter.

- Write a summary of what happens in the cardiovascular system when a person exercises. Remember to include explanations where you can.

- Write a summary of what happens in the respiratory system when a person exercises. Remember to include explanations where you can.

- Write a summary of what happens in the digestive system when a person exercises. Remember to include explanations where you can.

- Write a summary of how the three systems work together during exercise. (Hint: you should have already done the exercise in the previous 'think' question, although that was not particularly related to exercise.)

- Add into your paragraph an explanation of the part other systems in the body play in energy metabolism during exercise.

5.3 How homeostatic mechanisms operate in the maintenance of an internal environment

HOMEOSTASIS

The word **homeostasis** means 'staying the same'. It is important that the conditions inside the body remain relatively constant. The nineteenth century French physiologist Claude Bernard stated that 'the constancy of the internal environment is the condition for a free life'. He meant that we can be freed from the limitations of our external environment only if we can create a stable internal environment.

> ***Think*** We are able to live in both hot and cold countries because out bodies have the ability to regulate temperate. What would happen if we could not regulate our temperature?

179

Our internal environment is our tissue fluid (lymph) in which our cells are bathed. All substances must pass through this fluid as they move to and from our cells. We saw on page 168 that tissue fluid is derived from blood, so blood is also part of our internal environment. Our enzymes operate within very narrow ranges of temperature and pH. Only if these conditions are maintained at their optimum levels can efficiency of enzyme activity be assured.

CONTROL MECHANISMS AND FEEDBACK

The maintenance of stability requires control systems capable of detecting any deviation from normal and making the necessary adjustments to return to these conditions. Self-regulating mechanisms like this operate by means of feedback mechanisms.

The necessary parts of a control system, shown in the diagram, are as follows:

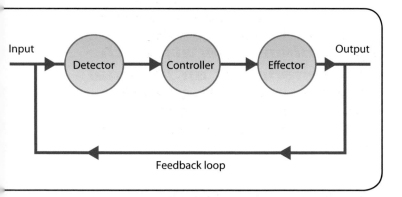

Figure 5.32 The components of a typical control system

- **Reference point** – the set level or normal level at which the system operates.

- **Detector** – detects or signals any deviation, and the extent of it, from the reference point.

- **Controller** – co-ordinates the information from the various detectors and sends out instructions that will correct the situation. In humans this is the brain.

- **Effector** – brings about change needed to return the system to the reference point.

- **Feedback loop** – informs the detector of any change in the system as a result of action by the effector.

This outline of how a control system operates can apply to any control system, biological or non-biological. It could apply, for example, to a house central heating system or to human body temperature control.

The mechanism to return the system back to the reference point after a deviation is called **negative feedback**. Note this might not necessarily be a reduction in, say temperature; it could be a rise back to normal following a fall in temperature. It is called negative feedback because it works in the opposite way to the original change from normal.

We shall now look at the homeostatic mechanisms that operate in different systems in the body. You need to know about the regulation of the following:

- heart rate

- breathing rate

- body temperature

- blood glucose.

CONTROL OF HEART RATE

You have already learned about the structure of the heart (see page 165) and heart rate (see page 166). We learned that the heart is composed of cardiac muscle. The cells of cardiac muscle are self-excitable or myogenic. This means that they can contract without any signal from the nervous system. Isolated hearts continue to beat for some time after they have been removed from an organism.

The contraction of the muscle cells must be co-ordinated, so that they all contract together. In order to do this the cells are arranged in continuous sheets of fibres. However, at the junction between the atria and the ventricles the sheet of cardiac muscle is interrupted by a layer of fibrous tissue. This controls the movement of contraction between atria and ventricles.

The rate of contraction is set by a specialised region of the heart called the **sinoatrial (SA) node**, also known as the **pacemaker**. The SA node is located in the wall of the right atrium, near the point where the anterior vena cava enters the heart. It is composed of specialised muscle tissue that combines the characteristics of muscle and nerve. It contracts like muscle, but in doing so it generates a wave of electrical activity. This wave of contraction radiates from the SA node across both atria until it reaches the fibrous ring at the AV junction.

At the AV junction there is another node, called the **atrioventicular (AV) node**. When the wave of excitation reaches the AV node, it is delayed for about 0.1 second, which ensures that the atria contract and empty completely before the ventricles contract. After this slight delay, the signal to contract is conducted to the tips the ventricles along bundle branches called the bundle of His, which spreads out into fibres called Purkinje fibres. From the apex of the heart, the wave of contraction passes upwards across the ventricles through these fibres.

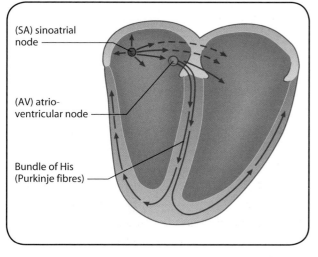

(SA) sinoatrial node

(AV) atrio-ventricular node

Bundle of His (Purkinje fibres)

Figure 5.33 The origin and control of the heartbeat

So, where does homeostasis come into this? You will be aware that your heart rate increases when you exercise or when you are frightened. That is perfectly normal and ensures that more food and oxygen is brought to respiring cells, so that more energy may be released. It also ensures that waste products, such as carbon dioxide, are removed quickly. You will also be aware that your heart rate returns to normal after you have finished exercising or have calmed down. We shall now see what causes the heart rate to increase and which homeostatic mechanism causes it to return to normal. This increase and decrease are both under the control of the autonomic nervous system and adrenaline from the endocrine system.

The autonomic nervous system

The **autonomic nervous system** controls the involuntary activities of smooth muscles and some glands. It is actually part of the peripheral nervous system and can be divided into two parts, the **sympathetic nervous system** and the **parasympathetic nervous system**. Both systems comprise motor neurones, which connect the central nervous system to their effector organs. The effects of the sympathetic and parasympathetic systems are antagonistic: that is they oppose each other. If the sympathetic nervous system is stimulated our heart rate increases. If the parasympathetic nervous system is stimulated our heart rate decreases.

The sympathetic nervous system

In general, stimulation of the sympathetic nervous system produces effects in muscles and glands that prepare us for stress, such as for shock, danger or exercise.

The following are examples of some of these effects:

- heart rate increased
- blood flow increased to muscles, lungs and brain
- blood flow decreased to gut and kidney
- arterioles in the skin contracted
- breathing rate increased
- bronchioles dilated
- glycogen converted to glucose in the liver
- peristalsis slowed
- iris in the eye is dilated
- sweat production increased
- muscles of hairs contracted
- bladder and anal sphincters contracted.

In addition, the adrenal glands produce more adrenaline, which has the same effect as the sympathetic stimulation.

> **Think** All these effects mean we are in the best condition to react to stress or to exercise. How might each of these effects contribute towards this?

The parasympathetic nervous system

The effects of stimulating the parasympathetic nervous system are the exact opposite of those produced by sympathetic stimulation. This would happen following a period of exercise when we are resting.

> **Think** What is the effect of stimulating the parasympathetic? (Hint: Look at the list of effects of stimulating the sympathetic nervous system.)

Control of heartbeat during exercise

The **cardiac centre** is in the medulla of the brain. It receives signals from chemoreceptors (receptors that detect chemicals). These receptors are located in the walls of the aorta and carotid arteries, which take blood to the brain.

When we exercise, increased respiration leads to a rise in the carbon dioxide in the blood. This is detected by the chemoreceptors. They send a greater number of nerve impulses to the cardiac centre than normal. The cardiac centre responds by sending nerve impulses along the sympathetic nerves to the SA node, the AV node and the ventricle walls, causing the heart rate to increase. The blood supply to the lungs is also increased so that carbon dioxide is taken to the lungs for quicker removal. We shall see that the increased blood flow helps us to cool down as we exercise. The control of the heartbeat during exercise is seen in figure 5.34.

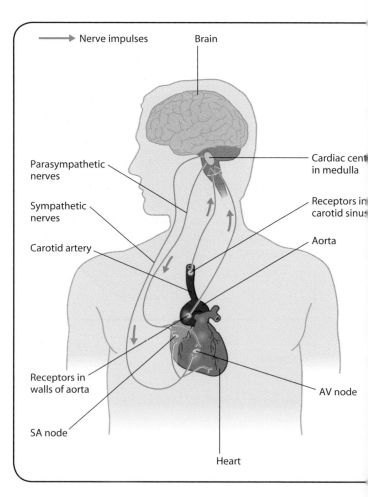

Figure 5.34 The control of the heartbeat during exercise

CONTROL OF BREATHING RATE

Our breathing rate is controlled by the nerves that are under the control of the respiratory centre in the medulla of the brain. The medulla has nerves going to the intercostal muscles and the diaphragm muscles.

When we breathe in the lungs become stretched. Stretch receptors in the lungs send nerve impulses to the respiratory centre along the vagus nerve. We already know that chemoreceptors in the aorta and carotid arteries are stimulated by carbon dioxide. There are also receptors directly in the medulla itself. The respiratory centre combines the information and controls the breathing rate via nerve impulses to the intercostal muscles and muscles of the diaphragm.

Breathing in and out

Our normal breathing could be thought of as a homeostatic mechanism. What stops us breathing in and makes us breathe out? What then stops us breathing out and start to breathe in again? The following steps should make this clear:

- We breathe in when the respiratory centre sends impulses to the intercostal muscles and the muscles of the diaphragm. These then contract and the lungs inflate.

- Inflation of the stretch receptors in the lungs and bronchioles send impulses to the respiratory centre, which then stops sending impulses to the intercostal muscles and the muscles of the diaphragm. This stops us breathing in.

- The intercostal muscles and the muscles of the diaphragm relax and we breathe out.

- The stretch receptors are no longer stimulated, so the respiratory centre sends impulses to the intercostal muscles and the muscles of the diaphragm once more-enabling us to breathe in again.

> **Think** How is breathing in and out an example of a homeostatic mechanism?

Control of breathing rate during exercise

The mechanism that controls breathing rate during exercise is very similar to that which controls heart rate during exercise. You must take care to ensure that you do not get the two mixed up.

As in the control of heart rate, it is the rise in the concentration of carbon dioxide levels in the blood during exercise that sets off changes. However, this time the changes are to the rate and depth of breathing. The chemoreceptors in the aorta, carotid arteries and the medulla detect higher levels of carbon dioxide during exercise. These chemoreceptors send an increased number of nerve impulses to the respiratory centre, which then sends an increased number of nerve impulses to the intercostal muscles and the muscles of the diaphragm. This causes the rate and depth of breathing to increase. These impulses travel down sympathetic nerves. The excess carbon dioxide is removed from the blood and the level returns to normal. This lowered level then stimulates the parasympathetic nervous system to decrease the rate and depth of breathing. The control of breathing during increased exercise is shown in Figure 5.35 on page 184.

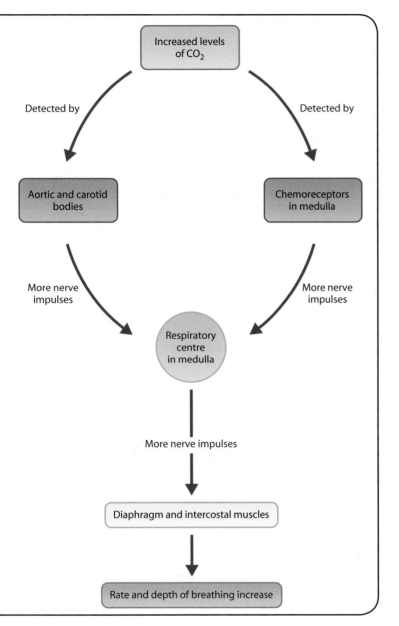

Figure 5.35 The control of breathing during increased exercise

CONTROL OF TEMPERATURE

Chemical reactions are very sensitive to temperature changes. For example, respiration increases with temperature up to a certain point, and then declines when temperatures are high enough to begin denaturing the enzymes (i.e. destroying the enzymes' structure). Therefore, in the interests of ensuring efficiency in chemical reactions, the temperature of cells must be maintained at an optimum level. Normal body temperature is around 36.8^0C, (ranging from 36.5 to 37.2^0C).

Table 5.7 shows what happens in the body if the temperature is outside the normal range.

Table 5.7 Effects of temperature

Temperature	Effect
Below 25^0C	low temperature that would lead to death
32^0C	hypothermia
$36.5 – 37.2^0C$	(normal)
Above 37.2^0C	fever
Above 38^0C	heat exhaustion
Above 43^0C	high temperature that would lead to death

Heat loss and gain

When we talk about our temperature, we mean the core temperature of the body. The surface temperature can fluctuate rapidly, but it is the internal or core temperature which is important when we are considering the operation of enzymes. We are continually losing and gaining heat. It is the balance between these which determines whether the core temperature falls, rises or stays the same. Babies who have a high surface area to volume ratio, tend to lose heat more rapidly than adults.

There are several ways in which an organism may gain or lose heat.

Heat is gained in the following ways:

- **metabolism of food** – heat produced by some reactions warms the core of the organism

- **absorption of solar energy** – directly, or indirectly, from:

  - heat reflected or radiated from objects

  - heat convected (rising) from the warming of the ground

  - heat conducted as we make direct contact with the ground.

Heat is lost by:

- **Evaporation** of water – this occurs during sweating. It can only occur if the air is not already saturated with water, i.e. the relative humidity is less than 100%.

- **Conduction** from the body – where heat is lost to the ground or by touching other cooler objects.

- **Convection** from the body – heat lost upwards to the cooler air.

- **Radiation** from the body – heat is moved outwards from the body in all directions to the cooler air.

Mechanisms of temperature control

Humans, like many animals, are endotherms or warm-blooded. We derive most of our heat from our metabolism. This is in contrast to ectotherms, such are reptiles, which warm their bodies mainly by absorbing heat from their surroundings. We lose heat through the respiratory surfaces, the gut and the skin. Heat loss cannot be prevented through the first two, but the skin is able to control heat loss. The skin is therefore the main organ of thermoregulation.

Structure of the skin

The skin covers the body and is the largest single organ. Figure 5.36 gives a generalised picture of human skin.

There are two main layers, the epidermis and the dermis. The epidermis is the outer layer and is an example of keratinised compound epithelium (see page 157). As new cells are made in the malpighian layer older cells are pushed outwards. They become more and more flattened, die and become cornified, forming a waterproof layer pierced only by hairs and the pores of glands. The dermis is the lower layer of the skin and it is composed of connective tissue made up of collagen and elastic fibres. The following structures are found there:

- Blood vessels – bring food and oxygen to cells, take away waste and help regulate temperature.

- Sweat glands – produce sweat, which is involved in lowering temperature.

- Nerve endings – sensory cells providing information on the external environment.

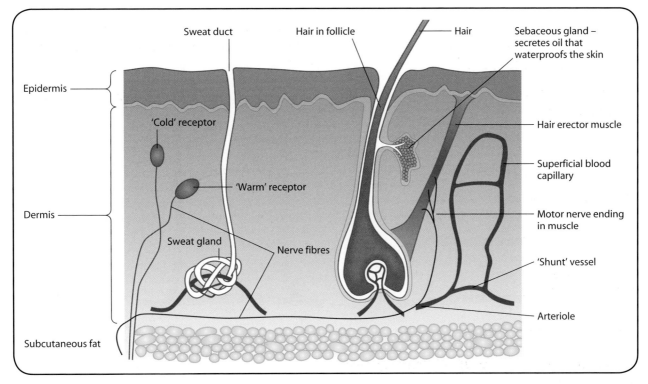

Figure 5.36 The structure of skin

- Hair follicles – muscles contract and relax to make hair erect or flatten to help raise or lower temperature, respectively.

- Sebaceous glands – produce an oily secretion called 'sebum' which waterproofs hair and the epidermis.

Response of the body to cooling

When we are in an environment at a temperature lower than normal body temperature, there is a tendency for heat to be lost. Heat loss can be minimised in the following ways:

- **Increasing metabolic rate** – any chemical reaction, such as respiration, produces heat.

- **Shivering** – involuntary rapid contraction and relaxation of muscles produce heat.

- **Vasoconstriction** – arterioles in the skin constrict and arteriovenous shunts come into operation. Blood is diverted through the lower skin layers. People with white skins who are cold appear very pale. Vasoconstriction and arteriovenous shunts are shown in the diagram below.

Figure 5.37 Vasoconstriction and arterio-venous shunts

Response of the body to heating

In the UK we are unlikely to encounter temperatures higher than body temperature of 37°C. However, our bodies may overheat through exertion or through a fever due to illness. Under these circumstances we need to lose heat rather than conserve it. Mechanisms to increase the rate of heat loss include:

- **Decreasing metabolic rate** – as the metabolic rate falls, activity slows to a minimum.

- **Sweating** – evaporation of water is a good way to lose heat. Sweat produced by dermal glands is released onto the surface of the skin, where it evaporates. The heat required to evaporate the sweat (the latent heat of vaporisation) is taken from the body, which consequently cools.

- **Vasodilation** – arterioles in the skin dilate, bringing warmed blood to the surface and increasing heat loss by radiation and convection. People with white skins who are hot appear flushed.

- **Insulation** – relaxation of the hair erector muscles lowers the hair, meaning there is less of an insulating layer of warm air next to the skin.

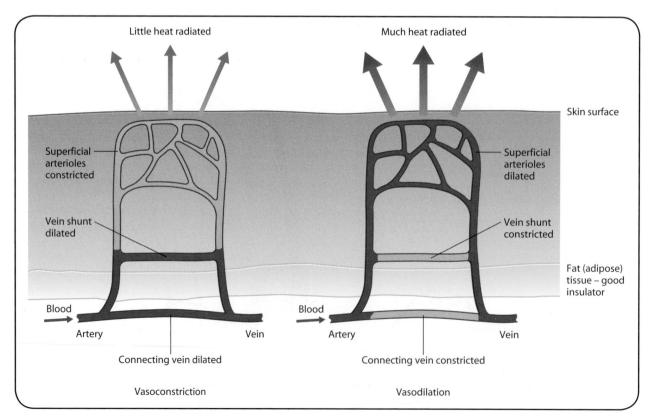

Control of body temperature

The skin contains thermo-receptors, which register changes in environmental temperature, but the skin is not the primary detector of temperature change.

Example

In a classic experiment, a naked man was placed inside a chamber with in which the temperature could be changed. Thermometers were placed against the subject's eardrum – the nearest point to the brain. The temperature inside the chamber was raised and the body of the man reacted as expected, e.g. vasodilation, he produced sweat etc. Then, while maintaining the high temperature in the chamber, the man was given iced drinks. Although the skin temperature remained high, the blood temperature fell because of the absorption of iced water. The body reacted as though the external temperature had fallen, e.g. vasoconstriction etc. So it would seem that the primary detector of temperature change is a region of the brain and not the skin.

The primary temperature detector region lies in the hypothalamus (in our forebrain). This region is sensitive to the temperature of the blood flowing through it. Within the hypothalamus is the thermoregulatory centre, which has two parts: a heat gain and a heat loss centre. The hypothalamus monitors the temperature of blood passing through it and in addition receives nervous information from the receptors in the skin about external temperature.

The hypothalamus has nervous and hormonal connections with a wide range of organs that contribute to the maintenance of body temperature. See Figure 5.38 below.

Control of body temperature, and other processes such as heart rate and breathing, involves the autonomic nervous system. This is the part of the nervous system which is not under conscious control. The autonomic nervous system consists of two components: the sympathetic nervous system, which in general increases organ activity; and the parasympathetic nervous system, which in general decreases organ activity.

> **Think** Make a table that summarises the key mechanism that operate when we are too hot and too cold.
>
> Figure 5.38 shows the higher centres in the brain linked to behaviour. What conscious decisions might you would make if you were (a) too cold or (b) too hot?

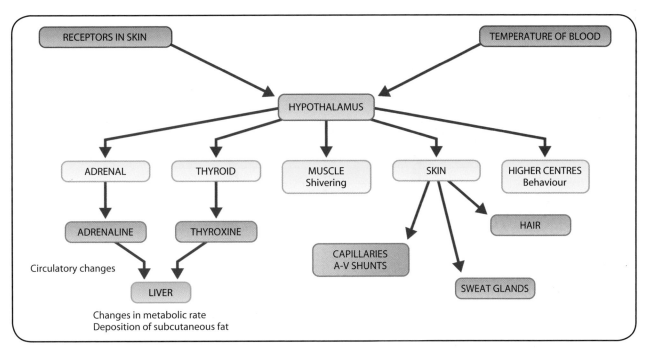

Figure 5.38 The role of the hypothalamus in the control of body temperature

CONTROL OF BLOOD GLUCOSE

The level of glucose in the blood, often referred to as the blood sugar level, is of great importance to the cells of the body because they use glucose for respiration. If the level falls too low, the cells are starved of energy. The cells of the brain are particularly vulnerable and a coma quickly results. Conversely, too much sugar affects the osmotic balance and water is lost from cells. The normal fasting glucose level in the blood is 3.5 – 7.5 mmol dm^3, or you may see it quoted as around 90 mg glucose per 100 cm^3 blood.

Throughout the day our supply of carbohydrates fluctuates because we do not eat continuously and the quantity of carbohydrate taken in can vary from one meal to the next. Thus, there may be quite long periods where glucose is not being absorbed from the small intestine. Cells, however, metabolise continuously and need a constant supply of glucose. It is therefore essential to have a system which can maintain a constant supply of glucose in the blood, despite intermittent supplies from the digestive system.

This is achieved by the interactions of several hormones with the glycogen stored in the liver. Two of the most important of these hormones,

insulin and **glucagon**, are produced by endocrine cells in the pancreas called the islets of Langerhans. Insulin is produced in cells known as gk beta cells and glucagon is produced in cells known as gk alpha cells.

- **Insulin** lowers blood glucose if the level goes too high. Excess glucose is converted to glycogen and stored in the liver.

- **Glucagon** raises blood glucose if the level goes too low. Glycogen in the liver is broken down to glucose and released into the blood.

The interaction of insulin and glucagon in controlling blood glucose is shown in the diagram below.

Diabetes

There are different types of diabetes. The most common is called diabetes mellitus. This occurs when the pancreas does not function properly and insufficient insulin is produced to control the level of glucose in the blood, or when insulin is produced but the receptors on the cells do not seem to recognise it. The end result is the same: blood glucose tends to be too high and sometimes glucose appears in the urine.

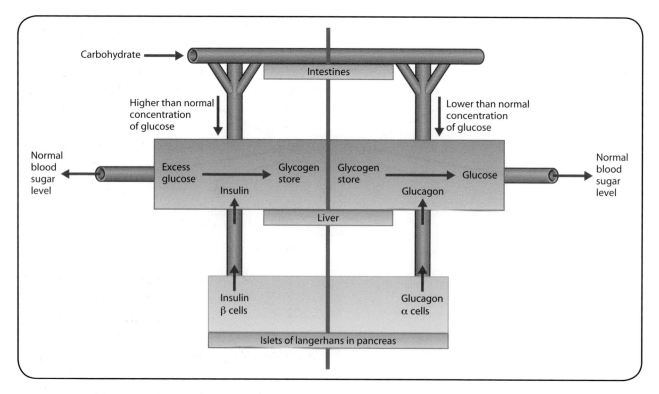

Figure 5.39 The interaction of insulin and glucagon in controlling blood glucose

If insulin is not produced in sufficient quantities by the pancreas, this is referred to as TypeI or insulin-dependent diabetes (mellitus). People with this type of diabetes have injections of insulin. If insulin is produced by the pancreas but it cannot be used, this is referred to as Type II or insulin-non-dependent diabetes (mellitus). People who have this have to control the amount of sugar they eat in their diet. There is no point in having injections of insulin as the body cannot use it.

There is another type of diabetes, called 'diabetes insipidus', which may occur as a result of kidney impairment.

EVIDENCE ACTIVITY

P5 – M2 – D2

For P5 you need to show that you understand the concept of homeostasis and give a description of the homeostatic mechanisms that regulate heart rate, breathing rate, body temperature and blood glucose levels. To gain M2, in addition, you need to explain how these homeostatic responses work. To gain D2, in addition, you need to relate these explanations to maintaining the healthy functioning of the body.

To help you to achieve this, consider each of the homeostatic mechanisms we have discussed in turn.

• Describe what happens when there is an increase in the level, i.e. of heart rate, breathing rate, temperature, blood glucose.

• Describe what happens when there is a decrease in each of the levels.

• While you are doing that, or after if you prefer, give an explanation of how the mechanism works; for example, how sweating helps to lower temperature.

• Consider, for each mechanism, what would happen if it was faulty; for example, if we could not sweat or there was a problem with the parasympathetic nervous system that linked to the heart or intercostal muscles.

5.4 *Interpreting data obtained from monitoring routine variations in the functioning of healthy body system*

GATHERING AND ANALYSING DATA

You need to be able to interpret data obtained from monitoring routine variations in the functioning of healthy body systems. You also need to investigate the effects of exercise. It is most likely that you will gather data from the people in your class, but you may use other subjects as well. The specification requires that you know how to take measurements of pulse rate, breathing rate and temperature. You may well have access to other equipment, such as sphygmomanometers for measuring blood pressure, spirometers for measuring vital capacity and peak flow meters for measuring peak flow. If you are going to use these, you need to make sure that you work with your teachers to follow safe practice. This is true of all practical activities.

MEASUREMENT OF PULSE RATE

Measuring pulse rate is a convenient way of measuring heart rate. The pumping action of the heart causes a regular pulsation in the flow of blood. Arteries have thick muscular walls (see page 167) that alternately expand and recoil with the flow of blood. This can be felt in arteries near the surface which lie over bone or other firm tissue. The most common places where a pulse is measured are:

• in the radial artery in the wrist

• in the carotid artery in the neck

• in the femoral artery in the groin.

A pulse should be measured by placing the second and third fingers over the artery and gently pressing it. The thumb should never be used as it has too strong a pulse of its own. There are no particular safety issues to consider when taking pulse rates. However, it is good practice to have the person seated and not to press too hard. Many people get anxious when they have measurements taken and this can sometimes make a result artificially high. A normal resting pulse is between 60 and 80 beats per minute. If someone has a resting pulse rate outside this range, there may be reasons for this. In general, the lower the resting pulse rate, the fitter the person usually is.

To work out the pulse rate, you can count the number of beats in a minute. You will need a stopwatch in order to do this. You could also count the number of beats in 30 seconds and multiply by two, or the number of beats in 15 seconds and multiply by four.

> **Think** Which of the above methods calculating a person's pulse rate you do think is the most accurate?

Sources of error

In general, the longer period over which the pulse rate is measured, the more accurate the answer is likely to be. Imagine if you counted the pulse for just 5 seconds and found that there were six beats. That would mean that the rate per minute is 72 (= (6/5) × 60). Suppose that you repeated the measurement and found that the second time the answer was seven beats. That would mean that the rate per minute is 84 (= (7/5) × 60). Think about that for a minute. Does this mean that a person cannot have a pulse rate of 74, 76, 78, 80, 82 etc.? We could not be sure because you cannot count in fractions of a beat.

To check the reliability of your method, you need to be able repeat the measurement, under the same conditions, and get the same result. Here there is some doubt about the reliability of this method. The first measurement gave an answer of 72 beats per minute and the second measurement gave an answer of 84 beats per minute. In general it is a good idea to repeat measurements several times, under exactly the same conditions. You may find that you have one result that is very different from the rest. This is called an anomalous

result. However, you are unlikely to find that a person's resting pulse rate is identical every time it is taken. This is because there are slight natural variations.

Example

Four boys, A, B, C and D, and four girls, E, F, G and H had their resting pulse rates measured. The results are shown below.

Resting pulse rate (beats per minute)

Measurement	A	B	C	D	E	F	G	H
1	72	74	82	68	75	78	67	84
2	74	71	78	70	73	92	68	82
3	79	68	80	66	77	73	69	80
Average	75	71		66	75	81	68	80

You will notice that there is a blank space in the table. This may be filled in by working out the average for Boy C. The separate values are added together, and then divided by 3 (82 + 78 + 80 = 240, 240/3 = 80).

Look at the table of results carefully. Pick out a result that is anomalous.

MEASUREMENT OF BREATHING RATE

Breathing is the process by which air enters and leaves our body. Our breathing rate is the number of breaths we take in one minute. One breath is considered to be one breath in and one breath out. Measurement should be over at least one minute as the normal range for breathing rate at rest is 15–18 breaths per minute. Measuring a person's breathing rate manually at rest is best done by the person themselves. This is because it is not easy to observe another persons breathing unless they are breathing deeply, for example during exercise.

Sources of error

The main source of error is the accuracy of measuring. We have discussed why a manual measurement is better done by the person themselves, but the fact of being aware of your breathing in itself tends to make you breath either faster or slower. Breathing is done unconsciously and is controlled homeostatically, but when we are aware of it, the rate can easily alter.

Errors may also be made if the time period for counting is too low. If counting is over, say, 15 seconds, a normal value for the resting rate would be around 4 breaths only. A measurement of 3 breaths in 15 seconds or 5 breaths in 15 seconds would mean that the breathing rate per minute was outside the normal resting value.

As with pulse rate, measurements should be repeated to ensure reliability.

MEASUREMENT OF TEMPERATURE

Core temperature may be measured in the mouth, in the ear or in the anus. Skin temperature may be measured directly on the skin itself. Our discussion of homeostasis (see pages 179–181) showed that it is the core temperature that is of main interest. Sometimes a person's temperature is taken under the arm. This may be for various reasons, such as they are not comfortable about having it taken in the mouth. Note that this does not strictly give a reading of core temperature.

Temperature is most usually measured by placing a thermometer under the tongue for a period of time. Increasingly electronic thermometers are being used because they give a more accurate reading and are safer to use. Thermometers containing mercury are being phased out. Mercury is a poison and someone may inadvertently bite on the thermometer and break it. Table 5.8 shows different types of thermometer along with their advantages and disadvantages. Infra-red thermometers work by measuring the infrared heat given off by the eardrum.

DATA PRESENTATION AND INTERPRETATION

Once you have collected your information you need to consider how you are going to present your data and interpret or analyse it. Data may be presented in tables/charts and/or in graphs. It is usual to present your data first of all in a table or chart.

You should always give your raw data, as well as your average data. Raw data is the data from each measurement; your first reading, second reading etc. Average data is derived by working out the mean or average from the raw data. You may present the average data in the same table, as in the example on resting pulse rate (on page 190). You may also wish to present summary tables that show your average data only.

Table 5.8 Types of thermometer

Type of thermometer	Where used	Advantages	Disadvantages
Clinical – coloured liquid in glass	mouth, armpit	cheap	may be difficult to read; disinfection required to help prevent cross infection
Electronic	mouth, rectal, armpit	clear digital reading; may be disposable cover over the probe	expensive
Infra-red	ear	easy to use; may be disposable cover over the probe	expensive
LCD strip	forehead	easy to use; cheap	just gives skin temperature; not precise

This worked example shows you how to analyse your data.

Example

A student carried out a project comparing fitness in boys and girls. The student decided to monitor the time it took for pulse rate to return to normal after exercise. Four people (subjects A–D) took part in the investigation. The subjects had their pulse rates taken at rest. Each subject then carried out the same exercise for the same length of time, and had their pulse rate taken immediately after the end of the exercise period and then each minute following that. The results are shown in the table below.

When pulse rate was taken	Pulse rate (beats per minute)			
	A	B	C	D
Resting	75	71	80	66
Immediately after exercise finished	94	94	99	78
1 minute after exercise finished	88	89	95	75
2 minutes after exercise finished	82	80	92	70
3 minutes after exercise finished	80	76	92	65
4 minutes after exercise finished	76	74	89	66
5 minutes after exercise finished	77	71	88	65

You could draw a graph of pulse rate against time after exercise for each person. Try this and see if you feel this makes your analysis easier.

Look at each of the people in turn.

- Person A's pulse rate has nearly returned to normal 4 minutes after exercise, but then is rises slightly from 76 to 77 beats per minute 5 minutes after exercise. This rise may not be significant.

- Person B's pulse rate returns to the resting value of 71 beats per minute 5 minutes after finishing exercise.

- Person C's pulse rate has not returned to the resting value of 80 beats per minute 5 minutes after finishing exercise. It is still high at a value of 88 beats per minute.

- Person D's pulse rate returns to the resting value of 66 beats per minute 3 minutes after finishing exercise.

This is a description of the results only. We now need to interpret them.

What do the results mean? To answer this you need to know that the quicker a person's pulse rate returns to normal following exercise, the fitter they are. This is because their homeostatic mechanism for heart rate is working efficiently. We also need to know that the lower a person's resting pulse rate, the fitter they are. (Note we do not know whether the values for resting pulse rate, or indeed any of the values, are single measurements or average values.)

Looking at the results, we can see that Person D is the fittest based on both these criteria. Their pulse rate returns to the resting value of 65 quickest, 3 minutes after exercise. Their value for resting pulse rate is the lowest, towards the lower end of the normal 60 – 80 beats per minute range.

Person C is the least fit based on both these criteria. Their pulse rate has not returned to the resting value, even 5 minutes after finishing exercise. Their resting pulse rate is at the very top of the normal range of 60 – 80 beats per minute. It is clear that their homeostatic mechanism is not working efficiently. The heart is still beating fast at 88 beats per minute 5 minutes after finishing exercise. This could be because their temperature is still high and they need to cool down. Think how you could check this. It could also be because the level of carbon dioxide in the body is still high. Think about why maintaining a higher heart rate for longer is helpful here.

SUMMARY OF VALIDITY, RELIABILITY AND ACCURACY

You always need to consider whether your data is valid, reliable and accurate. Data is valid if the method you use gives you the correct data. For example, does measuring pulse rate manually give heart rate? Does the thermometer you use give temperature? Data is reliable if the method used generates the same data under the same conditions. Are the results for a particular person the same or are there lots of anomalous results? If the latter occurs, then your method is not reliable. Data is accurate if the method or machine used gives the required precision. For example, does your thermometer measure to the nearest degree or tenth of a degree? The latter is more accurate than the former.

EVIDENCE

P6 – M3

For P6 you need to measure body temperature, heart rate and breathing rate before and after a standard period of exercise, interpret the data and comment on its validity. To gain M3, in addition, you need to analyse data to show how homeostatic mechanisms control the internal environment during exercise.

1. To help you to achieve this, read through the example again. Now generate some data of your own. If you are fit enough you could try the Harvard step test – to find out how fit you are.

• Step up and down onto a bench for 300 seconds (5 minutes)

• 1 minute after finishing the test count your pulse for 30 seconds.

• 2 minutes after finishing the test count your pulse for a further 30 seconds.

• 3 minutes after finishing the test, count your pulse count for another 30 seconds.

a) Use the formula to work out your fitness:

fitness =

$$\frac{\text{Time spent on exercise (secs) x 100}}{2 \times (\text{1st + 2nd + 3rd pulse counts})}$$

b) Use the fitness scale to work out your fitness:

Value from formula	Fitness scale
90 plus	super fit
80 – 89	very fit
70 – 79	fit
60 – 69	fair
less than 60	unfit

c) Repeat the investigation with some other subjects.

d) Repeat the investigation over a period of time and see if training makes a difference.

2. When you evaluate your results, consider validity, reliability and accuracy. In interpreting your results, draw on your scientific knowledge to discuss how well the various homeostatic mechanisms are working.

Personal and Professional Development in Health and Social Care

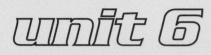

This unit brings together your learning from all the other units and highlights the vocational nature of this qualification. You will explore the different ways in which you can learn, as well as strategies for planning and monitoring your own professional and personal development. You will find out more about how your knowledge, skills set and experiences, both formal and informal, can help you get the job of your dreams.

Learning outcomes

By the end of this unit, you will:

6.1 Understand the learning process   page 197

6.2 Be able to plan for, monitor and reflect on own development   page 207

6.3 Understand service provision in the health and social care sectors   page 217

So you want to be a...

Midwife

My name Jennifer Lockhart
Age 25
Income £27,622

*If you're as cool as a cucumber yet compassionate to boot,
a career in midwifery could be just up your street.*

So, what do you do?

I provide advice, care and support for women and their families throughout their pregnancy, labour and birth, and for several weeks after the baby has arrived.

How did you get into it?

I did my three-year nursing degree and started practising as a community midwife two years ago, working both from a GP practice and the hospital.

Is work experience important?

It's not vital, but I would highly recommend spending time work shadowing midwives to see where you would be working and what you'd be doing. It also looks great on application forms as it shows a real commitment to the field.

What does a typical week involve?

I run an antenatal clinic at a GP practice. I take blood pressure, test urine samples, answer any questions the woman may have and give advice if they are suffering from any physical or emotional problems. The rest of my time is spent either at the hospital, helping women to deliver their babies and establish breastfeeding, or visiting new mums to make sure they and their babies are doing well.

> **“I provide advice, care and support...”**

Sounds pretty hectic. Are the working hours long?

They can be. Babies arrive at all times of the day and night and some take ages to appear! We work different shifts, but if you've been with someone throughout a long labour and she still hasn't given birth when your shift ends, it's always lovely to stay and see the end result!

What's the money like?

People who go into healthcare aren't usually driven by the desire to earn big bucks. However, newly qualified midwives earn around £19,166, while those in senior positions take home between £27,622 and £36,416 so it's not too bad.

What sort of person makes a good midwife?

All nurses have to be compassionate and a good listener, but especially midwives. You need good stamina to get you through long shifts, especially during the night. We take sole charge of the situation, unless the mother or baby gets into trouble, so you need to be comfortable with that amount of responsibility.

Where do you go from here?

When I'm more experienced, I'd like to work towards becoming a consultant midwife, where I could combine patient care with research.

Grading criteria

The table below shows what you need to do to gain a pass, merit or distinction in this part of the qualification. Make sure you refer back to it when you are completing work so you can judge whether you are meeting the criteria and what you need to do to fill in gaps in your knowledge or experience.

In this unit there are 4 evidence activities that give you an opportunity to demonstrate your achievement of the grading criteria:

page 207   P1, M1, D1

page 214   P2, P3, P4, M2, D2

page 216   P5, M3

page 227   P6, P7

To achieve a pass grade the evidence must show that the learner is able to...	To achieve a merit grade the evidence must show that, in addition to the pass criteria, the learner is able to...	To achieve a distinction grade the evidence must show that, in addition to the pass and merit criteria, the learner is able to...
P1 explain key influences on personal learning processes of individuals	**M1** analyse the impact of key influences on personal learning processes and on own learning	**D1** evaluate how personal learning and development may benefit others
P2 describe own knowledge, skills, practice, values, beliefs and career aspirations at the start of the programme		**D2** evaluate your own development over the duration of the programme
P3 produce and monitor an action plan for self-development and the achievement of own personal goals		
P4 describe own progress against action plans over the duration of the programme	**M2** explain how the action plan has helped support own development over the duration of the programme	
P5 produce and reflect on own personal and professional development portfolio	**M3** reflect on own experiences and use three examples to explain links between theory and practice	
P6 describe one local health or social care service provider and identify its place in national provision		
P7 describe the roles, responsibilities and career pathways of three health or social care workers		

6.1 Understanding the learning process

THEORIES OF LEARNING

Everyone has their own preferred way of learning, and this can affect the way they take in information.

American educational theorist David A Kolb explored the way in which learning takes place and identified four different stages. A **concrete experience** of a situation or event is followed by a personal **reflection** on that experience. This will then be followed by analysis and understanding of the experience or situation, which he called **abstract conceptualisation**. This enables you to make changes to the situation or experience the next time you are in it, through **active experimentation**. This then leads back to concrete experience again, and so the pattern continues. All this can happen immediately, over several days, weeks, months or years.

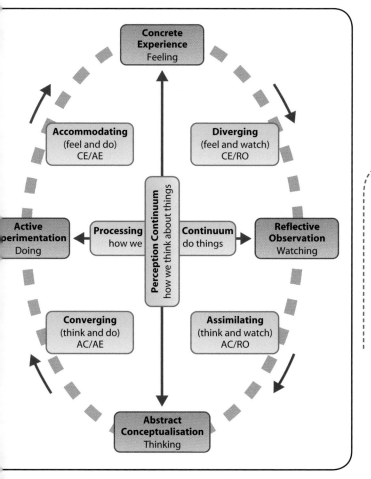

Figure 6.1 – Kolb's four stages of learning

[Source: Pearson Education]

Example

Anna was cycling to school on a very wet and rainy day. As she approached the traffic lights at a busy junction, she braked but her bicycle took a long time to come to a stop. Luckily she stopped before passing the lights, but the close call shook her. Anna thought about the experience for the rest of the way to school and how she could have done things differently to avoid the stressful situation. She realised her brakes took longer to work in wet weather and that she could have avoided the situation if she had slowed down or braked sooner. On the way home it was still raining heavily. She remembered the morning's experience and braked much earlier before reaching the set of lights.

Think How could you apply the four stages of Kolb's theory of learning to Anna's experience? How could you apply the stages to an experience in your own life?

You may find that one of these learning styles leaps out at you as matching your preferences. However, you might discover that while one type fits best, there are aspects of the others that apply to you too. This is fine: most of us have elements of more than one learning style.

Example

Susan is an experienced teacher who has taught Health and Social Care for many years. When she delivers a lesson on the experiences of racism to the class, she shows a video, asks students about their own experiences of racism and introduces them to some of the theoretical explanations on the issue. In the feedback session she asks the students what they found most helpful. One student liked the key messages from the video, another preferred to reflect on his own experiences of racism during his childhood and the experiences of the colleagues in the work setting. A third student preferred the theoretical explanations for racial discrimination and could not wait to apply some of the theory in practice.

Table 6.1 – Learning types based on Kolb's theory

Learner type	Likes/learns best	Dislikes/learns less well
Activist (common in people who are influenced by **concrete experience**)	• when 'doing' or 'experiencing' something • new experiences and challenges • working in groups • chairing meetings	• taking notes • working alone • listening to lessons
Reflector (common in people who are influenced by **reflective observation**)	• considering a situation from all angles before making a decision • producing reports in their own time • taking a back seat	• being a leader • acting spontaneously • being unprepared • working to deadlines
Theorist (common in people who are influenced by **abstract conceptualisation**)	• using skills and knowledge • tasks with a clear aim • questioning ideas	• situations requiring emotions and feelings • poor organisation • acting without knowing why or what is involved
Pragmatist (common in people who are influenced by **active experimentation**)	• likes to 'have a go' at something to see if it works • learning beneficial techniques (e.g. saving time) • copying something or someone they respect	• not seeing any obvious advantage to doing something • having no guidance • lack of rewards • too much theory and no practice

Think What is your preferred learning type and why?

INFLUENCES ON LEARNING

Learning is not just affected by your personal preferences and learning style. Many different factors affect the way in which you take in and store information.

Previous learning and experiences

Believe it or not, from the moment you were born you have been learning. Babies learn amazingly quickly through copying and listening to others; this is how they grasp basic language and communication skills. By the time you were ready for school, you were probably starting to be able to read and write, with some help from your carers.

Once at school, these skills will have gradually increased, with daily practice, to be at the level they are today. Of course, some of us will be stronger at reading than writing, for example, or better at talking and listening than studying from a book; and you will probably have discovered your strengths and weaknesses by now. The skills and knowledge you have developed from your previous learning and experiences will be the foundation for your future learning.

Research tip

The Campaign for Learning organisation provides excellent information on why learning is important, how you as an individual learn, and how you can improve your skills.

www.campaignforlearning.org.uk

Attitude and self-discipline

How well you take in information will partly depend on your attitude to learning. Even if you know you prefer a more 'hands-on' approach to study, you cannot use this as a valid excuse for not taking notes in a lecture! If you recognise that working on your own is not very motivational, try to think of ways to combat this: perhaps by teaming up with a study partner for some of the time.

Self-motivation is vital both in your studies and in the workplace. Most of us have aspects of our personal and professional lives that we would rather be without, but a positive attitude can work amazingly well to make even the more tedious aspects bearable.

> **Think** How self-disciplined are you? How could you improve on this?

Aspirations and motivations

Take a moment to consider the following questions:

- Why have you decided to do this course?

- What do you hope to gain from it?

- What is it about the health and social care sector that interests you?

- Is there a particular area you feel drawn to?

Often when you are studying, it can be hard to see where the reading, lessons, homework and assessments will lead you but thinking about these questions will help to give you some direction. Write out the answers if you like, and keep them as 'mission statements' in your notebook, or anywhere you are likely to come across them on a regular basis.

Studying can be hard work but if you keep your long-term goals in mind, rather than focusing on short-term frustrations, this will help you through any rough patches, both at school and at work. Think to your future whenever you find your present tricky.

> **Think** What areas of study do you find difficult? How could you make them more interesting or accessible?

Health, relationships and responsibilities

Often there are influences beyond the classroom that can affect your learning capabilities. Illness, problems with family and friends, and increased responsibilities can all put pressure on your workload and make studying a little harder as your concentration and motivation levels dip. If you are going through a rough patch, try to keep on track and remember that your problems are hopefully temporary. If the problem seems much more long term in nature, it might be worth talking about it with your teacher to see what support is available.

Access to resources

Although you are attending lessons and gaining information from teachers, you still need to do additional fact-finding work on your own. This can take the form of:

- internet research

- reading library books

- watching or listening to relevant programmes on the television and radio

- reading newspapers and industry-specific journals and publications.

Access to resources can affect how well you are able to research a topic and, therefore, how much information you can gather and store. Luckily, nearly 60 per cent of UK households have internet access, one of the main methods of research these days. If you do not have a computer at home, then you will probably be able to use one at college. Your college and town libraries should have the necessary books and publications for your topics and should be able to order them if they are not in stock. If you are having trouble locating a book or getting access to a computer, you could work with a friend to share the research.

SKILLS FOR LEARNING

The skills you learn and develop at school, in college and beyond will be of enormous benefit in the workplace.

Study skills

The kind of skills you develop when studying might not be immediately obvious to you, but they will be invaluable when you start work. Figure 6.2 is an example of how what you do at school could help in your future job.

Figure 6.2 – The study skills you develop now will help you in the future

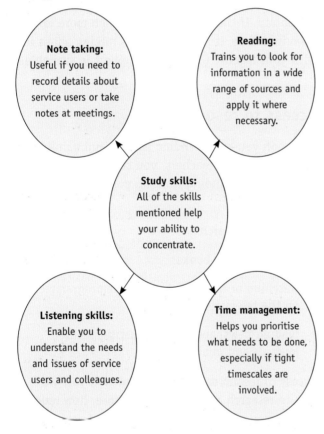

Note taking: Useful if you need to record details about service users or take notes at meetings.

Reading: Trains you to look for information in a wide range of sources and apply it where necessary.

Study skills: All of the skills mentioned help your ability to concentrate.

Listening skills: Enable you to understand the needs and issues of service users and colleagues.

Time management: Helps you prioritise what needs to be done, especially if tight timescales are involved.

Literacy skills

Despite the growing use of 'text speak' and other forms of quick, abbreviated language, proper spelling and grammar are still seen as important by employers. Your ability to write in a clear and concise manner will not only make your written communication more understandable, but it will also give a good impression of you as a person, and demonstrates attention to detail.

Reading skills are also important. You may be required to read documents of different lengths and complexity; this can seem daunting at first. If you feel unconfident about your reading skills, try reading a good-quality newspaper, books or magazines regularly. These are enjoyable ways of expanding your vocabulary and knowledge of spelling and grammar.

Numeracy skills

Some of us are better with numbers than others but you do not need to be Einstein to use numerical skills well in daily life. The following are ways in which you use numbers on a regular basis:

- budgeting to buy a new CD or pair of jeans

- working out if the change you have been given in a shop is correct

- saving up some of your allowance or money from a part-time job to go on holiday

- deciding if you have enough cash for the rest of the week to go to the cinema with a friend on Saturday night.

If you feel unconfident about your ability with numbers, or you have become a little rusty in this area, there are some easy steps you can take. Instead of using a calculator for basic adding up or subtracting, try doing this in your head or on paper then check your answer with a calculator.

By further developing these skills, you could be helping yourself in your future job, where you could be doing anything from working on expenses sheets to managing a budget on behalf of an organisation.

Research tip

Find out how good you are with numbers on the BBC's Skillswise site.
www.bbc.co.uk/skillswise

Information and communication technology skills

The world is becoming increasingly reliant on computers, and most organisations, companies and households have access to email, the internet and basic or advanced computer software. Therefore, these days the ability to use computers effectively is vital in the workplace. You may already have some of these skills, but others you will need to improve are:

- **Keyboard skills** – Typing quickly and accurately, using all your fingers and without looking at the keys (known as 'touch-typing'), will save time wherever you are working: at home, school or at work.

- **Report writing** – Letters, reports, assessments and projects are often written up as word-processed documents, then printed out or emailed to relevant contacts.

- **Spreadsheets and databases** – Spreadsheets and databases, often created using Microsoft Excel and Access software, are used to store, retrieve, analyse and compare sometimes quite large amounts of information.

- **Presentation packages** – The computer programme Microsoft PowerPoint is often used to help people create visually effective presentations.

- **The internet and email** – The internet offers organisations, companies and charities a vital web presence, where they can give visitors information and contact details. Email is a widely used method of communication, due to its speed and ability to send information such as attachments.

Research skills

You may already be something of an expert at knowing where to find out information; school and college projects often require you to go away and come back with an answer to a problem or prepare for a discussion on a topic.

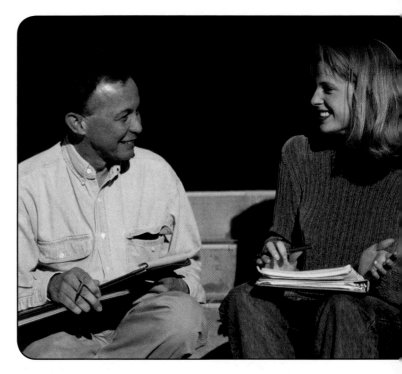

Figure 6.3 – Gain additional information about your subject by asking people in the know

You probably are also used to searching for information on the internet or looking for relevant books in the library.

However, research is not just about reading. Other good sources for research purposes include:

- **Questioning** – It can be effective to ask questions of people in the know. This includes your teachers, professionals working in a particular area and other people in your class doing the same work as you.

- **Observation** – Watching something being done by someone else, especially if this is your preferred way of learning.

You will use all of these research skills at work, and so developing them while you learn means they will have become second-nature for when you need them in the workplace.

Think What are your strongest and weakest skills?

Using feedback

Feedback from other people, both positive and negative, is invaluable when it comes to developing your skills base.

Positive feedback shows you:

- what your strengths are

- where your talents lie

- that you have skills worth shouting about!

Negative feedback enables you to:

- identify your weaknesses

- learn from your mistakes

- improve your skills in the future.

No one particularly likes getting negative feedback, but it can actually be a positive experience, certainly in the long term. Wherever possible, ask teachers, friends and family for honest opinions on your work, abilities and weaknesses so you can gain a better picture of yourself, academically and personally. Do not be discouraged by any negative feedback that you receive. Instead, view it as a positive opportunity to find out more about how you can develop your skills and knowledge even further.

Reflection

Reflection is a little like feedback but, instead of other people commenting on your performance, *you* are providing the criticism. Personal reflection is the ability to assess what you have learnt from any work or experiences you have completed and how you could do things differently next time. Sometimes it can be difficult being objective about yourself, but if you can be aware of the good and bad points of a situation, you will know what to repeat or avoid in the future. Take any errors in your stride: remember that we all learn from our mistakes.

> **Think** What have you learnt from negative feedback in the past?

You could use a table like the one below to help you identify your own strengths and weaknesses. These could be personal qualities, such as patience and self-discipline, or skills, such as numeracy and organisation. You could then ask someone who knows you well to add comments, giving their views about the things you have identified as strengths and weaknesses. It might be helpful to ask them to give you examples of situations in

APPRAISAL SHEET- 6 MONTH PERFORMANCE REVIEW	Date 3rd March
Staff Name - Joe Smith He came into this job with no previous experience and no particular training in communication issues.	**Job Role** Community support worker with people with high level support needs
Feedback - What is working well • Good team player • Organised • Punctual and reliable • Forming positive relationships with those who have mild communication difficulties • Developing positive relationships with extended family members of service users • Positive contributions to team meetings	**Development needs - Continuing professional development** • Learning other communication methods to communicate with hearing impaired service users • Not being over-reliant on verbal communication
Overall performance .... **Signed Supervisor** .... **Signed employee**	**Action to be completed by** 1st June 2007 Sign language training Observation and identification of service users' non-verbal communication signs and signals

Fig 6.3 Formal appraisals are one means of giving and receiving feedback

which they saw evidence of your strengths and weaknesses. If you keep a copy of the table you can review it regularly and consider whether you have improved on any of your areas of weakness.

Table 6.2 Assess yourself

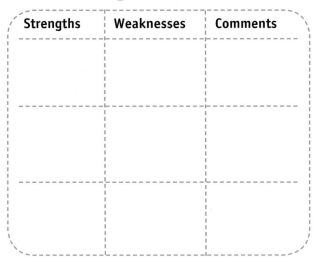

Strengths	Weaknesses	Comments

SUPPORT FOR LEARNING

Learning is not always a solitary activity. Sometimes the best ideas and solutions come from seeking the opinions of others and working as part of a team.

Discussion

There is only so much learning you can do from reading. While books and websites contain vital and useful information, it can sometimes be difficult to understand very complex facts just from reading. Talking to someone else can help to make matters much clearer, especially if they are able to put the information you have learnt into some sort of context.

- **Tutors** are often your first port of call, since they are delivering the subject you are studying. They will have knowledge of the area academically and know how this applies to your subject vocationally.

- **Supervisors and mentors** are people who you will probably meet in a vocational setting, perhaps during one of your work-experience placements. These people will understand

your training needs and potential areas of uncertainty. Supervisors and mentors are also responsible for your welfare, both professionally and personally, and can help deal with any problems you may encounter.

- **Peers** are people who are of the same age, status or ability as you. In your current environment these are the other students in your group. Since you are all working towards the same goal – a career in health and social care – these are ideal people with which to share information or discuss points that you do not understand. Talking together can sometimes make a tricky situation or topic clearer or shed a different light on a subject.

> **Think** When you ask other people for help, do you find that their input helps you to understand a topic better?

Meetings

When well managed, meetings can be extremely helpful in motivating a workforce and keeping them informed of changes and developments. If you have ever been on a committee at school or part of a club, you may have experienced a meeting yourself and be familiar with the structure and aims.

Meetings give people the opportunity to:

- get together with other like-minded individuals

- brainstorm ideas

- resolve problems and issues

- come up with a plan of action

- monitor the progress of a particular project or individual

- agree on working together as a team towards a common goal

- allocate jobs to different people on a joint project to reduce the time spent.

Participating in meetings can also benefit you on a more personal level because you learn how to:

- get across your point of view in a group setting

- listen attentively and patiently to other people, even if you do not agree with them

- use tact and diplomacy, (which means being sensitive to others) choosing when to listen, when to talk, and how to express yourself without offending anyone else

- stand up for your beliefs, which may be questioned by other people

- be a good leader, if you are chairing the gathering, by ensuring everyone is being heard and respected.

> ***Think*** Think back to a meeting you attended at school or in a social setting. What was your role? How did you get your voice heard? What was the atmosphere like? Was the outcome what you desired?

Increased self-awareness

The skills you use and develop in this course and the research and discussion you undertake, will help you to start forming ideas about where you see your future heading. We are constantly learning about ourselves, even if we are not aware of this! Take advantage of this insight into your emotions, motivations, and aspirations to consider what career areas might suit you best.

Once you have a shortlist of ideas, think about how you can access more information about them. The professional bodies of the various health and social care areas normally provide information on what qualifications they require in which careers, together with guidance on best practice. Do some internet research and check out their websites for further information.

LEARNING OPPORTUNITIES

Formal and informal learning

When we talk about learning, the immediate images that spring to mind might be a classroom, a library, or even an exam. These are all important methods of learning and assessing how well you have understood your studies but, important learning can take place in informal settings too. Informal learning can involve knowledge gained from experiences: something you have seen or participated in. You will have come away from the situation knowing something that you didn't know before. Often, in such circumstances, we do not realise that we are learning anything because the situation is not a formal one and information-gathering is not the primary aim. Figure 6.4 describes the differences between these two types of learning.

Figure 6.4 Key differences between formal and informal learning

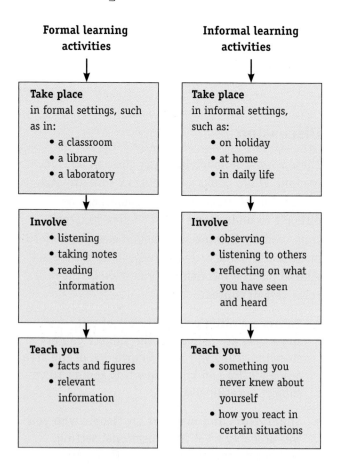

Example

The aim of the National Curriculum for children aged 5–16 years aims to give all children a set of knowledge and experiences in preparation for working life. Children learn lessons such as Science, Maths and English in formal environments, undertaking conscious learning. However, there is also a powerful learning tool known as the 'hidden curriculum'. Other messages are transmitted informally to children from the day they start school, giving them unconscious learning. Without being told, children soon learn that being good at maths is better than being good at art. Children are aware of the values placed on certain behaviours without any formal notification. If you talk to children they will quickly tell you who is seen as clever and who is bottom of the class. Gender behaviours are also a form of informal learning. Molly, aged 7 years, much prefers to read whilst Darren prefers to run around, exploring the environment as he goes along. Both children are acquiring subconscious feminine and masculine roles.

Independent studies

Your studies often teach you in a very theoretical way: you learn all the information and facts you need to know to pass an exam or write an essay, but you are not necessarily putting them into practice. This opportunity comes in your work-experience placements.

However, your studies also teach you about gathering information and then interpreting it. For example, a lesson on physiology might teach you the basics about the heart, but you might need to explore in greater depth how it works with other organs in the body. Once you have identified a good source of information, you can decide how many of the facts you need to know.

To get the most out of your studies:

- take any opportunities to ask questions and share your thoughts

- talk to your teachers and classmates about their opinions and views

- consider their views alongside your own: do they change your ideas or do they strengthen them?

Key words

Theoretical – based on ideas and information rather than practice; although you can put theory into practice!

Life experiences

One of the best ways to learn in life is to experience things for yourself. This need not be restricted to studying and careers. You can gain a great deal of knowledge from extra-curricular activities, responsibilities at home and holidays. These will teach you about:

- your likes and dislikes; for example, whether you like working with others or working alone

- what your personality is like; for example, whether you are outgoing or whether you prefer to be out of the limelight

- what your values and beliefs are; for example, are you passionately committed to helping others who are less advantaged?

Key words

Extra-curricular – events that happen outside of the normal school day and environment

Employment

Do you have a part-time job? Even if it is something that does not require much knowledge or skill, it does not mean that you have not gained anything while you have been working hard for a bit of extra cash! Part-time and temporary jobs give you skills that you can give as examples on your curriculum vitae (CV) and that you will be able to use in your future work. Table 6.3 gives a few examples.

Key words

Curriculum vitae (CV) – a brief account of your education, qualifications and previous jobs to date

---

Think What skills have you learnt from part-time or holiday jobs? How might they be useful in the workplace?

Table 6.3 Skills you can gain from part-time and temporary employment

Voluntary activities

Most employers in the health and social care sector prefer candidates for jobs to have done some sort of voluntary experience in a relevant setting, because it shows them that the candidate:

- is committed to working in the area

- has a knowledge of the field

- will have gained an understanding both of service users' needs and the demands placed on organisations

- has used the experience to decide that the area of work is right for them.

Research tip

To find out more about volunteering in the health and social care sector, visit the Community Service Volunteers website. www.csv.org.uk

Part-time/temporary jobs	Skills learnt
Delivering newspapers	• **time-management:** to deliver papers on time • **reliability:** people depend on you for their morning read • **commitment:** this is not an easy job due to the unsociable hours, particularly if you have to go to school afterwards
Shop assistant	• **interpersonal skills:** to deal with a wide range of customers and their queries • **numerical skills:** if you are handling money or working on the till • **presentation skills:** you need to be appropriately dressed at work
Waiter	• **stamina:** the ability to do physical work for long periods of time • **team work:** the ability to work well as part of a team • **technical skills:** using credit card pin machines and cash registers

EVIDENCE ACTIVITY

P1 – M1 – D1

Jane, Sasha and Brian are all students on a Health and Social Care programme at a local college, studying to become qualified care workers. They have different views about the types of work they do on their course.

- Jane finds the lectures stimulating and interesting. However, she finds the college environment a little boring and can't wait to put her newly acquired learning into practice.

- Sasha finds the practical sessions more fun and instructive and thinks she learns more by doing the job. Her favourite class is sociology because the lecturer is open, approachable and patient, and tries to put theory into context. She does find some lessons difficult as sometimes the theories are hard to grasp.

- Brian likes both the theory and the practice. He thinks that he makes good use of reflection to improve his performance in the work place.

1. Produce an information leaflet for the college to give to new students about the types of work they will do on their health and social care course, which explains the key influences on personal learning processes of individuals. (P1)

2. Now think about your own learning process and the ways in which you prefer to learn. Analyse the key influences on your own personal learning. (M1)

3. Think about the advantages of your personal learning on others, e.g. you may become more professional in your approach at work and care for people in a different way. Evaluate how your own personal learning and development during this course may benefit others. (D1)

6.2 *Planning, monitoring and reflecting on your development*

REVIEW AT START OF PROGRAMME

It may sound odd, but often you have to look back before you can look forward. This is certainly the case with career planning, as the skills, knowledge and experiences you have gained to date will, to some extent, determine your way forward. Reflecting on your previous experience will help you see what sort of person you are, your capabilities, your likes and dislikes, what is important to you and what you hope to achieve in life. Try to be as honest as possible about your skills and abilities. With this knowledge you can move on to consider career options that might suit you.

KNOWLEDGE

The *Oxford English Dictionary* has defined knowledge as 'information and skills acquired through experience or education'. It can be helpful to think about the knowledge you have gained throughout your life in the following categories.

- **at school** through the subjects and examinations you have studied to date

- **at home** through holiday and family experiences

- **at work** in part-time jobs or relevant work experience

- **through learning**, both formally and informally

- **through understanding** current issues affecting the health and social care sector, and the theories, principles and concepts involved

- **through opportunities** in the workplace, in college and beyond.

SKILLS

We all have a wealth of skills, but sometimes it is difficult knowing just what they are, or even that we possess them! The following information should help you identify when and where you have developed your skills, and suggest possible areas for improvement.

Communication skills

Communication skills are important in all jobs. They fall into two broad categories: verbal and non-verbal.

Verbal

Verbal skills are about how you talk to or with people, such as family, friends, colleagues, clients, service users and peers. Effective verbal communication is not just about the words you use, although it is important to ensure that your vocabulary suits your listener's ability to understand. It also involves how you adapt your tone of voice and even the volume at which you speak. Not everyone, for example, feels comfortable with someone who is loud and over-energetic. Equally, if you are too softly spoken, some people may lack confidence in your abilities. The ability to sense how to react to different people is a very useful skill in all aspects of life.

Non-verbal

Listening is as important a communication skill as speaking, particularly in the health and social care sectors. Clients in these settings often find it hard to explain themselves, perhaps because of embarrassment or fear, and sometimes need gentle encouragement. They might respond best to someone who is patient and shows that they are interested. In order to be able to react appropriately, it is important to develop your ability to read someone's body language, which will often give you a clue to how someone is feeling. For example, if someone's shoulders are hunched upwards, or if they are wringing their hands, they could be tense. If they are sitting or standing with their arms resting in their lap or at their sides, chances are they are feeling more relaxed.

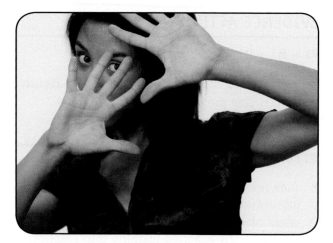

Figure 6.5 Body language can give you a clue to how someone is feeling

> **Think** Think about the conversations you have with friends and family. Do you dominate conversations or hold back? Next time, why not try the opposite approach to see what it feels like?

Working with others

In the health and social care sector, you almost certainly will spend a lot of time working with others. Whether you are dealing with service users on a daily basis or handling requests from other colleagues, you need to be happy regularly interacting with other people. The fact that you are already studying for this qualification means that you are probably a 'people' person. How you deal with people depends on your personality, and the reactions of those people around you. An ability to adapt to your audience and the situation you are in is very important.

Service users

Service users come from a range of ages and backgrounds, but they all need someone to understand the issues they face and have empathy for their problems. Developing these skills might involve research into socio-economic issues if you are working as a social worker, or the mental and physical effects of a person suffering from a chronic disease if you are employed as a healthcare professional. You will also need to understand why some service users might be mistrustful of a person in a professional role and be able to both acknowledge their feelings and gain their trust.

Key words

Socio-economic – relating to a combination of social and economic factors

Example

Sharmain is a single parent who has three children. Her flat is on a council estate in an area that is considered to be deprived. She has recently had a baby, but has no immediate family or friends to support her and her husband left her last month. She is finding day-to-day activities hard and shouting at her children more. Sharmain thinks she is suffering from post-natal depression, and is worried because as a child she remembers that her neighbours' children were taken into care.

Think What socio-economic issues do people in your area face? How might these affect their relationships with health and social care providers?

Professionals

In health and social care, you will work with lots of different professionals. Most health and social care professionals work within teams in order to ensure that service users and patients are given the best care possible, from the point of treatment and beyond. Your dealings with fellow professionals should be respectful, regardless of whether they are senior or junior to you. Most professionals enjoy a fairly relaxed and informal relationship once the ice has been broken! However, you must always remain willing to work as professionally and compassionately as possible.

Technical skills

Technical skills are highly valued by employers. Do you know what these skills are and whether you already have them?

IT

You can probably already use computers in a variety of ways, for example:

- surfing the internet
- emailing friends
- producing documents in word-processing packages.

All of these skills will be helpful in the workplace, but you might also be required to produce spreadsheets or manage databases to present certain types of information. Increasingly, IT is being used in health and social care to create, update and store patients' and service users' records electronically.

Equipment

The sort of equipment you are likely to use in a health and social care setting will depend on the area in which you work. Some equipment will be electronic or computer operated, so if you have used a computer, a digital camera or other electronic items, you should feel more confident learning how to operate this type of equipment in the workplace.

Creative and craft skills

You probably will not spend the day making paper aeroplanes or painting murals, but the skills you develop when drawing, painting or sculpting can be useful at work. All of these activities require manual dexterity and attention to detail, which is a desirable, and often compulsory, ability in certain jobs. Equally, if you are creative with words, this can help when writing documents that need to be easily understood by people.

Research skills

The research methods you use as a student can be described as either primary or secondary.

Primary research

Primary research uses new information that you collect yourself, rather than relying on other people to provide and analyse it for you. Information can be gained by interviewing people and asking them to describe how they feel about something (this is an example of qualitative research) or providing them with questionnaires with answers to choose from (this is an example of quantitative research). Carrying out primary research helps improve and develop skills such as information gathering, analysing, presentation and communication (both written and verbal).

Secondary research

Secondary research mainly involves using other people's observations and findings on a subject, rather than your own. It can be done through reading books, newspapers, specialist journals and information on the internet. This is the most common type of research used by students at school and in higher education to gain information. Doing secondary research helps develop and improve information-gathering and independent study skills.

Data handling

Once you have gathered information, whether it is for a school project or a professional document, you need to present it in a way that accurately summarises your findings. How you do this depends on the research methods used. Often both primary and secondary research is used within the same document.

Word-processing packages are helpful if you want to:

- write a lengthy report describing the outcomes of extensive research

- present evidence and arguments attractively.

Pie charts, tables and diagrams can be:

- used to represent statistical information in a clearer and more understandable format than just using words to summarise lots of 'bitty' information

- imported into word-processing documents.

Personal skills

Personal skills are one type of transferable skills that do not depend on you having any knowledge about a particular area. Table 6.5 lists some of the typical personal skills that employers look for.

Table 6.4 Skills often required by employers

Skill	What it involves
Teamwork	working together and using each other's strengths to solve problems and achieve a goal
Organisation	prioritising tasks according to importance, allocating appropriate time to each activity and reaching your goals
Initiative	being prepared to work independently, developing skills to deal with change swiftly as and when it occurs, and learning to anticipate and prepare for it
Leadership	listening, guiding and advising, as well as leading others; the ability to understand others and how to motivate them
Flexibility	the ability to react quickly and effectively to unforeseen circumstances; come up with alternative ideas and solutions, and deal with change as calmly as possible

Key words

Transferable skills – abilities that can be used equally well in one job or setting as in another

PRACTICE

Before you can start working in health and social care you need to understand certain important issues relating to practice. The most common are explained in the following section.

The value base of care

You must respect and understand an organisation's value base for care and develop your own values in order to support and promote good practice in whichever field you work.

The impact of legislation

You need to understand how legislation affects health and social care in general and the field in which you wish to work, as well as the impact on you as a future employee.

Key words

Legislation – a set of laws suggested by government and made official by parliament

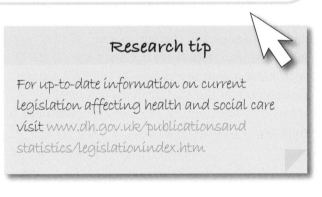

Research tip

For up-to-date information on current legislation affecting health and social care visit www.dh.gov.uk/publicationsand statistics/legislationindex.htm

Codes of practice and policies

Each organisation, and its members, must adhere to certain codes of practice and policies. You can research these online by looking at the websites of regulatory and professional bodies.

Personal values and beliefs

If you wish to remain professional at work, you need to understand what your values and beliefs are and how these could either help or hinder you in your job.

Working with others

In any health and social care field, working with others professionally and cooperatively is vital: could you do this well, knowing when to lead and when to take a back seat?

Your strengths and limitations

If you want to help your fellow colleagues, patients and service users you need to understand what your professional and personal strengths and limitations are. Play to your strengths but do be aware of your limitations.

VALUES AND BELIEFS

Many individuals go into careers in health and social care because they have very strong beliefs about how people in society should be treated. Perhaps they have been touched by the poverty in which many children live. Or maybe they have had a relative in hospital and want to become part of a team that provides such support to others.

It is vital to examine your values and beliefs when looking at possible areas of employment. While all health and social care areas are concerned with helping people, the ways in which this is done vary. For example:

- Would you prefer to work in an area like A&E, where you are treating people in one-off emergency situations or would you gain more satisfaction from dealing with patients who are battling long-term illnesses?

- Which do you feel more drawn to: mental or physical health issues?

- Would you prefer to support people in their own homes and communities or within a special setting?

Within the caring professions, you may come across difficult situations that conflict with your moral or religious beliefs, such as a GP who is against abortion having to refer a woman for one. If you hold any strong beliefs of this nature, be sure that you are aware of them and how you may react in a situation when they could be called into question.

Example

Frances works in a residential care home that has a diverse group of service users. She is not religious and finds it hard to accept that a room has been set aside for some residents to use for prayer. Frances believes that everyone should be treated the same and that services should be free of any religious or political persuasions. Her centre manager informs Frances that one of the values of the care home is to respect difference and meet the individual needs of all its residents regardless of race, religion or ethnic background. She gives Frances a copy of the Equal Opportunities Policy and organises a training session for Frances to attend on diversity.

Think Do you hold any moral or religious beliefs that could come into conflict in a health or social care setting? If so, could you help someone fairly in spite of them?

Value base of care

All health and social care workers need to adhere to a value base of care, which is an ethical code that determines how they should act in certain situations. This is designed to ensure that you do not discriminate against or are unkind to someone in need of your help.

Key words

Discriminate – to treat people unfairly and differently based on aspects such as skin colour, beliefs or background

CAREER ASPIRATIONS

When you were little, did you ever dream about a particular career? Being Spiderman perhaps?! Or maybe you always wanted to be doctor or nurse. It is important to have your dreams, as these often inspire us to go on to achieve great things in life. They can influence:

- our achievement at school and college
- our choice of subjects to study
- the sorts of activities we enjoy
- the kinds of jobs we undertake.

Unfortunately, we cannot always have the career of our dreams. We need to look at what we have achieved to date and how we can use our skills, knowledge, experience and beliefs in a setting that would suit us. At this stage in your learning, it is helpful to look at what you can offer employers, in which jobs your skills and knowledge would be required, and which of these appeal most.

You might find it helpful to use a table like the one below to help you think about your career options. Write down five career options you believe are open to someone with your knowledge, skills and qualifications in the left column. In the middle column, rate these options from 1 to 5, with 1 being your top choice. In the final column, make a note of the qualifications you need for these jobs, highlighting any areas you may need to work on.

Table 6.5 Your possible career choices

Career options	Preferred choice	Qualifications needed?

PLAN FOR OWN DEVELOPMENT

The Chinese philosopher Confucius once said 'A man who does not plan long ahead will find trouble right at his door'. The importance of planning for your career cannot be overemphasised. You should need to be looking into the future in order to know what you need to do now to get there. There are two types of plans you can prepare for this purpose:

- **Short-term plans:** normally last for up to six months and provide more immediate targets to attain, rather like a checklist of things to do. You can break these down even further by setting monthly goals.

- **Long-term plans:** should last for a minimum of 18 months to give you a better idea of the bigger picture of what you are trying to achieve. Some people draw up five-year plans, in which they state what they need to do each year to reach a desired goal.

CONSIDER PERSONAL GOALS

For a plan to work, you need to set yourself clear, specific and relevant targets that you stand a good chance of achieving with hard work and perseverance. Be realistic when setting your goals; there is no point aiming for the impossible as this puts undue and unnecessary pressure on you. When you meet your targets, not only will you help yourself professionally, but you will feel a great sense of personal and professional achievement. You can set yourself goals in the following areas:

- **knowledge** – by obtaining the qualifications you need

- **skills** – by improving on or gaining relevant ones

- **practice** – by learning about codes of practice and ethics in careers that interest you

- **values and beliefs** – by determining where your values and beliefs lie and where they could best be put to use

- **career aspirations** – by understanding where you hope to be working in both the short and long term.

MONITOR AND EVALUATE PLAN IN TERMS OF OWN DEVELOPMENT

It is important that you regularly monitor your plan to help you reflect on your own development. You should have a minimum of three specific goals in mind at all times, which you are actively working towards. Look at your plan on a regular basis and try to decide what progress you have made against the targets you have set yourself. If you have achieved some of your goals, set yourself new ones that will help you to develop your knowledge or skills further.

CHANGES

While Confucius was very astute in his observations about what happens without any plans in place, the Romans were also pretty clued-up on forward-thinking. One Latin proverb states that, 'It's an ill plan that cannot be changed'. This is absolutely true: plans are inevitably subject to revision.

Life does not always go to plan and we need to be able to adapt accordingly. Reasons for change include:

- a change in career preference

- identifying certain development needs that must be met

- realising that one of your priorities should be higher than another

- outside influences, such as family or study problems.

Sometimes, your studies will cause you to reflect not just on your academic ability, but also on your personal development. This may profoundly call into question previous choices you made based on what you thought were your likes and dislikes, and values and beliefs. This is a positive thing and one that should be welcomed: the more you learn about yourself, the more able you will be to make good decisions about your career.

CONTEXTS

All of this self-reflection and learning can take place in a variety of settings throughout the duration of your course, and beyond. Ideal contexts for finding out about your skills, strengths and weaknesses, and determining which career path should be yours, include:

- work experience placements, both related to this course and others

- visits to health and social care settings to speak to and shadow people doing the jobs you are interested in, and to experience their working environment

- study environments in which you can discover what kind of participation you feel most comfortable with, such as lively debates or written reflections

- life events in which you may have observed health or social care in action at a personal level

- other contexts such as employment opportunities in which you may have a chance to practise and improve your skills before using them in your chosen career.

EVIDENCE ACTIVITY

P2 – P3 – P4 – M2 – D2

1. Produce a profile of yourself at the start of your course which identifies your own knowledge, skills, practice, values, beliefs and career aspirations. You could use the example on the next page as a template.
Be as honest as possible and think hard about what areas you need to improve. (P2)

2. Produce an action plan for your own self-development and the achievement of your personal goals. You will need to monitor this regularly during the course. (P3)

3. Remember to update your action plan weekly, showing how you are gradually making progress in developing your skills further as you go through the programme. (P4)

4. At the end of your programme, look back at the profile of yourself that you completed at the start of the course. Explain how the action plan has helped to support your own development over the course. (M2)

5. Evaluate your own development from the start to the finish of the course. Remember to do this critically. What have been the highlights and lowlights? What could you have done better and what went well? Make sure that you link this to your practice in the work setting. (D2)

Table 6.6

Student Profile: James Stewart

Profile at beginning of Health and Social Care course

Knowledge	Skills	Practice	Values	Beliefs	Career aspirations
Understanding of policy and key legislation in social care area Principles of team work	Good listener Flexible Adaptable Good communicator	Be tolerant in work setting	Individuality Family life Marriage	Not religious	Social worker

My Strengths	My Weaknesses
• Good at team work • Good at communicating with service users • Hard working, reliable, tolerant • Can juggle lots of tasks at the same time	• Do not say no to a task even if I am busy • Shy and intimidated by other professionals
My Opportunities	**My Threats**
• Commitment from government to increase the number of social workers in the area • Have been successful in gaining three good GCSEs whilst at school	• Find it difficult to study due to family commitments • Own experiences of education mean that I do not see myself as able

Area for improvement	Target/Goal	Date for improvement	Feedback from tutor	Action following feedback
Week 1 Develop confidence at work and contribute ideas	To engage with other professionals without feeling intimidated	Meetings with three other professionals by the end of the month Submit plan of ideas for improvement to team meeting in month 2	This student is slowly developing his communication skills and now speaks confidently to all staff	Join and contribute to joint agency meetings which are held monthly in the local authority office
Week 2				
Week 3				
End of programme evaluation				

SUPPORT FOR DEVELOPMENT

Personal development does not have to fall just on your shoulders. Although you have to take responsibility for seeking out opportunities to improve your skills and knowledge, you can and should turn to others for help, advice and suggestions.

- **Other people** – Your tutors, peers, supervisors and mentors will be glad to give you feedback on how you are progressing and ways in which you can further develop your skills.

- **Meetings** – These will help to indicate any knowledge gaps you have, as well as inform you of how you perform in group settings.

- **Yourself** – The increased self-awareness and knowledge you gain from this course will highlight which areas you need to focus on in the future and where to find the support you need; for example, where to access information and support on knowledge and best practice.

REFLECT ON YOUR OWN DEVELOPMENT

Reflection is a very valuable process in lots of areas: professionally, personally and emotionally. It enables us to consider where we have been in the past, at what stage we are at in the present, and how this can affect our future. It is important to regularly make the time to reflect on your progress in order to see where your future may be heading and also to celebrate what you have achieved to date! You can do this in a variety of ways:

- **Linking theory to practice** – Think about how what you have learnt in the classroom can be applied to practical situations in the workplace.

- **Linking practice to theory** – Observe how something is done in practice (or do it yourself) and then try to understand the theory behind the practice.

- **Achieving personal goals** – Revisit Table 6.6 regularly to see which targets you have met for knowledge, skills, practice, values, beliefs, and career aspirations. Set yourself some new ones!

- **Accepting the influence of personal values and beliefs** – Consider how your current values and beliefs can help you choose an appropriate career and be aware if your views change during your studies or work experience.

EVIDENCE ACTIVITY

P5 – M3

1. Produce a personal and professional development portfolio. Revisit this regularly to reflect on the progress you have made and what you have achieved. (P5)

2. Keep a journal or diary while on your work placements to record your experiences and feelings. Choose three specific examples and explain how you used the theories that you have learned about in a practical context. (M3)

6.3 *Understanding service provision in the health or social care sectors*

PROVISION OF SERVICES

Health care is provided on a national, regional and local level in England, as shown in Figure 6.6.

NATIONAL PROVIDERS

The Department of Health

It is the Department of Health's job to help the government improve the health and general well-being of people in England, by setting the standards and working practices for both the NHS and local social services. The Department for Health also issues health and social care policies and standards in England, as well as modernising all parts of the NHS. Additionally, it provides health information to the public on topics such as the importance of eating five portions of fruit and vegetables a day and why immunising babies is essential.

Its main responsibilities are to:

- make appropriate changes in the NHS and social care

- improve standards of public health

- ensure the NHS works effectively with social care providers

- set standards to improve the quality of services nationwide

- obtain enough money from the Government to ensure that the NHS and social services can deliver their services

- work with other organisations, such as the Strategic Health Authorities, to ensure that the NHS and social care organisations get the support they need to deliver the best possible care.

The National Health Service

The National Health Service (NHS) manages and delivers the health and social care system in England, together with social services. It was set up in 1948 and is now the largest organisation in Europe, and rated as one of the best health services in the world by the World Health Organization. The NHS and its services are free to patients because it receives funding from the government from the taxes that we pay. Its key aims are to:

- promote health and prevent illness

- diagnose and treat injuries and diseases

- care for people who have long-term illnesses and disabilities and need NHS services.

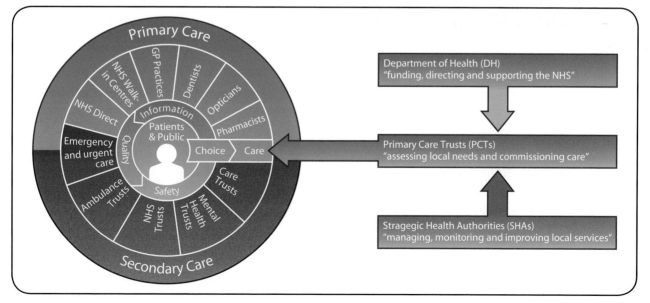

Figure 6.6 Provision of health care in the UK [source: www.nhs.uk]

CASE STUDY: NHS DIRECT

The NHS has always been committed to the development of patient-centred services. One of the most famous examples of this was the launch of the telephone advice service NHS Direct in March 1998 at three pilot sites. Two years later, NHS Direct became a national service.

NHS Direct is a 24/7 nurse-led helpline for people worried about common and unusual health complaints and concerns. In only five years, it became one of the largest e-health services in the world and currently helps more than 2.5 million people each month. The service spurred on a range of other convenient alternatives to GP services, including NHS Walk-in Centres, which offer treatment and advice for injuries and illnesses without an appointment.

People can access NHS Direct's services by several methods:

• NHS Direct website (www.nhsdirect.nhs.uk), which handles 24 million visitors every year.

• The telephone service, which receives seven million calls every year.

• NHS Direct Interactive, which includes 3,000 pages of health information available through TVs with Freeview or Sky Digital (about 16 million households).

The cost for the service to the taxpayer is very low: less than £2.80 per person each year. Around 80 per cent of those who contact NHS Direct are ill. Over a third of these are given home-care advice and about 16 per cent are told to visit their GP. In February 2007, NHS Direct launched a television campaign on their interactive channel, targeting young men and mothers in need of reassurance about their children.

Young men are often too embarrassed to see their doctor about health niggles, but NHS Direct hopes that their adverts on Freeview and Sky Digital will help provide them with information about problems that concern them. The adverts will also be in magazines such as *Nuts* and *Zoo*. Mothers are also being targeted so that they can find out the answers to common health issues faced by families. As well as on TV, the adverts will be in magazines such as *Bella* and *Chat*.

QUESTIONS

1. Why might patients prefer to access health information online, by telephone or via a television?

2. Why are young men embarrassed about going to the doctor? What else could be done to help overcome their shyness?

3. Are there any other groups who you think are reluctant to access health services? How could they best be reached?

4. Are there any patients who would find accessing the information provided by NHS Direct difficult?

Strategic Health Authorities

Ten Strategic Health Authorities were created in 2002 to provide a link between the NHS and the Department of Health, and to manage the NHS at a regional level. Their responsibilities include:

• assessing how well Primary Care Trusts (PCTs) and NHS Trusts (hospitals) are doing

• improving local health services

• recruiting more staff

• working with different organisations in local government, education, and the charitable and voluntary sectors

- making sure that any national priorities, such as improving cancer services for patients, are promoted locally

- coming up with immediate, short- and long-term plans for healthcare provision and improvements.

LOCAL HEALTH OR SOCIAL CARE SERVICE PROVIDERS

Health and social care is provided on a local level by several types of organisations: primary care, secondary care, tertiary care and social care.

Primary care

Community-based health services provide primary care. These are usually the first, and sometimes only, port of call for patients within the health service. The professionals working within primary care include:

- family doctors (GPs)

- nurses (in community and in GP surgeries)

- therapists (e.g. physiotherapists, occupational therapists)

- community pharmacists

- optometrists

- dentists

- midwives.

> ***Think*** What primary care services have you used in your area?

Primary Care Trusts

Primary Care Trusts (PCTs) control health care on a local level and are monitored by their regional Strategic Health Authority and ultimately report to the Secretary of State for Health. All of the 152 PCTs in England are free-standing and have

their own boards, staff and budgets. Overall, they control 80 per cent of the entire NHS budget and are responsible for:

- coming up with programmes that try to improve the local community's health

- deciding which health services the local population needs and ensuring they are provided and easily accessible (includes hospital care, mental health services, GP practices, screening programmes, patient transport, NHS dentists, pharmacies and opticians)

- integrating health and social care, enabling NHS organisations to work with local authorities, social services and voluntary organisations

- providing capital investment in buildings, equipment and IT.

Secondary care

Secondary care is provided by hospitals at a local level. There are 148 NHS hospital trusts throughout England, which work with the voluntary and private sectors, PCTs and social care providers to deliver services for patients who:

- cannot be treated by primary-care practitioners, for example those who require specialist care or who need emergency treatment

- are referred by their GP for further medical treatment or surgery in hospital.

Most of the NHS's workforce is employed in one of the many trusts, in a wide variety of both medical and non-medical settings. Some trusts are regional or national centres for more specialised care, while others are associated with universities to help them to train health professionals. Trusts can also provide community services through health centres or clinics or in people's homes.

Fifty per cent of patients treated in hospitals come in as an emergency, and the other half are either planned day admissions or require longer hospital stays.

Tertiary care

This is the most specialised stage of medical treatment and usually happens in a hospital centre that may not be near the patient's home. This sort of specialist care is offered to patients who have been referred by either primary or secondary care staff. The people employed within tertiary care will normally be specialists who work in centres or units that carry out specific investigations and treatments, such as diagnostic genetics laboratories, which test for such hereditary diseases as cystic fibrosis.

Example

David and Sue are Afro-Caribbean and have three children aged 1, 3 and 9. Sue's elderly parents also live with the family. Their nine-year-old has sickle cell anaemia and needs regular medical attention. Sue's father has a heart condition and Type 1 diabetes, and is finding it more and more difficult to get up the stairs. Both David and Sue have to make full use of the primary, secondary and tertiary care services available both locally and nationally. The family's primary care needs are met by attending the local GP surgery for general health care and their one-year-old sees the health visitor at the surgery. Secondary care at a local level is needed by her father, who is treated by the local hospital and is regularly referred for specialist treatment for his heart and diabetic conditions. Both David and Susan have received tertiary care in the form of genetic counselling due to their chances of having children with sickle cell. The nine-year-old also receives specialist care when he is experiencing a sickle cell crisis.

Key words

Tertiary care – medical treatment provided at a specialist clinic

Social care

Social care is one of the major public services and helps people to continue with their daily lives as far as is possible. A staggering 1.5 million people rely on social workers and other support staff at any one time. Currently, over 25,000 employers with over a million staff provide social care services for many users including:

- the elderly

- children

- people with physical and learning disabilities

- people with mental health issues

- substance abusers (e.g. alcohol, drugs)

- ex-offenders

- young offenders.

Social services work closely with:	People who work in social care aim to:
• the NHS • voluntary and private organisations • the education service • the probation service • the police • other agencies.	• support an individual's independence and respect their dignity • meet an individual's specific needs • organise and finance social care services fairly and consistently • ensure that children in care enjoy the same opportunities as other children • make sure that every user is not subject to abuse • provide a skilled, trained workforce and the best possible care.

Figure 6.8 The role of social services and social care

Local authorities spend £10 billion a year on social services. Nearly 70 per cent of the money is spent on community care services for adults, including the elderly, people with physical or learning disabilities, and the mentally ill.

Some social care users receive direct payments, through welfare benefits or social services funding, so they can pay directly for their services and remain financially independent. Over 70 per cent of the elderly living in care homes have all or some of their costs covered by their local council. Others pay for the services they use out of their own money.

Research tip
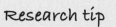

To learn more about the social services offered in your area, check out your county council's website.

Integrated care

In some cases both health and social care services work together to ensure individuals get the treatment and care that they need. Examples include nurses running care services for patients with diabetes or heart failure in a non-hospital setting, or a drug user who needs help with housing or education. It is up to the clinical staff involved to decide which health or social care support should be given. In England, there are 12 care trusts, which combine the provision of health and social care services for different client groups through better integration.

People working with service users follow the guidelines established in the January 2006 White Paper *Our Health, Our Care, Our Say* and their main responsibilities are to:

- identify different service users' needs

- know what is available within the service and how to access it

- work alongside other professional organisations

- provide access to the appropriate care or service when needed.

Key words

White Paper – a White Paper contains proposals and statements of government policy

Potential barriers to access

Sometimes health and social care is not accessed by the people who need it most. Table 6.7 summarises the reasons why this may be the case.

Table 6.7   Barriers to accessing health and social care

Barrier	Reason
Funding	If financial resources are stretched too thinly, people might not be able to access the health or social care provision that they need at the time when they need it most.
Lack of information	Some people might not be aware of the support and information available.
Misconceptions	With certain sensitive issues, such as mental health problems, people might be too frightened to approach a health or social care worker to ask for help.
Resources	Lack of staff in certain areas, such as midwifery, means that patients might not be getting the care and support they need.

REGULATORY BODIES

Regulatory bodies are appointed by the government to monitor and assess various organisations and their performance. The following bodies are the principal ones involved in health and social care in England.

The Healthcare Commission

The NHS is monitored by the Healthcare Commission, England's own health watchdog. The Commission makes sure that health-care services provided both by the NHS and by independent (private and voluntary) health-care providers meet acceptable standards in areas, such as safety, cleanliness and waiting times. In short, the Healthcare Commission aims to improve standards in both the NHS and independent health-care organisations (see Figure 6.9).

Key words

Watchdog – a group that monitors how other organisations are run

---

The Commission's main duties are to:

- assess the management, provision and quality of NHS health care and public health services
- review and rate each NHS Trust's performance
- regulate and inspect the independent health care sector
- publish information about England's health care
- consider unresolved complaints about NHS organisations
- investigate serious failures in health-care provision
- consider the access to, and the availability, quality and effectiveness of health care
- see whether health care is cost-effective and efficient
- ensure that the public is provided with good information about health care
- promote children's welfare and rights.

Figure 6.9 – Main responsibilities of the Healthcare Commission

Arm's Length Bodies (ALBs)

An unusual name for a regulatory body, ALBs actually play an important role in the health and social care system. These 38 standalone organisations, sponsored by the Department of Health, work closely with the local NHS, social care services and other ALBs throughout the country to:

- provide regulation
- set and improve standards
- protect public welfare
- support local services.

All ALBs report directly to the Department of Health, from whom they receive much of their funding. They also, sometimes, report directly to Parliament.

The Commission for Social Care Inspection (CSCI)

The Commission for Social Care Inspection (CSCI) assesses how well councils provide social services and helps them to improve their performance. Their four main aims are to:

- show social care service users that they can trust the CSCI to always act in their best interests
- be guided by what service users tell them, and help them live their lives independently and with dignity
- speak and act in ways that make sense and that respect people's rights and choices
- reward and promote good services and stamp out bad practice.

Research tip

To find out more about what the CSCI does, check out their website.

www.csci.org.uk

HEALTH AND SOCIAL CARE WORKERS

An amazing 1.3 million people work for the NHS, of whom half are medically qualified. There are approximately 1.2 million social workers across the UK. This figure includes the 250,000 social care staff working within the NHS, in roles such as occupational therapists and social workers.

The following are the main careers within the health and social care sector.

GPs and hospital doctors

Approximately 108,000 people work as hospital doctors and general practitioners (GPs). All doctors are responsible for providing medical care for their patients, diagnosing and treating illnesses and providing advice about preventative care. Table 6.8 shows the similarities and differences between the roles of GPs and hospital doctors.

Key words

Preventative – intended to stop or avoid something happening

Table 6.8 Comparison of the roles of GPs and hospital doctors

Nursing and related fields

Currently, there are around 386,000 nursing, midwifery and health visiting staff working in the NHS.

Nurses

A nurse's main responsibilities include providing patients with medical care, and helping them to recover from treatments or surgery. Like doctors, they are generally employed in one of two settings:

- **hospital:** working in general medical and surgical wards, intensive care, operating theatres and in special clinics.

- **community:** helping out in GP practices, health centres, residential homes, schools and hospices.

Nurses generally work as part of a multidisciplinary team but are often the professionals who deal with patients the most. Therefore, they need good interpersonal skills to be able to gain their patients' trust and confidence.

Key words

Multidisciplinary – involving different departments or specialisations

What GPs do	What hospital doctors do
work in a community setting in a general practice; sometimes seeing very ill patients in their homes	work in a hospital-based setting or clinic
train specifically in general medicine	specialise in a particular field, such as A&E, cardiology, audiology or surgery
see patients and deal with their problems sensitively, impartially and confidentially	monitor and provide general care to patients on hospital wards and in outpatient clinics
prescribe appropriate treatments, e.g. antibiotics, creams, etc.	admit patients to hospital who require special care, investigations and treatment
refer patients to specialist hospital services	examine and talk to patients to diagnose their medical conditions
provide specialist clinics for specific conditions or for certain groups, e.g. diabetes or new babies	make notes to record treatment given and to refer patients back to their GP
meet government-set targets for specific treatments, such as child immunisations	liaise with other medical and non-medical hospital staff to ensure quality treatment
carry out minor procedures such as removing warts or moles	treat patients using surgery or drug therapy
oversee and assess trainee GPs' work	oversee the work of trainee doctors

A nurse's daily responsibilities can include the following:

- drawing up care plans for patients

- preparing patients for operations and treatments

- recording pulse rate, blood pressure and temperature

- checking and giving drugs and injections

- responding quickly to emergencies

- organising staff and workloads

- training student and junior nurses

- setting up drips, blood transfusions and other treatments.

Midwives

Midwives provide care, advice and support for women and their families before, during and immediately after having their baby. The work involves antenatal health education, check-ups and care during the pregnancy, and medical and emotional support and advice during labour and for the 28 days following birth. After this time, care is then handled by a health visitor. Midwives mostly work independently in health-care settings such as GP practices and maternity hospitals, but will refer patients to doctors if concerns or problems arise with the mother and/or baby. They also frequently liaise with GPs, specialist doctors, health visitors and social workers.

Key words
Antenatal   before birth, during pregnancy

A midwife's typical duties include:

- monitoring women during pregnancy

- arranging antenatal tests

- referring patients with high-risk pregnancies to doctors and other medical specialists

- arranging and providing health education, such as antenatal and preparation for birth classes

- supporting parents through distressing events, such as miscarriage, termination, stillbirth and death

- supervising and helping mothers in labour, monitoring the baby's condition and supplying drugs for pain management

- advising mothers on how to care for their babies after birth, e.g. breastfeeding, bathing and bottle feeding

- working with other health-care professionals to ensure continuity of care

- training and supervising junior colleagues.

Health visitors

Health visitors are qualified and registered nurses or midwives, who have taken further training to enable them to promote good health to, and to prevent illness in, individuals, families and their local community. They work in a variety of settings, from special clinics in GP practices to visiting new mothers and children in their homes. They may also work with people who are considered at risk or who are socially deprived.

Typical duties include:

- listening to, advising and supporting people from all backgrounds and age groups

- delivering child health programmes and clinics

- running parenting groups

- identifying the specific health needs of certain community groups, often by working alongside them

- running support groups for specific health issues, such as giving up smoking

- counselling people who have mental health issues, such as postnatal depression, or have had a bereavement

- supporting and training new health visitors

- maintaining and updating patient records.

Ambulance staff

Approximately 15,000 people are employed as ambulance staff, or paramedics, in England. Their key role is to diagnose, treat and support patients in emergency situations, either where an accident takes place or where a person falls ill, or en route to hospital. Paramedics are trained to assess patients and start treatments, such as giving electric shocks to the heart, administering injections, and inserting a tube into a patient's throat to help them breathe. Paramedics are now recognised as state-registered professionals, in the same way as other health-care workers such as nurses and physiotherapists.

Their typical activities include:

- responding to 999 calls

- making quick diagnoses and giving emergency treatment to patients who are seriously ill

- bandaging wounds, applying splints to limbs and giving pain relief

- moving patients

- inserting drips and fluids

- caring for patients medically while they are being transported to hospital by ambulance

- driving and crewing their vehicles

- administrative tasks, such as writing up all case notes and passing on the patient's history, condition and treatment to hospital staff and coroners' offices.

Dentists

More than 20,000 people work as dentists in England, providing check-ups and dental treatments to their patients, as well as advice on how to care for their teeth and mouths. Most dentists are self-employed, but some provide dental care under the NHS and sometimes privately as well. Some work in other specialisms, such as hospital clinics, the armed forces, and teaching and research.

Ophthalmologists and optometrists

The 8,000 ophthalmologists and optometrists in the country test and deal with patients who have problems with their eyes, ranging from a short-sighted child to an adult with glaucoma.

Pharmacists

Pharmacists supply either hospital patients or the general public with medicine, through a doctor's prescription or through over-the-counter sales.

> **Key word**
> ---
> Over-the-counter – goods that can be bought without a prescription

Hospital pharmacists work in a hospital setting and are responsible for ensuring that the medicines used there are safe, appropriate and cost-effective. They can also use their specialist knowledge to supply drugs and to advise patients on any medicine they have been prescribed. They work alongside other health-care professionals, such as nurses and doctors, to come up with the most appropriate drug treatments for their patients.

Community or retail pharmacists normally supply medicine to the general public, in an independent pharmacy, a high-street chain or large supermarket. They can also provide people with advice on suitable medicines, the possible side effects and whether a drug could interact with any other treatment a person might be receiving. Some pharmacists also offer certain health-check services, such as blood-pressure monitoring and screening for diabetes.

> **Key words**
> ---
> Side effect – an unpleasant effect that a drug or medication can have on a person

Social workers

Social workers often work with people who are in difficult circumstances or who have been excluded socially. Their aim is to provide appropriate support to enable service users to help themselves; acting as a guide, adviser or friend. Social workers help individuals, families and community groups within a variety of settings, such as clients' homes, schools, hospitals and other public sector and voluntary organisations. More than 50 per cent of social workers deal with young people and their families, but they also work with young offenders, people with mental-health problems, drug and alcohol abusers, people with learning disabilities and the elderly.

Typical duties include:

- writing up assessments of individuals and their circumstances (often with medical staff)

- talking to service users and their families to assess and review their situation

- providing information and counselling support

- helping service users to lead the most independent life possible

- recommending and sometimes deciding on the best course of action for their client

- liaising with, and making referrals to, other agencies

- attending meetings on issues such as child protection

- maintaining accurate records

- preparing reports for legal action and giving evidence in court.

TECHNICAL SUPPORT PROFESSIONALS

The 122,000 scientific and technical staff employed in the health-care sector play a very important role in how patients are diagnosed and treated. Their role takes place behind the scenes, working in laboratories and does not generally involve interacting with patients. When you have a blood or urine test at your GP's, there will be someone in a lab looking for any sign of illness or problem.

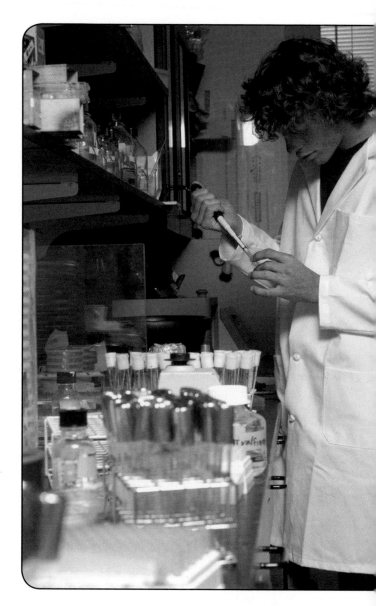

Figure 6.13 Lab technicians and scientists work mainly behind the scenes

Laboratory staff are normally divided into two job roles: technician and scientist.

- **Technicians** carry out tests on things such as blood and urine samples to determine if a patient has an illness, such as a genetic disease, or a health problem such as a urinary tract infection. A large part of this job involves using complex equipment to come to a diagnosis.

- **Scientists** conduct some tests on samples, but are more commonly involved with interpreting and analysing the results from tests and reporting back on these. They also have a development role such as working on new tests for diseases.

OTHER SUPPORT PROFESSIONALS

Health and social care organisations could not function efficiently without the support of other more general professionals. Within a hospital, a GP surgery, a social-care office and a laboratory, there are people keeping things running smoothly, ensuring that paperwork is being sent to the right people at the right time, that a department's IT needs are being met and that employees are getting paid! Around 199,000 people provide general support in such areas as IT, catering, finance and management.

Research tip

The NHS has a website where you can find out about the kinds of jobs available within the NHS, both medical and non-medical.

www.jobs.nhs.uk

THE ROLE OF PROFESSIONAL BODIES

Nearly every health and social care career you could think of is allied to a professional body: from optometrist to dentist, plumber to electrician. They have two main roles:

- to help provide the general public with information on what they can expect from a practitioner in their field

- to help people working in their field reach and maintain an agreed set of educational, professional and ethical standards.

Key words

Ethics – a set of moral principles

Briefly, professional bodies exist to:

- provide practice guidelines, which all members must adhere to

- advise on an appropriate code of ethics, particularly in health and social care

- give detailed information on careers within the profession and further development once members are qualified; this is called continuous professional development (CPD)

- run classes, training courses and seminars to help keep members up to date with various aspects of their profession

- keep members up to date with news on what is happening within the profession and factors that affect it; for example, government funding or changes in practice

- in some cases, help the general public to find a qualified professional in their area.

EVIDENCE ACTIVITY

P6 – P7

1. Choose a local health or social care provider in your local area that interests you. You are going to prepare a presentation for the rest of your group that identifies the place of this provider in national provision of health and social care services. Consider any current issues that have been highlighted by the media that might impact on this provider; for example, shortages of qualified workers, lack of funding, changes in local services or other policy issues. (P6)

2. You should now have some ideas about the type of career that you might want to pursue within health and social care. Choose three particular jobs that you would like to know more about. For each one, describe the roles and responsibilities the care worker would have, as well as the career pathway that you would need to take to achieve that position. The 'So you want to be a …' features in this book might be a good starting point. (P7)

Sociological Perspectives for Health and Social Care

unit 7

This unit is about sociology – the study of society and human social interaction. Understanding the basic principles of sociology is important for anyone working in health and social care. Practitioners need to be able to understand the influence of social factors and processes in order to recognise social problems, and to plan for and provide appropriate targeted care.

Sociologists analyse the ways in which people are influenced by each other and the group to which they belong. In this unit you will look at how various social factors and processes affect the lives of both individuals and groups. You will also examine the influence of social institutions and organisations.

Having explored the basic principles of sociology you will then look at how these can be applied to issues in health and social care, including how sociology influences our understanding of health, and the development of health and social care policies and services.

Learning outcomes

By the end of this unit you will:

| 7.1 | Understand sociological approaches to study | page 231 |
| 7.2 | Be able to apply sociological approaches to health and social care | page 242 |

So, you want to be a...
Social worker

My name Nadia Turner
Age 30
Income £ 22,000

If you are a patient communicator interested in helping all generations of a community then this is the job for you...

How would you summarise your job?
I work with families who are experiencing problems. My team is the Family Support Team within the social services department of the council.

What sorts of things do you do on a day to day basis?
I help run a centre for parents and children. Families are referred to the centre, where we make an assessment of the support that they need. We work with parents to help them improve their parenting skills and to give them practical support and guidance. We try to make the centre a fun environment for the children, far removed from the tensions at home.

What are the hours like?
The working week is 37 hours. Sometimes I have to do out-of-hours and weekend work too, in order to meet the needs of the families.

The work must be very demanding at times. What sort of personal skills do you need to be good at it?
You need to be patient, calm and adaptable to different situations. Being able to listen and observe what is going on is also really important. You need to be able to form effective relationships with a range of different people.

> **"We work with parents to help them improve their parenting skills..."**

It sounds like a really rewarding career. How did you get into it?
I did a vocational qualification in care, and after college I worked in a children's residential home; the hands-on experience was really helpful. Afterwards I went to university and did a degree in social work. Since qualifying, I've chosen to specialize in working with children and families, but I could have chosen to work with adults.

How easy is it to find a job in the sector?
My University provided a work placement. I also looked at the job adverts in specialist magazines and the Guardian on Wednesdays, and on websites such as www.communitycare.co.uk.

What about opportunities for further training?
My degree mixed academic study with work placements. Since joining my current team I have continued to receive training, for example, in child protection.

How good are the career opportunities in the sector? Where can you go next?
I am gaining experience and will soon have my own caseload. I would like to become a team leader. Managing the adoption or fostering processes are just two of the many different paths I could follow.

Grading criteria

The table below shows what you need to do to gain a pass, merit or distinction in this part of the qualification. Make sure you refer back to it when you are completing work so you can judge whether you are meeting the criteria and what you need to do to fill in gaps in your knowledge or experience.

In this unit there are 2 evidence activities that give you an opportunity to demonstrate your achievement of the grading criteria:

page 241   P1, P2, P3, P4, M1, M2, D1

page 257   P5, M3, D2

To achieve a pass grade the evidence must show that the learner is able to...	To achieve a merit grade the evidence must show that, in addition to the pass criteria, the learner is able to...	To achieve a distinction grade the evidence must show that, in addition to the pass and merit criteria, the learner is able to...
P1 use sociological terminology to describe the principal sociological perspectives		
P2 describe different concepts of health	**M1** use two sociological perspectives to explain different concepts of health	
P3 describe the biomedical and socio-medical models of health	**M2** explain the biomedical and socio-medical models of health	**D1** evaluate the biomedical and socio-medical models of health
P4 describe different concepts of ill health		
P5 compare patterns and trends of health and illness in three different social groups	**M3** use sociological explanations for health inequalities to explain the patterns and trends of health and illness in three different social groups	**D2** evaluate the four sociological explanations for health inequalities in terms of explaining the patterns and trends of health and illness in three different social groups

7.1 *Understanding sociological approaches to study*

SOCIAL STRUCTURES

Society and social behaviour can be studied by looking at the groups and organisations that people form. These are known as social structures. Through these structures people establish certain beliefs and ways of behaving; these make up their culture. Cultures can be very distinctive and vary from group to group or from country to country. In the following section we will look at three social structures that are particularly important to the practice of health and social care: the family, the education system and the health care system.

The family

The family is the first social structure that most people experience. Today, the family can take many different forms (see Figure 7.1).

The traditional image is of two heterosexual, married parents with a couple of children, a structure known as a 'nuclear family'.

However, there is a growing diversity of family types in the UK today. The number of single-parent families has increased for a variety of reasons, including marital breakdown and personal choice. There has also been an increase in the number of co-habiting couples who are living together without being married. Not all such couples are heterosexual; some may be in lesbian or gay partnerships.

Regardless of the type of family, all families share common features, linked to the family's social influence on family members.

> **Think** How would you describe your family structure?

The education system

Starting school marks an important step in a child's life. It introduces influences from outside the family. The purpose of the education system is to teach the knowledge and skills that society believes is necessary to function effectively within it. Sociologists are interested in how the education system tries to socialise pupils in certain key norms and values. For example, schools place value on achievement, competition and discipline. These values may be very different from the values young people have learned from their families.

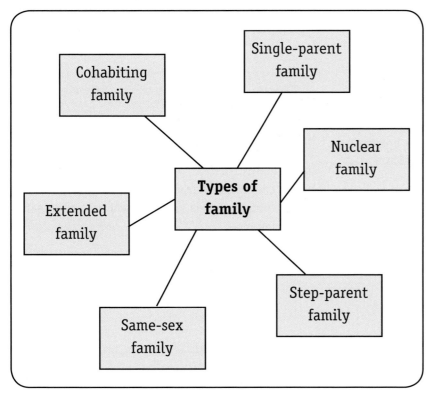

Figure 7.1 Some different family types

Cohabiting family
Single-parent family
Extended family
Types of family
Nuclear family
Same-sex family
Step-parent family

Key words

Beliefs – general feelings or opinions about the world
Culture – sets of beliefs and guidelines for how people behave in a society
Socialise – learning the ways of the society in which you live
Norms – expected patterns of behaviour that guide us in our everyday existence
Values – ideas about correct and fair behaviour that come from beliefs

Educational institutions are also important because young people are exposed there to another important social structure: the peer group. Peer groups have their own values and beliefs (not always the same as those taught in school!) and exert pressure on young people to conform to their values.

Health care services

Health care services are provided by both the public and the private sector. Public sector provision is funded by the state and ensures that all citizens receive the same basic standard of health services. In the UK, public services are provided by the National Health Service, which is part of the welfare state. The NHS was founded in 1948 to provide a system of health care that was free to all citizens.

In addition, individuals can access private sector services, for which they must pay. This creates inequalities in access to health care as privileged social groups are more able to pay for these services. There has been an increased use of the private sector to deliver health care in recent years.

Health care services are divided into three sectors:

- **primary health care** is the service provided by GPs, health visitors, dentists etc. This is the medical care a patient receives on first contact with the health-care system, before referral elsewhere within the system if necessary.

- **secondary health care** is provided by hospitals, clinics and other organisations to which a patient is referred.

- **tertiary health care** is highly specialised care that is available in regional centres, such as burns units.

Key words

Welfare state – a system in which the government takes resposibility for the welfare of citizens, for example by providing unemployment benefits, old-age pensions, medical care and education
Diversity – the differences between individuals and within social groups

SOCIAL DIVERSITY

All people are different: if you look around your group you will see that everyone has different social and cultural identities. These differences are a result of age, physical ability, race and ethnicity, religion, gender, sexuality and marital status. These differences are what create social **diversity**.

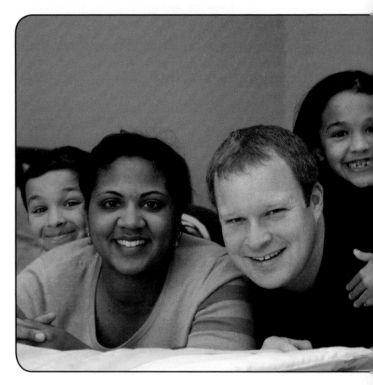

Figure 7.2 Diversity

> ***Think*** What examples of diversity are illustrated in Figure 7.2?

Sometimes these differences may affect how an individual is treated. When some people receive better treatment than others, inequalities in society result. This is an important area of research for sociologists.

Social class

Differences between individuals and groups in society can lead to social stratification. One of the main forms of stratification is when people are ranked into different social classes or socio-economic groups according to differences in their social and economic status.

Traditionally, social classes were defined as upper, middle and lower (working) class, but now it is more common to talk about socio-economic status. The Office for National Statistics uses a scale consisting of eight social classes (see Table 7.1).

Key words

Social stratification – the ranking of different social groups into a hierarchy

This was first used for the analysis of the 2001 census of England and Wales to reflect current

Research tip

The website of the Office for National Statistics is an excellent source of data about the UK. www.statistics.gov.uk

types of employment, including those who are not in paid employment.

Those in the same socio-economic group may share some of the same characteristics; for example the same educational background or similar housing. Most importantly, for health and social care practitioners, they also tend to have similar experiences of health and illness. Analysis of patterns of ill health shows a clear link with socio-economic group, highlighting the fact that there are inequalities. For example, individuals in the lower socio-economic groups are more likely to die prematurely.

Number	Socio-economic classification	Examples of job types
1	higher managerial and professional occupations	managing director, judge, solicitor
2	lower managerial and professional occupations	nurse, teacher, journalist
3	intermediate occupations	clerical worker, secretary, airline cabin crew, auxiliary nurse
4	small employers and own account workers	self-employed builder, taxi driver,
5	lower supervisory and technical occupations	employed craftsman, plumber, train driver
6	semi-routine occupations	shop assistant, postman, security guard
7	routine occupations	cleaner
8	long-term unemployed	unemployed

Table 7.1 Classification of employment types (Source: Office for National Statistics)

Gender

Sex is the biological state of being male or female. Gender is based on society's expectations about the differences between males and females. There are certain actions and thoughts that are seen as 'feminine' while others are seen as 'masculine'.

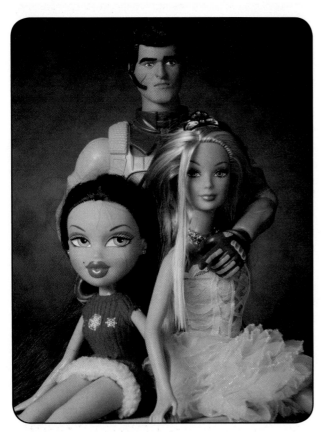

Figure 7.3 Toys reflect society's views of gender roles

> ***Think*** What can you learn about what society expects boys and girls to be like from toys like the ones in Figure 7.3?

Traditionally, home-making and the care of children have been seen as feminine activities, whereas risk-taking behaviour, for example, driving at high speed, has been seen as masculine. Sociologists are interested in gender as an explanation of inequality, for example, in health and illness.

Culture and ethnicity

People's ethnicity is linked to their genetic inheritance, culture, behaviour, language, rituals or religion. In the UK, the majority of the population is classified as white British, but there are also significant numbers of people from other ethnic groups. Some of the largest of these groups are Indian, Pakistani, Black Caribbean, Black African and Chinese. These are known as 'minority ethnic groups'. Studies of the experience of health of a range of ethnic groups has shown marked differences between them.

Age

People are frequently classified by age because every age group has different expectations and needs. For example, for the majority of people, health care is most needed at the beginning and towards the end of their lives.

The view of people of different ages varies between societies. In some societies older people are considered of greater worth because they are seen as wise and are therefore respected. In our society, the elderly have lost much of their status as they are generally poorer and have less influence and power. This is particularly significant because the UK has an ageing population as the birth rate has fallen. Inequalities in the experience of health care can be linked with an individual's age.

Locality

The places where individuals live and work have different environmental and social influences. If people live in an area where there is pollution, industrial hazards or poor social surroundings, these can have very serious effects on their health. Individuals' access to health care services is also determined by their locality, and this can lead to inequalities if certain services or treatments are not available to an individual for this reason.

SOCIALISATION

The first social structure that individuals experience is the family. Babies do not know the expected ways of behaving when they are born, but learn these from their family. This process is known as socialisation. It starts at birth and continues throughout life.

Key words

Socialisation – the way people learn to adopt the behaviour patterns of the community in which they live

Primary socialisation

The family is the main influence in socialising a child (see Figure 7.4). From their family, most children learn speech, basic health and hygiene, beliefs and values. They also learn moral or religious concepts, for example, the difference between right and wrong. This is known as primary socialisation. Much of what is learnt through primary socialisation stays with an individual for life.

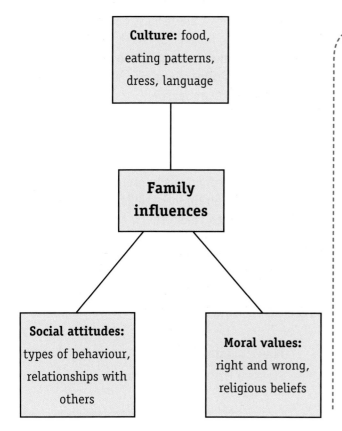

Figure 7.4 Influences of the family on a child

Secondary socialisation

Individuals are also socialised by influences outside their immediate family. Through this secondary socialisation people learn social rules and ways of behaving with others. This occurs through institutions or organisations such as school, the workplace and the mass media. Individuals are also influenced by the attitudes and values of their peer groups, teachers, work colleagues and even television personalities and celebrities.

Norms, values and beliefs

Socialisation allows individuals to learn the norms, values and beliefs of a cultural or social group. **Norms** are accepted rules about what behaviour is appropriate or expected in a particular social situation. **Values** are ideas or beliefs that are seen positively or thought to be important: a particular social group might value not having sex before marriage. **Beliefs** are the feelings or ideas about what is true on which values can be based. Shared norms, values and beliefs help groups and societies to live and work together effectively.

Example

Talia and Anoushka have become good friends at school and have visited each other's homes. Talia stayed at Anoushka's house one Friday night. Anoushka lives with her mother, father and one older brother. Each Friday her father and brother play football then go out with their mates. Anoushka and her mother spend the evening doing the shopping and household chores. Anoushka complains that her brother is never required to help in the house. He and their father see it as 'women's work'. They usually eat their evening meals while watching the television.

Talia lives with her parents, two older brothers and two younger sisters. The family is Jewish – they observe Jewish customs and celebrate the Shabbat or Day of Rest. Talia explains to Anoushka that this is a family occasion that starts on Friday night with a family meal together and continues through until Saturday. Her family observe their traditions and try to do things together over that day.

> ***Think*** In what ways do Anoushka's and Talia's families demonstrate different values and beliefs?

Most people in society behave as they are expected to behave and conform to society's norms. To function successfully, society relies on people conforming. However, there are always some individuals who do not conform, for a variety of reasons. Their behaviour may be classed as deviant. Individuals whose behaviour is deviant may reject some of the beliefs and values of society and behave in ways that are unacceptable to many people; for example by breaking laws. Society's view of what types of behaviour are deviant can change over time or in different circumstances. For example, having a baby before being married was seen as deviant behaviour in the 1940s; today many children are brought up by single mothers and this is seen as a norm.

Key words

Conform – to behave in the way that most people in a society or social group behave
Deviant – behaviour that is seen as unacceptable or strange

Roles

Most people behave as society expects them to behave. They adopt a role that is appropriate to their situation. The roles that people are expected to play in life are learned through socialisation. Gender roles are often learned in this way. For instance, girls learn how to be daughters, sisters, wives and mothers. In addition, they may learn about the types of occupational roles that society expects them to take on.

Key words

Role – a position or relationship within society or a group

Individuals play a number of different roles depending on the situation and it can be difficult to balance these. For example, a woman may have roles as a wife and mother, but also as a manager in the workplace. Tensions frequently arise when people try to combine different roles, particularly if society has certain expectations. On the whole, a woman is still expected to take responsibility for childcare while the man earns the higher salary. Sometimes the roles people play are the opposite of what is expected – this is known as role reversal; for example, if a man takes on the role of house husband.

> ***Think*** Care of children...DIY... cooking... cleaning...paying the bills...gardening. Do you associate these roles as being either 'male' or 'female' roles? Do the other people in your group agree with you?

Example

Some feminists argue that medicine is a predominantly male profession that marginalises women. Although 75 per cent of NHS workers and 90 per cent of nurses are female, only 14 per cent of consultants are female. In recent years the role of women in medicine has begun to change. Now over 50 per cent of those entering medical school to train to be doctors are female.

Status

The position of individuals in society is known as their status. Certain jobs, skills or actions are more highly valued than others, and therefore individuals associated with these are respected. Status can come from the social position into which someone is born, but can also be gained through achievements, which may be academic, financial, sporting or cultural.

Key words

Status – the relative position or standing of a person in a society

PRINCIPAL SOCIOLOGICAL PERSPECTIVES

Societies change, some more quickly than others. Sociologists describe patterns in social relationships and develop models that can help to explain and, in some cases, predict social change. They may be able to suggest actions or interventions that might improve an individual's life chances. Over the years people have tried to explain and analyse the way in which societies work from a range of different perspectives.

Functionalism

Functionalists argue that social institutions have a wider function for society as a whole. They claim that social institutions are interdependent and work together to create what society needs; for example social stability. Functionalists have likened society to a human body – for the body to function well, all of the organs and systems need to work together, and the same is true of social institutions.

French sociologist **Émile Durkheim** (1858–1917) was one of the first people to define different parts of a society by the function they served in keeping the society healthy and balanced. He argued that traditional societies were held together because everyone was more or less the same and held common beliefs.

In modern industrial societies, people have more differentiated and specialised roles. This results in a division of labour. People are forced into interdependence since they can no longer fulfill all of their needs by themselves: workers earn money and must rely on buying essential products from others to meet their needs.

Example

John's grandparents lived on a small farm in the north of England. They kept a cow, pigs and some chickens. A well supplied their drinking water. They would collect wood for their fire. His grandmother used wool from the sheep to knit warm jumpers. They only visited the nearby town once a month to buy a few supplies. They were often snowed in, but had enough of everything to keep warm and to eat well. Their friends were other farmers who lived very similar lives to them.

John lives in the centre of a city. He relies on his local supermarket and other nearby shops for all his needs. He is a highly skilled IT technician and is in great demand by firms who need him to sort out their complicated IT systems. He buys expensive clothes. He employs a cleaner to clean his flat and iron his shirts. When he meets his friends he visits the local pub.

In 1956, Talcott Parsons suggested that the nuclear family was an example of a structure that has developed to meet the functional needs of an industrial society. As society became more industrialised it required people to take on more specialised jobs, which led to the need to be more geographically mobile. Previously people had lived in extended family groups, but smaller nuclear families were able to move more easily to go where the jobs were.

Marxism

Marxist theories focus on the inequalities of wealth that are created by a capitalist economic system and the effects that this system has on individuals and society.

Figure 7.5 Karl Marx

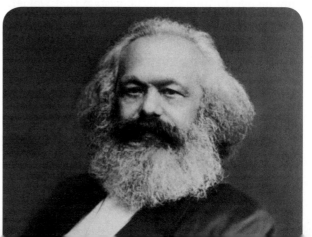

Karl Marx (1818–1883) disagreed with the idea that society meets its basic needs through people working together. He argued instead that the structure of society is based on economic power and wealth. In an industrial or capitalist society, the workers no longer control the means of production because the manufacture of goods is financed and controlled by the owners of private wealth. This leads to large inequalities in wealth, power and social status between the workers and the capitalist owners, creating class conflict in society. Marx expected that eventually groups of workers would rise up against the capitalists who exploit them in order to overthrow them.

Marx's views have continued to be supported by some sociologists. Marxists argue that the value of labour is continually being downgraded by the increased use of mass production techniques. The introduction of new technologies deskills the workforce, meaning that many people have to undertake tasks that require little skill. This gives the owners even more control over the process.

Key words

Capitalist society – a society where property and wealth are owned privately, rather than controlled by the government

Means of production – the machinery, equipment and materials used by workers to make products

Feminism

Feminists believe that society is structured in a way that leaves women at a disadvantage and argue that women deserve equal rights and opportunities to men.

Marxist feminists believe that the capitalist system is responsible for the inequalities between men and women in society. They argue that it is only by overturning the social system that women will stop being oppressed. Under capitalism, it is claimed, women are oppressed because it serves the interest of those who control the means of production. For example, they would argue that women benefit male capitalists by taking the role of unpaid housewives and having low-paid part-time jobs. In doing this they take responsibility for producing and rearing the workforce for the next generation without cost to the capitalist class.

Radical feminists believe that society is patriarchal, with men exercising power over women and children; this may include violence. Originally men had power over women because of women's reproductive role. Frequent pregnancies meant that women could not make the same contribution to the labour market and society as men. However, women now have much more control over when and if they have children through the introduction of the pill and other modern reproductive technologies. Radical feminists argue that changes in beliefs about a women's role in society have not kept pace with these reproductive changes.

The mass media is seen as supporting a patriarchal society by creating stereotypical images of women; for example, by depicting women as sex objects. Some radical feminists believe the solution is separatism: men and women should be helped to go their separate ways in society; for example by developing lesbian partnerships.

Key words

Patriarchal – ruled or controlled by men

Separatism – a belief in seeking independence

Liberal feminists believe that women and men are becoming more equal in society, but that more needs to be done through legislation and social processes to achieve equal opportunities. Changes in divorce laws, the introduction of the Sex Discrimination Act and the greater number of women in the workforce all support the view that there is now greater equality. However, liberal feminists believe that it is important to continue to challenge gender role stereotyping and the impact that this has on socialisation. For example, within the family children may be given toys that are gender-based: dolls and domestic toys for girls and cars and trains for boys.

The mass media also has a powerful role in creating male and female stereotypes, and liberal feminists point to the changes that have come from the increasing number of female journalists, writers and presenters. Schools and other educational establishments also have many opportunities to promote equality of opportunity for both sexes through resources which challenge gender stereotypes. Courses that have traditionally attracted only one gender now often have targets to challenge this; for example by attracting men into childcare and women into engineering.

> ***Think*** Look at some current magazines. What gender stereotypes do they portray?

Interactionism

Interactionists try to understand society by analysing the behaviour and actions of individuals in small-scale social situations, such as in conversations. They argue that behaviours and norms develop as a result of these types of interaction between individuals. For example, interactionists might observe a class in a school and analyse how the students and teachers interact, rather than looking at the whole education system.

George Mead, an American sociologist, argued that social life consists of people interacting with each other and that we learn from the ways that individuals react to and behave towards us. This allows norms to be established and then acted on.

CASE STUDY: FEMINISM AT WORK

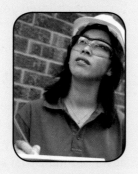

Jenny is now a high-flying career woman. At school she studied physics, maths and chemistry. She found that she was in the minority in her classes as there was only one other girl studying these subjects. She was determined to study engineering at university, so did some work experience with a major construction company, which she enjoyed. However, several of the managers suggested that she would find it difficult to succeed in her chosen career because 'it's a man's world'.

Jenny chose to go to a university where there was a female professor of engineering, and while she was there she met a group of other girls who were equally as determined to qualify in traditionally male careers. They kept in touch after university and have provided support to each other. At their yearly reunions they discuss problems that they believe they have encountered. Some believe that they continue to face discrimination because they are female. This led two of them to set up a consulting company that employs only women.

Jenny joined a national company, where she has risen through the company to be sales manager. She has had to work hard but has been promoted several times, often in competition with male applicants. There are several other women who have senior positions in the company. She feels that the situation is improving and that opportunities are now more equal. When she visited her old school recently there were many more girls studying science subjects.

The job that Jenny has involves her working long hours and travelling around the country, often spending nights away from home. Her husband is a busy GP and has never been interested in the running of the house or doing any shopping or cooking. Jenny is worried about what will happen if she has a baby, and is concerned that she will lose her status in the workplace as well as losing out financially.

QUESTIONS

1. What views about the role of women are illustrated in this case study?

2. How could Jenny's situation be explained from a feminist perspective? How would the different types of feminists differ in their analysis?

Interactionists argue that, in order to make sense of the world, we use a process of labelling to define certain categories; for example, 'criminal', 'insane' or 'heterosexual'. It is through this process that stereotypes are developed. People make assumptions about how to behave towards individuals who have been labelled.

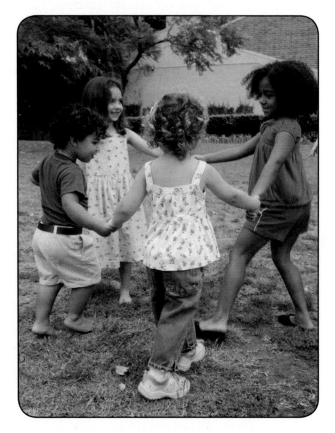

Figure 7.6 Interaction between children

> **Think** How do young children learn to behave through their interaction with one another, for example, in playing? Think of any time you have observed young children in a new setting.

Collectivism

Collectivists believe that collective goals are more important than individual goals because society as a whole has more value than separate individuals. Collectivists focus on the importance of community and society, and give priority to group goals over individual goals. Collectivism is the direct opposite of individualism. Collectivism rejects the importance of individual happiness or ambition unless it contributes first and foremost to the good of the group, which could be the nation, society, community or a gang.

Communist states organise themselves according to collectivist principles. In China, the state adopted a one child policy, taking the decision about the number of children to have away from individuals and families. The reasoning was that it would restrict population growth, so this policy would be for the good of the whole society. Communes, such as Israeli kibbutzim, also follow collectivist principles, as children are cared for by the community rather than families, and production of food is shared collectively.

> **Think** What are the implications for an individual if society restricts the number of children you may have?

Postmodernism

Postmodernists argue that many of the previous sociological theories have been superseded because the nature of society has changed in contemporary advanced industrial societies. They argue that class identity is no longer as important as it was. There are a larger number of factors, including gender, age and ethnicity, that influence people's lives. They also argue that people are now able to exercise more choice over what they want to be.

The role of the media in influencing society is also highlighted in postmodernism. It is claimed that the media increasingly suggests how people should behave and what they should buy, for example.

> **Think** How does the mass media influence the choices that you and your family make?

New Right

The 'New Right' is a descriptive term for various forms of conservatism that emerged in the mid to late twentieth century; for example, in the UK under Margaret Thatcher and in the USA under Ronald Reagan. It is largely a political perspective that makes claims about how society should be organised, rather than providing a way of analysing existing social structures.

The New Right argued that the rising costs to government of the welfare state were preventing economic growth and that individuals had become increasingly dependent on the state. Traditional roles in society were thought to have been undermined by the permissive values of the 1960s and 1970s. For example, they argued that the nuclear family is very important to society and that the rise in the number of single parents and same sex couples is bad for society. The New Right also argued that the welfare state creates a dependency culture and that individuals should take more responsibility for themselves.

> ***Think*** In what ways do individuals depend on the provision of the welfare state? What changes have there been since the 1980s to reduce an individual's dependency on the welfare state?

Key words

Permissive – allowing behaviour, especially sexual behaviour, that other people disapprove of

EVIDENCE ACTIVITY

P1 - P2 - P3 - P4 - M1 - M2 - D1

1. Create a presentation that describes the seven principle sociological perspectives. This could be in the form of a poster, leaflet or PowerPoint presentation. For each perspective you must use the correct terminology and give examples linked with health and social care. (P1)

2. You need to describe the different concepts of health and ill health and the biomedical and socio-medical models of health. Produce a table that includes all this information. (P2, P3, P4)

3. Identify a case study of an individual or family, for example:

- An elderly couple who have health problems and can no longer look after themselves

- A single mother with two young children living in high rise flat

- A young man who is depressed and living alone.

Use your case study to:

a) Apply two sociological perspectives to different concepts of health. (M1)

b) Explain the biomedical and socio-medical models of health (M2)

4. Write an evaluation of the biomedical and socio-medical models of health. You should comment on the strengths and weaknesses of each model and draw conclusions. You may wish to do this in the light of the case study you have considered. (D1)

7.2 Applying sociological approaches to health and social care

CONCEPTS OF HEALTH

What is meant by health? Different people and organisations have tried to define the concept of being healthy or having good health (see Figure 7.7).

> **Think** What does being healthy mean to you? What is the difference between 'aspects' (views) of health and 'concepts' (ideas) about health in this context?

As you can see, there are a number of different aspects to health. As an individual goes through life they are likely to gain a greater understanding of what health means to them and to society.

Negative concepts of health

A negative definition of health is one that concentrates on the absence of disease or illness. It suggests that you can only be regarded as being healthy if you have no disease or illness; for example, 'I don't feel ill – I don't have a cold'. This is the definition that is used in the biomedical model of health which we will explore in more detail later in this unit.

Positive concepts of health

Positive concepts view health as a state of well-being. An individual might 'feel' well even if they have a disease. An individual might say 'I feel great today – fit for anything'.

Lay concepts of health

Before the rise of scientific medicine people tried to explain concepts of health and illness in non-scientific ways. Many of these beliefs still exist and are known as lay concepts.

Here are some of the things people say about health:

> *'Feed a cold and starve a fever'*
>
> *'An apple a day keeps the doctor away'*
>
> *'Early to bed and early to rise makes a man healthy, wealthy and wise'*

> **Think** What do these sayings suggest people think about health and illness?

People's understanding of what it means to be healthy varies widely and is influenced by many different factors. The cultural heritage of individuals might affect their views, such as traditional Chinese medicine, which uses herbal medicine and acupuncture as treatments.

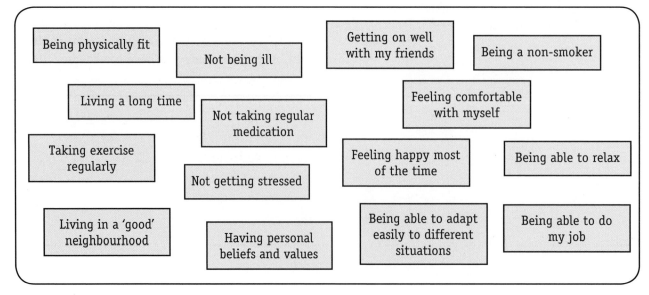

Figure 7.7 Some definitions of good health

Holistic concepts of health

Holistic concepts of health take account of all the different dimensions of health. These dimensions were classified by Ewles and Simnett in 1992 as:

- physical: the functioning of the body

- mental: the ability to think clearly and make judgements

- emotional: the ability to recognise and express feelings appropriately

- spiritual: an individual's beliefs and values, which may include religious beliefs, and how they put them into practice

- social: the ability to have satisfactory relationships with other people

- sexual: the acceptance and expression of one's own sexuality

- societal: the way individuals are treated within society; for example, access to basic necessities or the existence of racism, political unrest, war or inequalities between men and women

- environmental: the standard of the physical environment in which individuals live, including housing, sanitation and pollution.

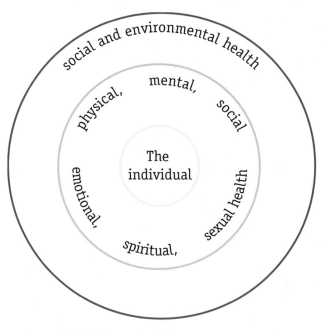

Figure 7.8 Holistic health

Although health can be divided into these different aspects, it is clear that many of these are interlinked. When individuals are physically ill, they often become depressed, which affects their emotional and mental health (see Figure 7.8). This is the basis of the holistic view of health. This view means that health professionals need to understand the importance of treating individuals as a 'whole' and not merely concentrating on one aspect of their health.

World Health Organization definition of health

The World Health Organization is a specialised agency of the United Nations, founded in 1948. Its objective is to help all people achieve the highest possible level of health. The WHO's original definition of health was:

> 'Health is a state of complete physical, mental and social well-being, not merely the absence of disease or infirmity.'

This definition is based on a broad concept of health. It is a holistic definition because it encompasses all aspects of health. It has been argued that this definition is too idealistic and therefore unattainable. However, it is a clear attempt to define health in its broadest sense.

In 1984 the WHO published a further definition:

> 'Health is the extent to which an individual or group is able on the one hand, to realise aspirations and satisfy needs and on the other hand, to change or cope with the environment. Health is, therefore, seen as a resource for everyday life, not the object of living: it is a positive concept emphasising social and personal resources as well as physical capabilities.'

Health should be understood as a social construct. Many people think of health as freedom from disease, but this can be interpreted in different ways. For example, some people may believe their lifestyles are healthy when medical evidence might demonstrate otherwise. In addition to this, different cultural groups have different attitudes to health.

Social constructs of health have changed over time. Before the 18th century, illness was thought to be the result of sinful behaviour by the victim, but scientific advances have proved this view wrong. However, in recent times, there has been a tendency for some illnesses, such as HIV/AIDS, alcoholism, lung cancer and obesity, to be blamed by some on the behaviour of the sufferer.

Example

Mr and Mrs Torres are both in their thirties. They live in a flat on the top floor of a high rise building on a large council estate. The lift has been out of order for the past few weeks. They have two young children who are frequently ill with chest infections. Mr Torres rarely works and they rely on Mrs Torres's part-time job at the local supermarket for their income. The flat is damp and they are behind in paying their rent. They live over 100 miles from their extended families.

Think Are Mr and Mrs Torres healthy according to the different definitions of health? What would need to happen for Mr and Mrs Torres for them to be seen as healthy?

CASE STUDY: AHMED AND KATE

Ahmed is 29 and lives with Kate, age 26. They live in the north west of England. They have a 15 month old daughter, Mia, and plan to marry next year.

Ahmed was born in Pakistan and came to England with his parents when he was three years old. He lived in a mainly Asian community and grew up understanding the culture of his parents.

Kate was born in London and is white. Her father left home when she was five years old and she was brought up by her mother. Kate is very close to her grandmother, who helped look after her when she was young. Her father 'does not approve of mixed marriages'.

Kate and Ahmed met while they were at college. After school, Ahmed studied psychology and, following postgraduate training, is now a social worker. Many of his clients have mental health problems. He is part of the crisis intervention team, which seeks to keep individuals in their own homes and avoid admission to hospital. The last emergency he had to deal with was when one of his clients was threatened with eviction from his home because he had been neglecting himself while he was ill. He finds the work very interesting and rewarding, but at times stressful.

Kate is a community midwife. She took a health studies course at a further education college before training as a nurse. She then undertook midwifery training. Since having Mia she works part time and also tries to support her grandmother who is suffering from the early stages of Alzheimer's disease. In her job she covers two distinct areas near her home. One is an affluent part of the town and the other is a run-down estate. She has noticed that the mothers and babies from the two different areas have different experiences of health. There are differences in behaviour, such as smoking during pregnancy, attendance at antenatal classes and rates of breast feeding.

QUESTIONS

1. What different aspects of health are shown in the case study?

2. What might cause the differences in the health of the mothers and babies that Kate cares for in the different areas of the town?

3. Explain why Ahmed might be involved in trying to prevent one of his clients being evicted from his home.

MODELS OF HEALTH

As we have seen, there are a number of different concepts of health, including negative, positive and holistic. These different concepts have led to the existence of alternative models of health which seek to address the main factors that contribute to health in different ways.

Biomedical model

The biomedical model is an approach to health that focuses on the structure and functioning of the body. It is based on the Western scientific approach to medicine and has the following main characteristics:

- it focuses on abnormalities in the body

- disease or illness is explained by biological factors

- it seeks to diagnose the cause of ill health through observations, examinations and tests

- doctors and medically trained staff are regarded as the only people who are trained to identify and treat disease and illness

- it emphasises treatment, such as surgery, medication or other interventions

- treatment is expected to take place in an appropriate environment, such as a hospital

- illness is regarded as a temporary state that can be changed by the intervention of medical expertise.

The biomedical model does not consider the social factors that affect health. This model remains very powerful in Western medicine. If an individual cannot be diagnosed with a specific medical condition they may be labelled as 'malingering' (pretending to have an illness in order to stay off work or collect insurance benefits, for example).

Example

Tejus had had a cough for several weeks. It had started after he had been doing some particularly dusty work in his house. He had been very anxious about the work and often coughed nervously when worried. As the cough had not improved he went to see his GP. She examined him and arranged a series of tests. She asked him to provide a specimen of his sputum (the phlegm that he coughed up). He went to the hospital for a chest X-ray and she also gave him a course of antibiotics. The doctor asked him to return to the surgery in two weeks' time so that his progress could be reviewed. The GP did not think that the dusty house was the cause of the infection.

Socio-medical model

Not all of the factors considered by a holistic concept of health will be considered under the biomedical model, and thus no interventions will be made to address some problems. The socio-medical model is based on the idea that health can be improved by making social conditions better, as these affect the health of particular groups.

Looking at the history of health improvements, McKeown concluded in 1974 that improvements in sewerage systems, clean water supplies, and better nutrition and diet had dramatically affected life expectancy. There had been a decrease in child mortality well before the introduction of biomedical techniques, such as vaccination. In the past health problems such as malnutrition were associated with poverty and poor housing.

The main causes of preventable death in modern Western societies are linked to personal behaviour or lifestyle choices, such as smoking, diet and drug use. In countries in the developing world, lack of access to clean water is still responsible for the high numbers of deaths in childhood. The United Nations reports that 4000 children die each day as a result of diseases caused by drinking dirty water.

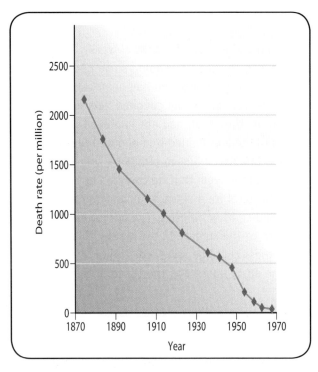

Figure 7.9 Decline in deaths from tuberculosis in England and Wales

> **Think** Look at Figure 7.9. When did death rates start to fall? When was medical treatment introduced? In what ways could child health be improved without the use of medical intervention?

Example

Orla is 65 years old and about to retire. She has smoked for all her adult life and now finds that she gets out of breath very easily. She enjoys her food and has become very overweight. This has meant that she has found it difficult to exercise, particularly as she says her knees 'keep giving way'. However, Orla is looking forward to retiring and plans to spend more time on her hobbies, which include gardening and bowls. She and her husband are planning a cruise together to celebrate her retirement and are confident that their pensions are sufficient for their needs.

> **Think** How might the lifestyle choices that Orla has made be affecting her health? What measures could she take to improve her health?

The biomedical model does not address the social and psychological factors that contribute to maintaining good health. The socio-medical model builds on the biomedical model by considering these aspects of health. These include:

- how well individuals care for themselves

- how able they are to function in their social role

- how they feel about themselves – this gives an insight, for example, into a person's emotional life, pain, social integration and physical mobility.

The socio-medical model has opened up the treatment of mental illness. Although some types of mental illness are physiological, such as Alzheimer's disease, others are not. A greater understanding of the patient's experience is gained through the socio-medical approach. For example, the Government issued the following recommendations to improve mental health:

- Unemployed people are less likely to suffer depression and have better success finding work if they are given social support and help in developing job-seeking skills.

- People caring for relatives with dementia are less likely to suffer from depression if they are given practical information about the disease.

- People caring for relatives with schizophrenia benefit from practical information and social support.

- Support groups supplying a combination of practical help, social networking and advice on parenting have been proven to have a dramatic impact on the mental health of young isolated mothers and on the cognitive and emotional development of their pre-school children.

- Rapid treatment for depressed mothers can prevent harm to children, who may otherwise experience cognitive and emotional damage.

- Self-help support groups have proved beneficial for widows, where they can offer each other one-to-one support alongside other practical help and small group meetings.

- Children at school with unrecognised learning difficulties, including dyslexia, will benefit from appropriate school programmes for assessment and help.

Example

At a get together, some members of a family have been discussing their health over the past year:

- Tom, aged 59, has had chest pain and has been diagnosed as having angina.
- Jane, aged 45, has lost her job and has felt depressed.
- Mike, aged 20, had an accident on his motorbike and broke his leg.

Think What are the main causes of each of their illnesses? Which approach is likely to ensure successful treatment or prevention of health problems?

The socio-medical model recognises the effectiveness of the promotion of health through social policies and legislation to improve the environment and help individuals make healthier lifestyle choices. For example, legislation to ban smoking in public places makes it easier for individuals to choose not to smoke. The socio-medical approach highlights the fact that changes made beyond the health and social care sector, through the law, education and local government, for example, also have a part to play in creating good health.

As we saw earlier, New Right thinkers are concerned about the role of the welfare state in creating dependency. They emphasise the need for individuals to take more responsibility for themselves, and this applies to their own health, putting increased emphasis on people making the 'right' lifestyle choices.

In 1999, the Government published a White Paper entitled *Saving Lives: Our Healthier Nation*. This will be examined in more detail later, but the following information was included to encourage individuals to take personal responsibility for their own health:

'There are many ways that an individual can take responsibility for improving their own health. Many of them are to do with choices that they make about their own lifestyle; for example, whether they choose to smoke or take exercise.'

Look at the ten tips from the White Paper for better health.

1. Don't smoke. If you can, stop. If you can't, cut down.

2. Follow a balanced diet with plenty of fruit and vegetables.

3. Keep physically active.

4. Manage stress by, for example, talking things through and making time to relax.

5. If you drink alcohol, do so in moderation.

6. Cover up in the sun, protect children from sunburn.

7. Practise safer sex.

8. Take up cancer screening opportunities.

9. Be safe on the roads: follow the Highway Code.

10. Learn the First Aid ABC – airways, breathing, circulation.

Think To what extent are individuals responsible for their own health? Are there any causes of diseases that are outside individuals' control?

CONCEPTS OF ILL HEALTH

Having looked at what it means to be healthy, we will now look at how individuals and society view ill health.

Illness and disease

Ill health is the absence of health and the presence of disease or illness. It is possible for individuals to be diagnosed with a disease even though they do not have any symptoms or feel ill. For example, a routine screening may show the presence of a breast cancer of which a woman was totally unaware. On the other hand, individuals may describe themselves as feeling ill, but investigations may fail to identify any specific disease to account for their symptoms. Figure 7.10 looks at this in more detail.

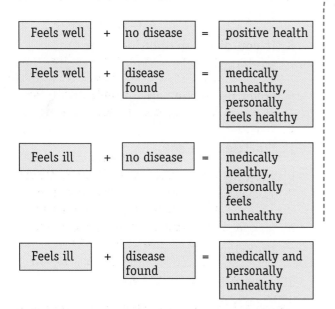

Figure 7.10 Results of different combinations of illness and disease

Key words

Disease – the presence of some abnormality in the body that can be detected and identified
Illness – the feeling associated with loss of health

Disability

A disease may lead to impairment. The impairment may affect a psychological, physiological or anatomical structure or function. A disability is any restriction or lack, resulting from an impairment, of ability to perform an activity normally. A dysfunction is a disadvantage for individuals that results from an impairment or disability; for example, something that prevents them from fulfilling their normal role, taking into consideration age, gender, social and cultural factors.

Key words

Impairment – a deviation from the norm through a loss or abnormality

Example

Basia is a 20 year old woman. As a child she had a serious accident when her leg became trapped in some farm machinery. After a series of operations, her leg had to be amputated. She has had a false leg fitted, which attaches below her knee. She and her parents were determined that she should participate in the same activities as her friends. She swims, skis and runs. However, she is sometimes unable to keep up with her able-bodied friends, as she cannot go at the same pace as them. She needs to use specially-adapted equipment. Basia feels that nothing can hold her back from doing what she wants in life.

The biomedical model argues that disease and illness stem from abnormalities or malfunctions in the human body. However, some believe that medical definitions of disease are constructed by society. Some diseases, such as mental illness, attract a stigma. Some sociologists have argued that there is no such thing as mental illness, but that by labelling certain behaviours as an illness society can control unacceptable behaviour.

Key words

Stigma – when a person is labelled in a way that sets them apart and links them with an undesirable stereotype

There are sometimes differences of opinion as to what behaviour might be regarded as 'normal', 'bad' or 'mad'. People's views may also change over time and in different circumstances. In some societies, individuals who have wanted to stand up to the state have been labelled as mad and put into psychiatric hospitals. It is therefore suggested by some that mental illness is partly socially constructed.

Iatrogenesis

In 1976, Ivan Illich argued that not all medical interventions were successful and that the practice of medicine could lead to what he called 'iatrogenic ill health'. This is a disease or illness induced by medical treatment or diagnosis. He identified three types of iatrogenisis:

- **Clinical iatrogenesis** is ill health caused by medical intervention, such as an unwanted reaction to a prescribed drug or an infection acquired while under medical care. An example of this is the rise of hospital acquired infections such as MRSA (methicillin-resistant Staphylococcus aureus).

- **Social iatrogenesis** is the loss of the ability to cope. This may be linked to the medicalisation of everyday life or the institutionalisation of individuals in medical settings, such as psychiatric hospitals.

- **Cultural iatrogenesis** is the loss people experience from the unrealistic expectations raised by modern medicine.

> **Think** Give examples of the way in which clinical, social and cultural iatrogenesis have occurred.

The sick role

Talcott Parsons developed a theory of how society views those who are ill. He argued that society sees illness as deviant because it interferes with the normal social roles that an individual is expected to perform. Therefore, it is necessary for rules to be applied to those who are sick and those who care for them. In 1951 Parsons suggested the following as the main expectations of sick people:

- **Sick people are allowed exemption from the performance of their normal social roles.** This means that, relative to the severity of the illness, individuals are no longer expected to undertake their normal social roles. So, for example, pupils are not expected to go to school. These exemptions need to be confirmed by appropriate people in order that they should be seen as legitimate; for example, children might need a note from a parent or doctor.

- **Sick people are not responsible for their own condition.** People who are ill are not expected to get better by themselves. There is not an expectation that the illness is within their control and they should 'pull themselves together'. It is expected that they will need to be cared for.

- **Sick people should try to get well as soon as possible.** It is expected that individuals should want to get better. Any suggestion that they may not want to improve may be labelled as malingering. It is assumed that illness should be seen as a temporary situation and that individuals should not use illness as a way of avoiding normal social roles.

- **Sick people should seek technically competent help and co-operate with medical experts.** Doctors are seen as important 'gatekeepers'. Patients are expected to consult doctors who can legitimise the diagnosis of being sick and officially label the condition.

> **Key words**
>
> Deviant – different from the norm

> **Think** In what ways might parents lose their social roles if they are ill? What effect might this have?

The clinical iceberg

It is thought that a large proportion of the population is in need of medical care, but is not consulting a doctor or seeking treatment. This is known as the clinical iceberg and represents a large unmet need (see Figure 7.11).

Like any iceberg, most of its bulk is below the water line. The submerged section represents the part of the general population who does not go to a doctor. Some of these people have symptoms and some self-medicate. In this model, those people interacting with health-care services are above the water line. The largest proportion of these are seen in primary care and smaller numbers in secondary and tertiary care.

Think Why might an individual not go to a doctor, even if they are feeling unwell?

Figure 7.11 – The clinical iceberg

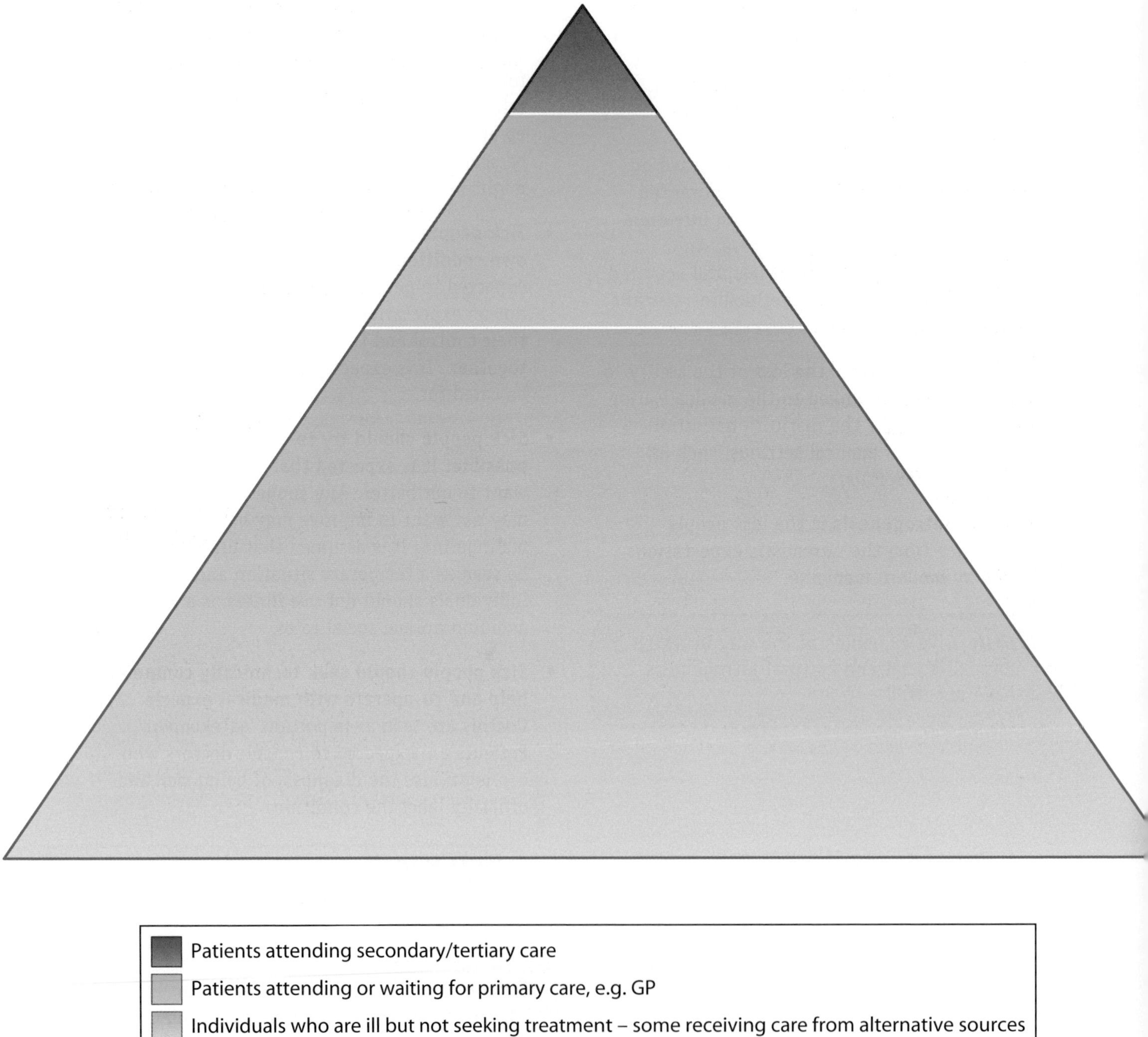

■	Patients attending secondary/tertiary care
▨	Patients attending or waiting for primary care, e.g. GP
▢	Individuals who are ill but not seeking treatment – some receiving care from alternative sources

UNDERSTANDING PATTERNS AND TRENDS IN HEALTH AND ILLNESS AMONG DIFFERENT SOCIAL GROUPINGS

Measurement of health

The study of how disease and illnesses are spread through society is called **epidemiology**. This plays an important part in providing the scientific basis for assessing health. Data is also collected on the risks associated with certain lifestyles or patterns of behaviour.

It is important for health and social care professionals to understand some of the terms that are used by epidemiolgists:

- **morbidity rate**: the proportion of people who get a certain disease

- **mortality rate**: the proportion of people who die from a disease

- **prevalence**: the number of cases of a certain disease at any one time

- **incidence**: the number of new cases occurring in a given period of time

- **health surveillance**: the monitoring of individuals for the purpose of identifying changes in health status.

Information about disease and illness may be collected internationally, nationally and locally and is presented in a variety of statistical formats. The information collected can help to answer important questions, such as how many people are or could be affected by an illness, who is most at risk and whether certain groups are more vulnerable than others.

Example

One of the early pioneers in the field of the study of disease was Doctor John Snow. In 1854, London was in the grip of a cholera epidemic. People had no idea about how cholera was spread or what they could do to avoid becoming ill. Snow thought that the cause was probably drinking water and so conducted research, which resulted in him being able to isolate the contaminated water pump responsible. For the further specifics of the case please refer back to Unit 4, page 133.

What this study demonstrated were the advantages of reviewing disease amongst certain groups, including its social and environmental aspects. This led to the development of epidemiology.

There are many types of data that can be used to gain information that helps to measure health. These can include:

- childhood immunisation rates

- health statistics

- the uptake of screening services

- main causes of admission to hospital

- accident rates

- socio-economic data, including unemployment rates, crime statistics and leisure facilities etc.

- mortality statistics.

> **Think** Look at Figure 7.12 on page 36. Which age group is most at risk of developing malignant melanoma? Can you suggest what social reasons might influence this?

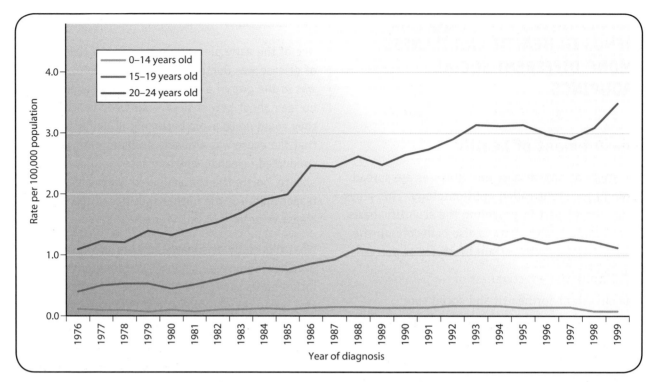

Figure 7.12 Age specific incidence rates of malignant melanoma

Another method of collecting data on health is through surveys, which can be used to show lifestyle decisions and attitudes towards health, such as smoking and participation in exercise.

Think Look at Figure 7.13. Which social group is most motivated to give up smoking and which least? Can you give any explanation for these findings?

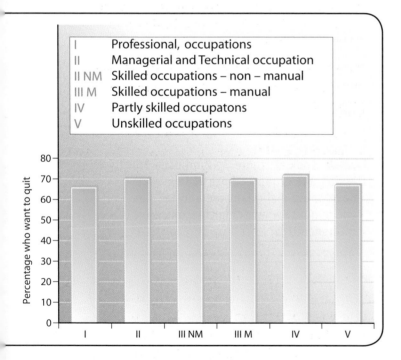

Figure 7.13 Motivation to quit among adult smokers by socio-economic group

[Source: Jarvis 2001]

Using data to analyse the health of a society can be very helpful, as it will give a scientific reason for interventions or provision of services. It also gives a baseline that can be used as a comparison to evaluate the success of the intervention. It is, however, important that the data used is up to date.

In order to make comparisons between societies, some form of agreement is needed about how diseases are classified. The World Health Organization publishes the *International Classification of Diseases*, which has 20 main categories and many subsections. Each disease has its own code and these are used when completing records, such as hospital admissions forms and death certificates. Some diseases are classified as 'notifiable'. These include infectious diseases such as measles, meningitis and tuberculosis, as well as such diseases such as malaria and rabies.

Think Why are some diseases classified as 'notifiable'?

Difficulties in measuring health

With so many different definitions of health, it can be difficult to measure it. However, there are several reasons why it might be considered important to do so:

- In order to plan, it is necessary to have evidence of the needs of a population. It is important have a standard against which to measure the effectiveness of interventions.

- It is important to understand the composition of a population in order to assess the meaning of health and disease statistics. For example, a population that is made up of a large number of older people is likely to have a higher incidence of age-related illnesses, such as cancer or heart disease. For this reason, demographic data showing the size and age profile of a population is used alongside health data to allow meaningful comparisons. For example, when working out death rates, a standardised mortality rate is used, which shows how many deaths should be expected.

Other problems in measuring health are such concepts as the clinical iceberg, discussed in the previous section, which can mask the true picture of health in any community

Key words

Demographics – statistics about an area's population, such as age, sex, income and education
Standardised mortality rate – the ratio of the number of deaths observed in a specific population to the number of deaths that would be expected if that population had the same mortality rate as a standard population

Patterns and trends in health and illness

Epidemiological and demographic evidence confirms the view that there are many inequalities in society with regard to health. If health and illness occurred randomly across the whole of society, everybody would have an equal chance of experiencing ill health. However, certain groups have greater rates of disease and illness. The main factors that cause these higher rates are socio-economic status, gender, ethnicity, age, locality and certain risky behaviours.

In 1980, the Black report was published. It had been commissioned approximately 30 years after the founding of the NHS and provided a commentary about how the UK had done in providing for the health of its population. The report concluded that there was a poorer health experience for the lower occupational groups at all stages in life. Examples included:

- Men and women in occupational class V had a two and a half times higher chance of dying before reaching retirement age than those in occupational class I.

- At birth and during the first month of life, the risk of death in families of unskilled workers was double that of professional families.

- Boys in class V had a ten times greater chance of dying from fire, falls or drowning than those in class I.

- The difference between the health of men and women indicated that the risk of death for men in each social class was almost twice that for women.

- Differences in the health experiences of different racial and ethnic groups were also identified.

Since the publication of the Black report there have been many other studies which continue to identify inequalities in society. The Acheson Report (1998) was asked to review health inequalities and make recommendations for policy developments that would reduce these inequalities.

They found that the scientific evidence supports a socio-economic explanation of health inequalities, which are caused by factors such as income, education, employment, environment and lifestyle. The report made three key recommendations to the government:

- All policies likely to have an impact on health should be evaluated in terms of their impact on health inequalities.

- A high priority should be given to the health of families with children.

- Further steps should be taken to reduce income inequalities and improve the living standards of poor households.

In *Saving Lives: Our Healthier Nation,* evidence still persisted of inequalities based on social class, gender, ethnicity and locality.

Coronary heart disease (CHD) and stroke

- The death rate from CHD in people aged under 65 was almost three times higher in Manchester than in Kingston and Richmond.

- Death rates for CHD for those born on the Indian sub-continent were 38 per cent higher for men and 43 per cent higher for women than rates in the UK as a whole.

- The death rate from CHD was three times higher among unskilled men than professionals and the gap had widened sharply in the previous 20 years.

- Stroke death rates in people born in the Caribbean and the Indian subcontinent were one and a half to two and a half times higher than for people born in the UK.

Accidents

- Children up to the age of 15 years who came from unskilled families were five times more likely to die from unintentional injury than were those from professional families.

Mental Health

- Suicide was three times more common in men than in women.

- Women living in England who were born in India or East Africa had 40 per cent higher suicide rates than women born in the UK.

Cancer

- 40 per cent of unskilled men smoked, compared with 12 per cent of men in professional jobs.

- Bangladeshi women were less than half as likely as other women in this country to come forward for cervical screening.

Many of these findings can be further analysed to link them with social factors, ethnicity or geographical area.

> **Think** Look at Figure 7.14. Which ethnic groups are most at risk of having high blood pressure?

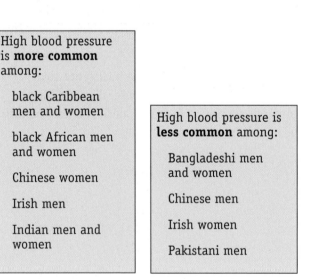

High blood pressure is **more common** among:

    black Caribbean men and women

    black African men and women

    Chinese women

    Irish men

    Indian men and women

High blood pressure is **less common** among:

    Bangladeshi men and women

    Chinese men

    Irish women

    Pakistani men

Figure 7.14 High blood pressure in ethnic groups in England [Source: Health Survey for England: The health of ethnic minority groups '99]

Think Look at Figure 7.15. According to this chart, what is the influence of living in different localities on an individual's experience of cancer? What reasons can you suggest for this?

Figure 7.15 – Effect of locality on survival
[Source: Office for National Statistics, 1999, www.statistics.gov.uk] .

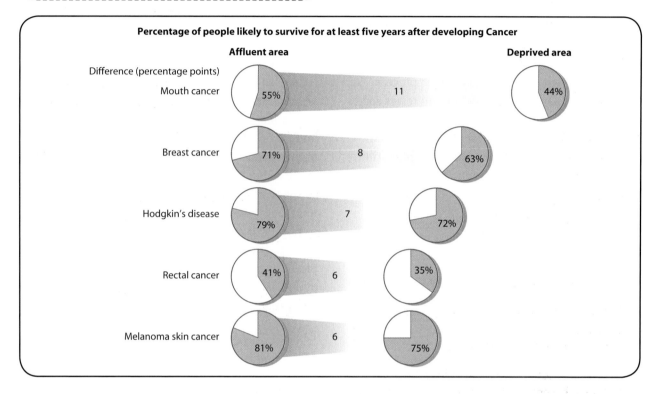

Percentage of people likely to survive for at least five years after developing Cancer

	Affluent area	Difference (percentage points)	Deprived area
Mouth cancer	55%	11	44%
Breast cancer	71%	8	63%
Hodgkin's disease	79%	7	72%
Rectal cancer	41%	6	35%
Melanoma skin cancer	81%	6	75%

Figure 7.16 Child pedestrian deaths in Europe in the mid 1990s [Source: Department of the Environment, Transport and the Regions]

Think Look at Figure 7.16. What are some of the main causes of childhood pedestrian deaths? Why might England have one of the worst records in Europe?

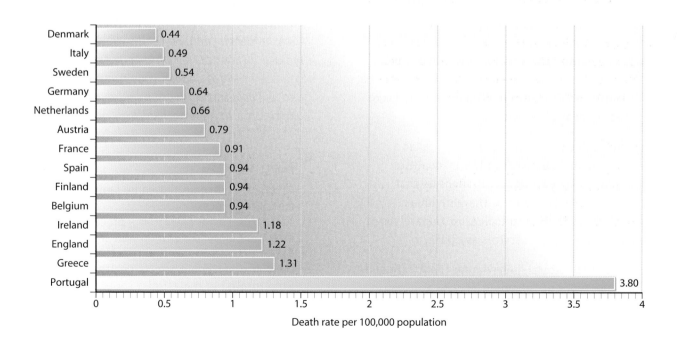

Country	Death rate
Denmark	0.44
Italy	0.49
Sweden	0.54
Germany	0.64
Netherlands	0.66
Austria	0.79
France	0.91
Spain	0.94
Finland	0.94
Belgium	0.94
Ireland	1.18
England	1.22
Greece	1.31
Portugal	3.80

Death rate per 100,000 population

Sociological explanations for inequalities in health

Different explanations have been put forward to explain the existence of such striking inequalities in health.

One view is that the evidence for inequalities is a sociological artefact. This view suggests that inequalities in health are not real inequalities, but occur as part of the measurement process. For example, the gap between higher and lower socio-economic groups is seen not as a true picture, but as a result of the way the data is collected. The Black report did not accept this explanation and there has been little convincing evidence to support this argument.

Natural or social selection was a theory put forward as early as 1855. It suggests that people who are fitter and in better health are likely to get better jobs and will therefore be in a higher socio-economic group. According to this theory it is likely that those in lower socio-economic groups will suffer more illness.

Other sociologists put forward a cultural/behavioural theory. They suggest that inequalities in health are a result of cultural differences and lifestyle choices. For example, those who smoke, eat unhealthily and take little exercise are more at risk from ill health and disease than those who make healthier lifestyle choices. There is also evidence to show that members of lower socio-economic groups do not take advantage of preventative health-care services, such as immunisations, antenatal care or cancer screening. Members of some ethnic groups may be disadvantaged as language difficulties may make the use of medical facilities difficult.

The cultural/behavioural perspective takes a 'victim blaming' approach to the inequalities that individuals experience. It suggests that inequalities are the fault of the individuals themselves for failing to look after themselves or to take advantage of services available.

Critics of the cultural/behavioural theory argue that some types of behaviour may be a response to poorer economic circumstances. They offer a structuralist or materialist theory that lifestyle choices made by individuals are determined by social structure and that it is social inequality that is to blame for health inequalities. For example, those in lower socio-economic groups may be less able to afford healthy food, more likely to have poor housing and be unable to access sports or health-care facilities.

Research has shown that doctors spend more time with patients from higher socio-economic groups. Health inequalities can also be caused by poor allocation of NHS resources. Areas with a large number of people from lower socio-economic groups often have fewer and worse health-care facilities, in terms of primary care and hospitals. GPs may not want to work in poor and run-down neighbourhoods. The NHS has also been accused of failing to meet the needs of ethnic minority communities by neglecting to teach health-care professionals the different cultural norms and by failing to provide information in appropriate languages.

The response to the issue of health inequalities has been to develop strategies and services that meet the needs of different groups. In *Saving Lives: Our Healthier Nation*, a commitment was made to seek to improve the health of the nation.

'In securing better health we reject the old arguments of the past. We believe that the social, economic and environmental factors tending towards poor health are potent. People can make individual decisions about their and their family's health which can make a difference. We want to see a new balance in which people, communities and the government work together in partnership to improve health.'

Key words

Artefact – outcome caused by faults in the measuring process
Natural or social selection – process in which the fittest are most likely to do well socially
Cultural/behavioural theory – the way in which individual behaviour affects health
Structuralist or materialist theory – emphasises the role of the external environment on health

Research tip

The Kings Fund website has a useful section about health inequalities.
http://www.kingsfund.org.uk/resources/briefings/health.html

Example

Middlehampton is a large town in the UK with a diverse population spanning the whole range of socio-economic groups. Some areas are very affluent, whereas others have many properties in bad condition.

The Links housing estate mainly contains poor housing stock, occupied disproportionately by single older people, with young unemployed couples and minority ethnic groups making up the rest of the residents. In contrast, Cavendish Park is a highly desirable housing development occupied by professional families, some of whom have children educated at boarding school or university. The Broadlands is a new development under construction with a proportion of affordable housing. Some young families have already bought or rented properties in this development, but, because of health and safety considerations, it has no play facilities for the young children living there.

Think How could the artefact, social selection, cultural and behaviourist approaches help to explain the differences?

Research tip

You can find *Saving Lives: Our Healthier Nation* at the TSO website.
www.official-documents.co.uk

EVIDENCE ACTIVITY

P5 – M3 – D2

1. You have been asked to prepare a report detailing the patterns and trends of health and illness in three different social groups of your choosing.

a) Compare the differences between the three different groups, making sure that you keep a list of the sources that you use when getting your information.

b) Display your findings for the three different groups in either a report, leaflet or Power-Point presentation. (P5)

2. Explain the possible sociological reasons for the differences in the three groups (M3)

3. Using the four sociological explanations for health inequalities evaluate their strengths and weaknesses in explaining the patterns and trends in the three different groups. (D2)

Psychological Perspectives for Health and Social Care

unit 8

Psychology sets out to explain how people think and feel, how they learn and develop, and why people behave in the ways they do. A knowledge of psychology can be really helpful to health and social care workers. It influences the way we think about our service users and the issues and problems they face. In addition, it gives give us the means to help them with their lives.

In this unit we will look at six psychological approaches that are relevant to work in health and social care. This unit explains the key points of each approach, and also shows how these approaches can be used in a work context. You will explore lots of examples that give you the chance to listen in on conversations between health and social care workers and their service users. All the examples are based on real situations, but of course they are anonymous.

Learning outcomes

By the end of this unit, you will:

8.1 Understand psychological approaches to study   page 261

8.2 Be able to apply psychological approaches to health and social care   page 280

So you want to be a...

Mental Health Nurse

My name Jonny Epstein
Age 29
Income £27,000

If you are motivated by the thought of bettering the everyday lives of people suffering from mental health problems then read on...

What do you do?

I have a really rewarding job! I work with young children who have autism, and I work with their parents. I'm employed by the local NHS Trust.

What responsibilities do you have?

I work as part of a specialist team. We have a consultant psychiatrist and a clinical psychologist in the team, along with a speech and language therapist, an occupational therapist and a teacher. Young children are referred to us by family doctors. We carry out assessments, and then work with parents to find practical ways of helping them to promote their child's learning and development. The team is based in a hospital but I do a lot of my work in the families' homes.

How did you get into the job?

I did a vocational qualification in health and social care at college and then went on to train in nursing. I wasn't sure what branch of nursing I would go into, but I've always been interested in mental health. I started off working with adults were depressed and phobic, others were schizophrenic, and needed long term support.

How did you find your current job?

I'd always been keen to work with children and their families in a community setting. http://www.jobs.nhs.uk/ is a good resource for finding a variety of roles within the NHS.

> **❝ I have a really rewarding job! ❞**

What training did you get?

After college I went on to university to do a nursing degree. This was a three year course which had a common foundation programme, followed by specialist training in mental health nursing. This part of the course covered a lot of sociology and psychology, and it also helped us to acquire the interpersonal skills we would need in our jobs. Like other nurses I have to do on-going training to keep my skills up to date.

What are the hours like?

Our working week is 37½ hours.

What skills do you need?

In my job you need be able to empathise with people, you need to be a good listener, and you need good communication skills. You also need to show warmth and caring. Some of the people we work with in adult services can be very challenging and we need to be able to spot when things are getting tense and be able to defuse them. Mental health nursing is a complex and demanding area of nursing and you do need a strong personality of your own.

What about the future?

For now, I would like to gain more experience of people with autism. One day I'd like to be a team leader.

Grading criteria

The table shows what you need to do to gain a pass, merit or distinction in this part of the qualification. Make sure you refer back to it when you are completing work so you can judge whether you are meeting the criteria and what you need to do to fill in gaps in your knowledge or experience.

In this unit there are six evidence activities that give you an opportunity to demonstrate your achievement of the grading criteria:

page 283   page 284

page 285   page 287

page 289   page 290

To achieve a pass grade the evidence must show that the learner is able to...	To achieve a merit grade the evidence must show that, in addition to the pass criteria, the learner is able to...	To achieve a distinction grade the evidence must show that, in addition to the pass and merit criteria, the learner is able to...
P1 describe the application of behaviourist perspectives in health and social care		
P2 explain the value of the social learning approach to health and social care service provision		
P3 describe the application of psychodynamic perspectives in health and social care	**M1** analyse the contribution of different psychological perspectives to the understanding and management of challenging behaviour	
P4 describe the value of the humanistic approach to health and social care service provision	**M2** analyse the contribution of different psychological perspectives to health and social care provision	**D1** evaluate the roles of different psychological perspectives in health and social care
P5 explain the value of the cognitive perspective in supporting individuals		
P6 describe the application of biological perspectives in health and social care		

8.1 Understanding psychological approaches to study

Before we go any further, let's look at the idea of a theory.

Key words

Theory – a set of ideas that we use to understand and explain things. Some theories also allow us to predict and control what will happen next

Think about theories you have learned about in science lessons. Science has theories to explain why things fall to the ground, how electricity passes along wires, and how we get energy from food. Theories in psychology do the same sort of thing. They explain how we think and feel, how we learn and develop, how we behave and what we aspire to.

Theories are built up from careful observations of how one thing is linked to another. In your science lessons, these observations probably included practical experiments and analysis of what the results told us. Theories in psychology are also based on observations and on what people tell us about themselves. Some areas of psychology also make use of experiments.

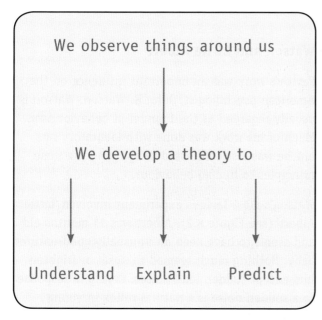

We observe things around us

↓

We develop a theory to

↓   ↓   ↓

Understand   Explain   Predict

Figure 8.1 Developing and using theories

Theories should explain things. Some theories, but not all, can be put to practical use in a work situation, for example by helping us to understand people's behaviour and giving us the tools to sort things out for people. Other approaches help us to think about our service users' needs, but they don't tell us what to do to help them.

Why are there so many different theories in psychology all trying to explain human behaviour? One answer is quite simple: different theories try to explain different aspects of behaviour. Some theories, such as behaviourist approaches, are very broad and try to explain everything. Other theories set out to explain a more limited range of things, for example personality development or language development. And other theories are more specialised still, such as theories about how children learn to read or how adults deal with post-traumatic stress.

Another answer is a bit more complicated: different theories have different ideas about the evidence – the raw material that psychologists work with. Here are three examples that illustrate this.

- The **humanistic** approach accepts what people say about themselves and thinks that's all there is to it.

- The **psychoanalytic** approach hears what people say, but tries to interpret it. The analyst looks for underlying meanings that the person is not aware of.

- The **behaviourist** approach has no time for what people say. They simply look at what people actually do.

As a result, health and social care workers have a large number of theories to draw on. At this point we can say that all these theories have areas where they work well, and areas where they don't work so well. We'll see how this works out in practice later in the unit.

Think How can theories help us to offer more than just common sense in health and social care work?

PRINCIPLE PSYCHOLOGICAL PERSPECTIVES

Behaviourist approaches

Behaviourist, or behavioural, approaches are easy to understand. Behaviourists are only interested in our behaviour – in what we actually do. They are not interested in anything that might be going on inside our heads. Behaviourists apply scientific principles to studying behaviour. They don't think it is important to ask and analyse what people might be thinking or feeling. All that matters is what we see them doing.

Key words

Behaviour – to a behaviourist, behaviour is what we see someone do

Behaviourist approaches are really theories about learning and are easy to apply in a health and social care context. If we understand how people learn, we can help them to learn new skills. We can also help them to unlearn old habits that are unhelpful to them. Behaviourist approaches are used by a wide range of practitioners; for example:

- clinical and educational psychologists

- physiotherapists, occupational therapists, and speech and language therapists

- teachers and learning assistants

- nurses and care workers.

> **Think** Behaviourists believe that, apart from a few reflexes that we are born with, everything we are and everything we become is the result of learning. What do you think of this idea? Can you think of any aspect of your own behaviour or personality that is not the result of learning?

Pavlov and conditioning

The first person who studied behaviour scientifically was the Russian physiologist, Ivan Pavlov. Pavlov was actually studying digestive processes in dogs at the time, but in doing this he discovered the phenomenon we now call **classical conditioning**.

When dogs are presented with food, they drool (or salivate). This is a natural reflex: the food is a stimulus, and salivation is the response. Because this is natural, we describe the food as an unconditioned stimulus and salivating as an unconditioned response.

In the course of his work, Pavlov noticed that the dogs began to salivate before the food actually arrived. For example, they started to salivate at the sound of someone approaching the kennel. This was inconvenient because it interfered with his experiments on digestion, but it intrigued Pavlov. He decided to introduce a new sound to the dogs. This was a neutral stimulus, the sound of a bell. It had no effect on its own, but, when it was paired with food, the dogs began to salivate as before. After hearing the bell before food arrived just a couple of times, learning began to take place: the bell on its own was causing the dogs to salivate. The bell had now become a conditioned stimulus and the salivating had become a conditioned response. This is a very simple form of learning and is known as classical conditioning.

Watson and Little Albert

Pavlov's work was an important influence on the American psychologist, John B. Watson. Watson is usually regarded as the founder of behaviourism. Much of his work was done with laboratory rats, but he was also interested in applying the same principles to human behaviour.

Watson's most famous experiment involved 'Little Albert' (see Figure 8.2). Albert was 11 months old and seems to have been an unusually good-natured baby. Nothing much seemed to upset or frighten him except sudden loud noises. Crying in response to a sudden noise is a natural reflex in young children. Watson would stand behind Little Albert, strike a steel bar with a hammer, and Albert would begin to cry!

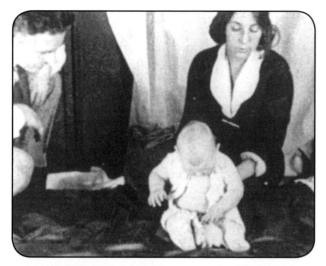

Figure 8.2 Watson conducts his experiment with 'Little Albert' and the white rat

Watson then looked for something that Albert enjoyed. He used to play with one of Watson's white rats, so Watson and his assistant decided to condition Albert to be afraid of it. The assistant sat with Albert while he played with the rat, while Watson sneaked up behind him and hit the steel bar hard with the hammer. Albert naturally began to cry. Watson repeated this a number of times until Albert began to cry whenever he saw a white rat. Watson didn't have to frighten him with the noise, seeing the rat was enough to make him cry. The white rat had now become a conditioned stimulus and the crying was now a conditioned response.

Can you see the similarities with Pavlov's work?

Before conditioning:

• the white rat was a neutral stimulus

• the loud noise was an unconditioned stimulus

• Albert's crying was an unconditioned response.

After conditioning:

• the white rat became a conditioned stimulus

• Albert's fear became a conditioned response

• Albert became fearful of anything that resembled the white rat.

Think What do you think about this experiment? Was it scientifically justifiable or simply cruel?

Skinner and the role of reinforcement

Another American psychologist, B. F. Skinner, developed the work that had been done on classical conditioning. His work is useful to health and social care workers. Classical conditioning is concerned only with reflex, or automatic, behaviour, like salivating or crying in response to noise. Skinner believed that his theory could explain all of people's behaviour, and that it could also give us the tools to change people's behaviour. These tools came to be known as **behaviour-modification programmes**.

Put simply, Skinner believed that most of our behaviour is learned. Learning occurs as a result of rewards, or what Skinner called '**reinforcement**'. If a piece of behaviour is rewarded or reinforced, we tend to repeat it next time round under similar circumstances. Once we understand these principles, we can use reinforcement to teach people new behaviour. We can also encourage clients to use behaviour that they have already learned, and we can use reinforcement to get rid of behaviour that is inappropriate or unhelpful (see Figure 8.3).

Key words

Behaviour-modification programmes – applying behaviourist principles in a systematic way in order to change someone's behaviour
Reinforcement – a reward of some kind which happens after we have done something, and which makes that behaviour more likely to happen again

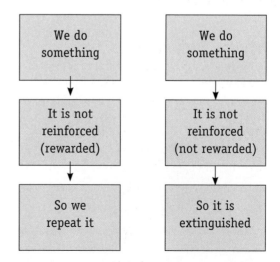

Figure 8.3 How reinforcement can be used in behaviour modification

Skinner did most of his experimental work on animals and often used food pellets as a form of positive reinforcement. Other forms of positive reinforcement might include:

- treats of some kind

- the chance to do a favourite activity

- certificates or stickers

- praise or attention.

Skinner also used negative reinforcement in his experiments. Remember this is not the same as punishment. Negative reinforcement is when something unpleasant stops happening. This might be something like:

- losing your smoker's cough when you quit smoking

- worrying less about your health when you start an exercise programme

- getting sent out of class – if pupils find the work too hard and get sent out for disrupting the lesson, an unpleasant experience has stopped.

Key words

Positive reinforcement – positive reinforcement takes place when something pleasant happens

Negative reinforcement – negative reinforcement occurs when something unpleasant stops. People often confuse negative reinforcement with punishment

Social learning theory

Social learning theory developed out of the work of an American psychologist, Albert Bandura. Although it is similar in some respects to the behaviourist approach, it has some important differences.

Behaviourists argue that we learn from our own actions. We do something, and if it is reinforced we are likely to do it again under similar circumstances. Bandura didn't disagree with this, but argued that learning must take place in other ways as well. If we had to try everything out for ourselves and wait for reinforcement, it would take a very long time to learn everything we need to know!

Bandura said that we also learn by observing other people and modelling our own behaviour on what we see others do (see Figure 8.4). If the behaviour we observe seems to work for another person, if it seems to be reinforced, then we think that perhaps we will be reinforced if we imitate their behaviour.

Like Skinner and the other behaviourists, Bandura believed in studying behaviour experimentally. He is probably best known for his Bobo doll experiment. In this study, a group of children were shown a video of a young woman attacking a Bobo doll – a large inflatable doll which rolls and returns upright when it is knocked over. The young woman punched and kicked the doll, hit it with a hammer and shouted at it aggressively.

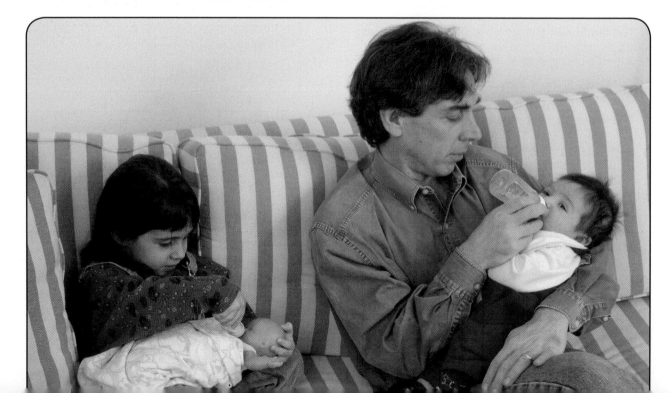

Figure 8.4 Children often imitate their parents

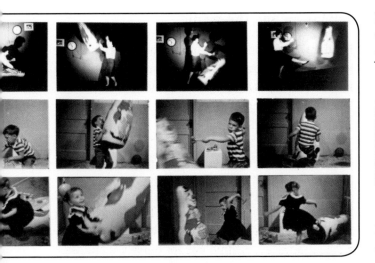

Figure 8.5 After watching the violent video (top), the children attacked the Bobo doll

The children were then taken into a playroom where there were a number of toys, including a Bobo doll. About 90 per cent of the children ignored the other toys and began to attack the Bobo doll with a hammer and shouted at it as the young woman had done. When Bandura brought the same children back eight months later, 40 per cent of the children showed that same behaviour again.

What was going on in this experiment? The children hadn't learned to do this through a process of shaping and reinforcement. This was an example of observational learning: learning from watching someone else and modelling their behaviour on what they observed. Bandura's theory became known as 'social learning theory'.

Key words

Shaping – building up a complex piece of behaviour through reinforcing attempts that get closer and closer to it

Bandura was interested in why people behave aggressively. Modelling helps to explain this. For example, if a child grows up with a violent parent, they might come to model their own behaviour on the parent's, especially if they see this behaviour

being reinforced in some way. If their father is violent, for example, their mother might do things just to please him.

> ***Think*** List some other examples of observational learning; for example things that younger children might learn, or that you have learned from watching other people.

Bandura said that there are four components to observational learning:

- **attention** we need to pay attention to the model, and our attention is better when something about the model catches and holds our attention

- **retention** we need to retain (or remember) the behaviour we have observed

- **motor reproduction** we need to be able to replicate or reproduce the behaviour we have observed

- **motivation** we must be motivated to reproduce the behaviour.

Peer group

Our friends and our peer group have a powerful effect on our behaviour, particularly when we are young. We are also influenced by the people we would like to have as friends – people we look up to and admire. They become models for our behaviour, and if we start to imitate and behave in the same way as they do, a group culture begins to take shape.

Groups

We often behave differently when we are in a group than we would if we were on our own. Groups often have norms, or expectations, about how group members will behave.

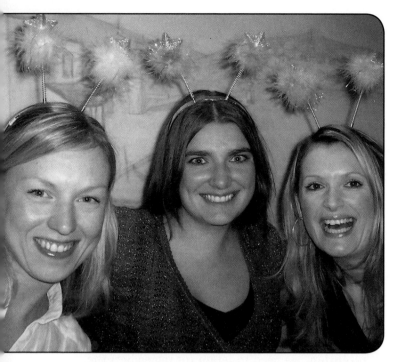

Figure 8.6 A group of friends on a hen night

Think You are out on the town on a Saturday night, with a group of people you know well. Are there group norms that affect the way you behave? Do you behave differently if you are with a group of friends from school than when you are with a group of older people?

Culture

The beliefs, traditions and values that are passed on from one generation to another form a culture. A person's culture may be based on geography. Do people from Yorkshire have the same beliefs and values as people in London? Do people in the United Kingdom have the same beliefs and values as people from Italy? There will be lots of similarities, but there may also be some differences. Culture may also be based on the ethnic and religious groups people belong to.

Think Consider two groups you know something about who are defined by where they live, by race or by religion. Can you identify any beliefs that are strongly held by one culture, but not by the other?

Television and the media

Bandura's work on modelling and observational learning raises some questions about the role of the media. Television is a big part of many children's lives, so what kind of models does it provide?

Think Can you think of any positive models on TV which might encourage children to behave well? Who are the models? Why would imitating their behaviour be reinforcing for young children?

Many people believe that watching aggressive and violent programmes on television can influence children to behave more violently. Social learning theory might predict this: people will imitate violent behaviour if they see it being reinforced and if there are no negative consequences. An example of this is 'copy cat' crimes, where people imitate in real life an unusual crime shown on TV. However, the relationship between aggression on TV and aggressive behaviour is not so clear cut. Some people disagree with social learning theorists and argue that watching violent programmes on TV, or playing violent video games, allows people to get rid of their aggressive feelings in a socially acceptable way. This is the sort of argument that a psychoanalytic theorist might make.

Think How would you design a study to look at the effect that violence on TV has on young children's behaviour?

Role theory

Role theory gives us another way of understanding people's behaviour. Role theory says that we act out different roles in our daily lives. You might act out a number of different roles during the day, such as friend, student and volunteer care worker; these roles guide the way you behave in each of these contexts. Certain behaviour is expected in your role as a friend, which is different from the behaviour you would show as a volunteer worker in a care home. If roles guide our behaviour, we can understand a lot about what people do if we know something about the roles they are playing.

Think What sort of behaviour would be expected from someone taking the role of a nurse? How would that be similar, and how would it be different, from someone in the role of a teacher?

Role theory recognises that there are times when we have difficulty carrying out the roles we have. We might experience **role confusion**. This happens when we don't know what behaviour is expected in our role. For example, someone who has just started a new job as a learning assistant may not know how far they ought to go in controlling an unruly group of children. We might also experience **role strain**. This happens when we have difficulty doing what is expected of us in a role. For example, newly appointed learning assistants may not have all the training they need to carry this role out as well as they would like to do.

Role conflict comes about when we occupy two roles that come into conflict. Imagine, for example, a learning assistant, Nina, who has been in the job for some time. She experiences no role strain as she is doing the job well, but then a new child joins the nursery. The child has challenging behaviour, which she can deal with in her role as a learning assistant. However, if the child was her nephew she would have a second, conflicting role as the child's aunt.

Self-fulfilling prophecy

It is often difficult for people outside of a group to understand group norms, and this may lead them to stereotype people in the group. For example, think about the attention given to 'hoodies' by the media. Is that really a useful way to refer to young people? Can we come to any sensible conclusions about how they will behave from the clothes they choose to wear? People often come to conclusions based on stereotypes, and by speaking to and treating people in a certain way, because of a stereotype we hold, we can set up a self-fulfilling prophecy. If we expect people to behave badly, they often do so.

Psychodynamic approaches

Psychodynamic approaches to understanding behaviour are the earliest of the approaches we are looking at in this unit. They began with the work of Sigmund Freud. Freud was a doctor who worked in Vienna. In 1886 he set up a clinic to treat patients with nerve and brain damage; he would become known as the 'father of psychoanalysis'.

Freudian theory

Freud's theory was very complex and was developed over his whole working lifetime, but there are a number of key ideas that allow us to see how it works.

How much are we aware of? Freud believed that there are three levels of awareness (see Figure 8.7).

- We have thoughts and feelings which are in our **conscious** mind. We call these conscious because we are aware of them.

- Other thoughts are **preconscious**. Although we may not be aware of them now, we can easily bring them into our conscious mind.

- Most of our thoughts and feelings, Freud said, are in our **unconscious** mind. Our unconscious mind contains all the things that have ever happened to us, and we are unaware of these 'hidden thoughts'.

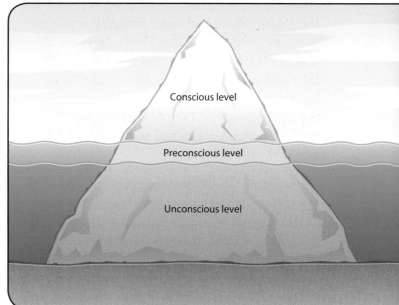

Conscious level

Preconscious level

Unconscious level

Figure 8.7 Fraud's three levels of awareness

The importance of the unconscious mind

The unconscious mind is very important in Freud's theory. He believed that many of the things in our unconscious mind have been forgotten by us, and others are being actively repressed. However, they continue to have a major influence on our feelings and our behaviour. Freud used special techniques in psychoanalysis to bring these unconscious thoughts into consciousness. Psychoanalysts use this technique to help people deal with tensions and conflicts in their past, so that they can reach a better state of mental health.

The id, ego and superego

Freud believed that the mind works as three systems that are linked to each other. He called these systems the id, ego and superego. These systems don't exist as physical structures in the brain, but they give us a useful way of thinking about how our personalities develop and why we behave as we do.

Id is a Latin word which means 'that thing'. The id is an unconscious mass of powerful instincts and drives. These are very basic, such as the drive for food, sex or self-preservation. The id provides us with motivation and energy, but it is completely self-centred. It is only interested in pleasure, operating according to the pleasure principle, and it demands immediate satisfaction.

Obviously the id has to be controlled. We share the world with other people and this ruthless pursuit of our own interests wouldn't get us very far. This is where the ego comes in. Ego is the Latin word for 'I' and it refers to our conscious self. The ego operates in the real world and works according to the reality principle. The ego tries to keep the id in check by finding safe and acceptable ways to satisfy the id's demands.

The superego is a bit like our conscience. While the ego is realistic and tries to get along in the real world, the superego is idealistic and always wants to do what is right. This creates another tension: the superego tries to persuade the ego to follow its idealistic goals. The superego operates according to the perfection principle. It is partly conscious and partly unconscious so we are not always aware of its influence.

The id and the superego are always in conflict with each another: one has no sense of what is right and really doesn't care, and the other is impossibly moral! The ego is in the middle and has to find a way of resolving this conflict so that we can get on with our lives in the real world.

If the id is stronger than the ego the impulses from the id push through, which could lead to destructive and immoral behaviour. But if the superego is more dominant, we could become too concerned with doing what is right, and deny ourselves ordinary and acceptable pleasures. This might lead to anxieties, phobias and neurotic behaviour in later life. If, however, we have a strong ego, we can find ways of allowing both the id and the superego to express themselves in appropriate ways. Freud would say that having a strong ego makes for a balanced and healthy personality.

> *Think* Can you think of any historical or fictional characters who had an id or a superego that seemed to dominate their personality?

Freud developed his theory by listening to the accounts his patients gave of their lives. He didn't take what they said as being true, however. Freud believed that much was buried in his patients' unconscious and that his patients were not aware of this. Anything they told him would have reached consciousness only after it had been filtered through their ego's defence mechanisms. This meant that what they said had to be interpreted or analysed, and so his technique for helping people became known as psychoanalysis.

The importance of early experiences

Freud believed that people's personalities are formed from a very early age, and he thought that some processes, including breast feeding and toilet training, were key to this. Freud believed that children who were told off for filling their nappies grow up to be anally retentive. In adult life they become rigid, obsessive, and show a meticulous attention to detail. Children who are praised for their bowel movements come to enjoy them. They are anally expulsive and grow up to be self-confident and generous, if a little disorganised!

CASE STUDY: PSYCHOANALYSIS IN ACTION

In order to help patients understand what has been going on in their lives, psychoanalysts have to do two things. They must find ways of getting in touch with people's unconscious and then analyse (interpret) what this means. Let's look at how this might work in practice.

Brandon is six years old. He has had a difficult childhood and is in the care of the local authority. He seems angry and destructive. His social worker has referred him to the Child and Adolescent Mental Health Service where he meets Hannah, a clinical psychologist. Hannah often uses psychodynamic approaches in her work with children.

Hannah plans to ask Brandon about himself and she will listen carefully to see if there are any themes in what Brandon says. If there are things he wants to talk about, or things he seems to be avoiding, she will get some idea of what the issues are for him. Brandon, however, refuses to speak to her. Hannah isn't sure if this is because Brandon doesn't have the language skills to express himself, or because the issues are just too hard for him to deal with.

Hannah needs to try something else. Freud used free association with some of his patients. He would say a word, and the patient would say whatever came into their head. Some words he used, such as 'holiday' would be quite safe, but other words, such as 'father', would have more of an emotional loading. Hannah rules out this technique as she doesn't think Brandon would co-operate, and it seems a bit risky this early in their meetings.

Freud also asked his patients to talk about their dreams. He believed that dreams are our unconscious mind at work, and the things we dream about represent people and situations we are trying to deal with in our waking lives.

We are not aware of the connections, but if the psychotherapist can interpret our dreams, they may be able to understand the working of our unconscious mind. Brandon won't respond to questions about his dreams; he says he doesn't remember any.

Hannah decides to try something safer. She gives Brandon some toys and watches him at play. His play is violent, with lots of fighting and people dying. She wonders if this represents his earlier life. Was his father violent? Nobody in his life actually died, and so could this be Brandon's way of representing the loss of people who were important to him, such as his mum or dad?

This gives Hannah something to think about. At their next meeting she asks Brandon to draw some pictures. Brandon enjoys this and one of his pictures shows a group of people who might be a family. Hannah asks Brandon who is in the picture. In the centre is a little boy. Could this be Brandon? And next to him is a woman. Could this be the mummy that Brandon wants back in his life? Standing at the edge of the picture is a man. This could be Brandon's representation of his father. The man is small – does that mean he's not important? Hannah isn't sure. And is the man coming in to join the group, or is he walking away? Perhaps Brandon will tell Hannah as they will only be talking about a picture and Brandon hasn't said this is his mum and dad. In fact, if this is his unconscious mind at work, he won't be aware of the connection between his picture and his life.

In the end Hannah used play therapy to help Brandon act out his feelings about his father, who was violent and deserted the family. In doing this Brandon lost most of his anger and became able to trust and form attachments with other people. After a while he left care and went to live with his mum.

Some of Freud's other ideas were even more surprising. Listening to his patients, Freud came to believe that little boys, from age three to about five, go through a process called the Oedipus complex. They realise that they are competing with their father for their mother's love and attention. They become intensely jealous of their father and desire his removal, so as to have the mother all to themselves.

His thinking on girls was even more startling. Freud believed little girls blamed their mothers for te fact that they didn't have a penis: their mother didn't give them one, or perhaps they cut it off out of jealousy. In any case, the girl experiences what Freud called penis envy. Without a penis, she can identify with her mother, but she can also be her mother's rival for her father's affections, or a 'Daddy's girl'.

People don't remember having these feelings, but Freud would say they are examples of your id at work and as such, all this is buried deeply in your unconscious. Many pychologists today use the theories of Freud, but others (paricularly feminists) dismiss them.

Key words

Oedipus complex – The story of Oedipus comes from Greek mythology, about a boy who unwittingly kills his father and marries his mother

Penis envy – The idea that females envy and desire the penis is a controversial theory and disputed by feminists

Erik Erikson and our later experiences

Erikson was a German developmental psychologist who worked in the USA from the 1950s. He is a more recent psychoanalytic theorist than Freud and his work is considered important in health and social care. Whereas Freud thought that people's personalities were well formed by the age of five or six, Erikson argued that people continue to develop and change over the whole of their life. Erikson's work helps us to understand the issues that people face in adolescence, adulthood and in their later years.

Erikson identified eight stages in our lives. At each stage there is a particular conflict that has to be overcome if our ego is to develop.

- **Age 0–1: Learning basic trust (and not mistrust)** Children learn a sense of trust in the world. If this stage is badly handled, they become mistrustful and insecure.

- **Age 1–3: Learning autonomy (and not shame or doubt)** Children learn to act independently of parents. People often refer to this age as the 'terrible twos'. Children make mistakes, for example a toilet accident, which can lead to shame or doubt. Gentle but firm parenting helps them through this period.

- **Age 4–6: Learning initiative (and not guilt)** Children are now able to explore the world and should be learning to play and co-operate with others. However, if they are treated as though they are a nuisance, they might develop a sense of guilt.

- **Age 7–12: Learning industry (and not inferiority)** Here children learn the more formal skills they will need in life. In Western culture, that may be things we learn at school, and the more formal rules for co-operating and living together. If children don't learn these skills, they may feel themselves to be inferior.

- **Age 12–18: Learning identity (and not identity confusion)** The key task for young people now is to work out what kind of person they are going to be. They experiment with different roles until they find one most suitable for them. If they do not, they experience identity confusion.

- **Age 19–25: Learning intimacy (and not self-absorption)** Young adults can now experience truly intimate relations with another person. If they are unsuccessful in this task, they might become isolated, lonely and self-absorbed.

- **Age 26–40: Learning generativity (and not stagnation)** 'Generativity' was Erikson's word for taking an interest in the next generation. We do this through our children, and if we don't have children we often do this through our work. If we don't achieve this, we fall into a state of stagnation.

- **Age 40+: Achieving integrity (and not despair)**
  In this last phase of our lives, we may be able to look back and feel happy at what we have done and what we have achieved. Erikson called this 'integrity'. If we are unhappy, we look back on our lives with regret, or despair.

Humanistic perspectives

Humanistic psychology, which is also known as person-centred psychology, is concerned with the way we grow and develop as people. Unlike other approaches, this approach is not particularly concerned with what has happened to us in the past. It is more concerned with what we will become in the future.

Self-actualisation

A key idea in humanistic psychology is that we all have an inbuilt drive to grow and develop as people. This is known as the tendency for self-actualisation. If conditions are right, we will grow well. We will have a strong sense of who we are, a positive self-concept, and will feel able to direct our own lives. We will also achieve a sense of wholeness and fulfilment in our lives.

Key words

Self-actualisation – an inner drive to grow and develop
Self-concept – our own view of the kind of person we are

Maslow's hierarchy of needs

There are lots of things we need to achieve growth in our lives. We need food and shelter, we need friends, and we need to feel valued. American psychologist Abraham Maslow thought that some of these needs are more basic than others and said that we have a 'hierarchy of needs'. Lower-level needs have to be met first, then needs at the next level ... and so on. If the highest level of needs is met, we then become fully complete as a person.

There are six levels in Maslow's hierarchy of needs.

1. **Physiological needs.** We need air, water and food. These are our most basic needs.

2. **Safety needs** Next we need to be safe, and to avoid pain and harm.

3. **Belongingness.** Next, we need to feel secure and that we belong. This need will be met first within our family, and later by other groups we belong to.

4. **Love needs.** Once we feel secure and belong, we need to be loved and to love other people in return.

5. **Self-esteem needs.** Once we feel loved, we need to feel that we are worthwhile people.

6. **Self-actualisation needs.** This is the highest level in Maslow's hierarchy. If our love needs and our self-esteem needs have been met, we are on our way to becoming a whole and integrated person, and we reach the stage of self-actualisation.

To be a self-actualised person doesn't mean that you have to be very clever and famous. We do have to feel comfortable with who we are, to have a strong and positive self-concept that works for us, and we need to make the best of the talents and opportunities we have in life. This might involve developing our understanding of ourselves and other people. It might be something creative or athletic, or it might be through achievements in our education or careers.

As we move up Maslow's hierarchy of needs, we find fewer people at each level. In our society, most people's physiological needs are met. Many people, however, do not experience a sense of belonging, and even fewer reach the stage of self-actualisation. Maslow thought that perhaps two per cent of people reached this final level in the hierarchy.

Carl Rogers

Rogers developed the approach we call **person-centred counselling**. This is a way of helping people who have social or emotional problems, but it is quite different from the approach a psychoanalyst would use. Person-centred counselling is **non-directive**. The counsellor does not try to interpret people's unconscious thoughts. Instead, the counsellor works with the words and the thoughts that we use ourselves. The counsellor does not give advice or tell people what they ought to do. Instead, the counsellor helps people to find the answers for themselves, which allows people to take charge of their own lives.

An important idea in person-centred counselling is the **locus of control**. 'Locus' is a Latin word meaning place. People are said to have an internal locus of control if they believe that they have the power, within themselves, to make things happen. People have an external locus of control if they believe that they don't have the power to change things. They might blame fate or other people. The counsellor may need to help the client develop an internal locus of control.

Unlike other approaches, such as psychoanalysis or cognitive behaviour therapy, person-centred counselling does not use any special techniques. It works through the relationship the counsellor achieves with the client. According to Carl Rogers, there are three key features in this relationship:

- unconditional positive regard
- empathy
- genuineness.

Unconditional positive regard

Unconditional positive regard is similar to acceptance. A counsellor will demonstrate this by showing warmth and respect for the client and by avoiding making any kind of judgement, including approval or disapproval.

> **Think** In what circumstances might it be difficult to show unconditional positive regard for a service user?

Empathy

Empathy involves trying to see things from another person's point of view, and trying to understand what they might be feeling. This is not easy. You need to concentrate, listen carefully and actively, and avoid making any immediate judgements. Person-centred counsellors need to have empathy with their clients, and they need to demonstrate this to the client. They often do this using non-verbal signals, for example by leaning forward slightly when listening, to signal to the other person that they are paying attention. They might also copy the other person's mannerisms, such as folding their arms, touching their chin or crossing their feet. We do this quite naturally, and the counsellor will do this too.

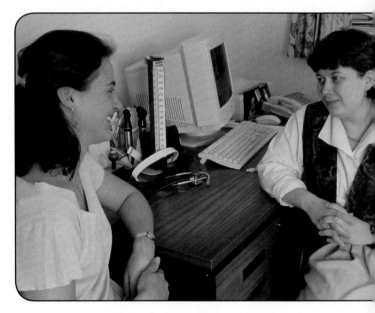

Figure 8.8 Mirroring another person's body language is a sign of empathy

> **Think** What other signals can we use to show we are listening carefully?

Counsellors also express empathy through what they say. One way of doing this in a non-directive and non-judgemental way is to summarise what the other person has said. This shows the client that the counsellor is listening, and also allows the counsellor to check that they have understood.

Example

Habib is a counsellor. He is working with Emma who is a client.

Counsellor So, your mum told you off in front of your friends?

Client Yes.

Counsellor Sounds like you were really embarrassed by that.

Client Yes. She's always doing stuff like that.

The counsellor might simply repeat something the client has just said.

Counsellor Always doing stuff like that?

Client (pause) Yes. Treating me like I'm a kid. Showing me up and stuff.

Here the counsellor, Habib, has shown that he is listening. He has also prompted the client, Emma, gently to go on and say a bit more, to explain how she is feeling. Remember that this is a non-directive approach, so the client doesn't have to say anything unless she wants to. Notice that there was a pause before the client started to speak again. Counsellors sometimes use silence to signal empathy. It's respectful, they don't want to break the client's train of thought; they are simply waiting until the client feels he or she wants to go on.

Genuineness

This is the third feature of the counselling relationship, and it involves being yourself and acting as a real person with thoughts and feelings, which can be expressed when it is appropriate to do so.

According to Rogers, if a counselling relationship is built on these three features, nothing more is needed. There are no other counselling techniques. The counsellor creates a safe and accepting space in which the client can explore and express their feelings. The client begins to feel accepted and valued, they develop their own insights into how they feel and they make better sense of their lives. Over time, they come to learn that they do have the power to make choices and changes in their lives … if they want to do so. Rogers rejected the idea that the counsellor was an expert who could tell the client what to do. The counsellor is an expert listener, but their relationship with the client is based on equality.

Cognitive or information processing perspectives

Cognitive theories are concerned with how people think. Some of the other theories this unit has covered so far don't have a place for thinking at all. Cognitive theories are interested in what goes on inside people's heads and the link between what they think, and what they feel and do.

Psychologists are interested in the way people pick up and process information from what is going on around them. We are surrounded by a huge range of sights, sounds and smells, but we don't pay attention to most of them. Something might grab our attention; for example, if our own name is mentioned among a lot of background noise we are more likely to hear it than another name spoken at random. Most of the time our attention is selective and what we notice depends on what we think is important at the time.

Jean Piaget and the development of children's thinking

Piaget, a Swiss philosopher and psychologist, was one of the first psychologists to show how children's thinking develops from infancy through to adolescence. For example, Piaget showed that babies have to learn the idea of object permanence, that things continue to exist even though the child cannot see them, whereas older children take this for granted. He would show a desirable toy to an infant, then cover it with a cloth. Some of the children showed signs of confusion or upset, which were interpreted as showing that they thought the toy had disappeared.

One of Piaget's most famous experiments was about conservation. A child would be shown some liquid in a clear container. The container is short and wide, and the child can see the liquid in the container. The experimenter then pours the liquid from the short, wide container into a tall thin container and it rises higher. Children under the age of seven are likely to say that there is now more liquid than there was before. After around the age of seven, children are likely to say that the amount hasn't changed.

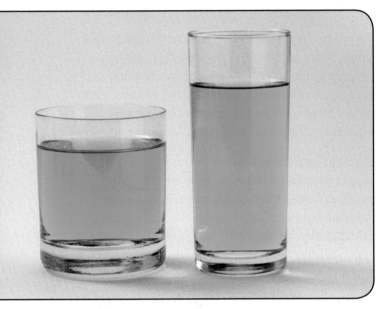

Figure 8.9 Two containers with the same amount of liquid in.

Piaget said that children go through four stages in developing their thinking. Everyone goes through these stages in the same order, and each stage lays the foundations for the next.

- **Age 0–2: Sensorimotor stage** Here children begin to explore the world, largely through their senses and through movement. Children at this stage haven't developed object permanence.

- **Age 2–7: Preoperational stage** Children are now beginning to use mental representations. However, their thinking is not logical and it can be very centred on themselves. For example, a child might shut their eyes tight. The child can't see us, and so they think that we can't see them! Children in the preoperational stage haven't mastered the idea of conservation.

- **7–11: Concrete operations** Children's thinking is becoming less rigid and more logical.

For example, children can now sort things into order of size and they can also classify things in terms of their similarities and differences, e.g. big red bricks, small red bricks, big and small blue bricks. They are also beginning to grasp the idea of conservation. Their thinking is not yet abstract. It is based on things that are real (concrete), which might be objects or actual experiences.

- **11–16: Formal operations** This is abstract and logical thinking. The children or young people are not limited to concrete thinking. They can form ideas that are not based on their own experiences and they can run through ideas in their heads. They can consider alternatives and can also think deductively, drawing conclusions about particular cases from general principles.

Piaget's theory has been very influential in education, particularly in nursery and early primary. Piaget stressed that young children are active learners. You cannot tell them what they need to know, instead they need to work this out for themselves. So Piaget's theories are often used to support the idea of active, play-based learning.

Other psychologists take a different view. Bruner, for example, said that Piaget underestimated the role that language plays in helping our thinking to develop. The Russian psychologist Vygotsky drew attention to the importance of 'scaffolding' in helping a child to learn the next new thing. He said that you should not leave children to discover something by themselves, but that you should help them by, for example:

- simplifying the task so they can focus on the important parts of the problem

- providing a structure of clues or prompts

- thinking aloud for the child

- building carefully on what they already know.

As the child begins to learn this new thing, the scaffolding can gradually be removed.

Outside of education, Piaget's theories have not been applied in health and social care. He has, however, left us with the idea that children and adults are active learners who try to make sense of their experiences.

George Kelly and personal construct theory

The idea that people actively make sense of their experiences is central to George Kelly's theory. Kelly likened people to scientists, constantly observing the world and building up theories about how it works. This involves creating categories that help make sense of our experiences; for example, 'people I like' and 'people I don't like'. Kelly called these categories 'constructs' because we build them for ourselves. We all have hundreds of these constructs. Some will be very big and hold lots of things, such as 'things I like' and 'things I don't like'. Others will have a limited range of application; for example 'things that are good for my complexion' and 'things that give me spots'.

Our constructs are very individual, which is why Kelly called them 'personal'. The set of constructs that you have will be different to your friend's. Sometimes you might use the same words, for example, 'people I like' and 'people I don't like', but within these constructs you will like and dislike different people, for different reasons. You might like people who are quiet and thoughtful (another construct), but your friend might like people who are extrovert and outgoing.

Constructs help us to simplify and make sense of our experiences and also help us to anticipate what might happen next. This is why Kelly thought of people as being like scientists: they use theories to explain and predict things.

Example

If you meet a person, let's say Ruth, for the first time who seems quiet and thoughtful, you might think you are going to like her. If you get to know her better and find that you do like her, this supports your theory that you like quiet, thoughtful people and you become more confident in your theory. If you find you don't like her, then you begin to doubt your theory. If this happens often, you may come to change your theory.

A case study showing how George Kelly's theories can be applied in a health and social care setting can be found on page 30.

Biological perspectives

The theories this unit has looked at so far explain human behaviour in quite different ways:

- behaviourist approaches look at how our own actions are reinforced

- social learning theories are concerned with the influence of other people

- psychoanalytic theories stress the importance of our unconscious mind

- humanistic approaches stress the progress towards self-actualisation

- cognitive theories explore the links between thinking, feeling and behaviour.

At this point you might be thinking that something is missing. We all have a brain and that's where our thinking happens. So if we understand how the brain works, maybe we can understand more about people's behaviour.

Gesell and maturational theory

Arnold Gesell used the term 'maturation' to describe the process of change that takes place during our lifespan. These might be changes in what we are able to do: babies sit up, they walk, they begin to talk. These might also be physical changes, as our bodies grow and develop from childhood into adulthood.

Maturational changes are biologically programmed and come about as a result of our genes, said Gesell. But how can we distinguish maturational changes from other sorts of changes that occur over our lives? If a change takes place as a result of maturation, it should be:

- **universal**: it will happen in all people

- **sequential**: it will follow the same predictable pattern

- **biological**: it does not need any environmental influences to make it happen.

If changes occur in all children, in the same order, and as a result of some kind of biological unfolding, it should be possible to map this process out.

We can work out developmental norms – the ages at which children normally are able to sit up, walk and begin to talk, for example. A map might help us to understand more about the process of development, and would also allow us to look at how individual children are developing.

CASE STUDY: REPERTORY GRIDS

Kelly developed a tool called a repertory grid, which can be used to help us discover and understand people's personal constructs.

Marcel is a community mental health worker. He wants to find out why Sandra has such low self-esteem, so decides to use the repertory grid technique. Marcel starts by asking Sandra to give him a list of people who are important to her. He then selects three of these at random and asks her, 'Can you think of a way in which two of these are alike, and different from the third?' Sandra replies, 'I like these two people, but not that one so much.' Marcel has uncovered one of Sandra's constructs, one of the categories she uses when she's thinking about people. Marcel continues in this way, taking people at random, and Sandra continues to provide Marcel with her personal constructs. Marcel finds that she is using a wide range of constructs, including:

- people I like   and   people I don't like
- people who   and   people who are shy
  seem confident
- people who   and   people who are
  dress smartly   scruffy
- optimistic people   and   pessimistic people
- people who   and   people who skive a
  work hard   lot

They continue until Sandra seems to be running out of ideas. It looks as though Marcel may have uncovered Sandra's most important constructs. These are Sandra's own ways of thinking about people and they are expressed in her own words. Marcel then asks Sandra to look at the first construct, 'People I like and people I don't like', and invites her to put all the people on the list in rank order, from the person she like most to the person she likes least. But Marcel has been a bit sneaky. He's introduced two other people to

the list: Sandra as she is now, and Sandra as she would like herself to be.

Sandra does the ranking task with all her constructs, putting the people into order, and Marcel puts this in a table. Here is a simplified version of the table with only some of the people and constructs.

Rank	People I like	People who seem confident	People who dress smartly
1	Mum	Me as I'd like to be	Me as I'd like to be
2	Me as I'd like to be	Priya	Priya
3	Priya	Mum	Joe
4	Joe	Joe	Mum
5	Victoria	Victoria	Victoria
6	Me as I am now	Me as I am now	Me as I am now

With Sandra, Marcel can now look at how she has ranked these people on the different constructs. He sees that Sandra doesn't like herself very much. The repertory grid suggests that she seems to like people who seem confident, and the people who seem confident are people who dress smartly, she thinks. Sandra has provided a lot of information about how she sees herself and people around her, and Marcel is beginning to wonder whether Sandra's poor self-esteem has something to do with how she thinks about her own appearance.

If she felt she looked smarter, would she feel more confident and like herself more? Sandra hasn't felt able to say this for herself. Perhaps Marcel will raise this later, and see where that takes them.

If they seem to be slow to develop motor skills or language skills, for example, we might think about involving an occupational therapist or a speech and language therapist to help stimulate their development in these areas. Developmental screening may be carried out routinely by health visitors on babies and young children. Some children may be screened again, perhaps before they start school. The aim is to discover any areas where children's development might be falling behind that of other children; they might then be referred on for more detailed assessment and intervention.

> **Think** Why might it be a good idea to screen children before they start school?

The Gesell Development Schedules aim to chart the development of a number of skills in children up to six years old. The areas covered are:

- **motor skills** fine and gross motor skills

- **language skills** understanding and using language

- **personal-social skills** skills involved in interacting with others

- **adaptive behaviour** the ability to learn from past experiences.

Gesell's early work was criticised because it was based on observations of only a small number of white, middle-class children who all lived in the same American city. Since then, however, psychologists have got much better at devising ways of measuring children's development.

Although Gesell believed that he was observing a biological process, many of the items in developmental schedules depend on both biological and environmental factors. For example, children will be slow to learn to walk if they are seldom taken out of their cot, and they will learn to speak more quickly if they are exposed to good models of language. In the health and social care sector it is important to recognise that children's development is not fixed by their biology. If it was, there would be little point in trying to find ways of helping them to catch up if they were delayed.

Importance of genetic influences on behaviour

People often say things like 'You know, Julie's just like her Mum' when they are describing someone's behaviour. Perhaps Julie has learned this behaviour from her mother (remember social learning theory) or perhaps the behaviour is inherited, and passed on genetically in some way. We also say things like, 'That runs in the family' to suggest a genetic link over a number of generations. In many cases it is impossible to tell whether a characteristic is genetically determined, but science can help.

Psychologists argue about how far our intelligence is determined by our genes or by the environment we grow up in. Intelligent parents often seem to have intelligent children, but why is this? Psychologists explore how far people's scores on intelligence tests are determined by our genes or by our environment.

Most people believe that it is a combination of genes and the environment, but how do we know this? Psychologists often use twin studies. Identical twins have identical genes and non-identical twins have similar, but not identical, genes. Because twins usually grow up together, the environment they grow up in is also likely to be similar. So if we compare their IQ scores, what do we find?

Table 8.1 Relationship between IQ scores and genes

Pairing	Correlation
Identical twins growing up together	0.86
Non-identical twins growing up together	0.60
Non-twin siblings growing up together	0.47

Table 8.1 suggests that scores in intelligence tests are strongly influenced by genes. The closer the genetic match, the closer the IQ scores are. However, it could also be argued that the environments for identical twins are more similar than for non-identical twins: parents often dress

them the same and treat them in the same way, to a greater extent than non-identical twins or siblings. These findings might therefore say as much about environmental factors as about genetics.

There are some cases of identical twins who have grown up in different environments; for example, if they are adopted by different families. In these cases the genetics are the same, but the environments are different. Researchers have found these children through adoption records and investigated whether their scores in intelligence tests match.

Table 8.2 Effect on twins of growing up in different environments

Pairing	Correlation
Identical twins growing up together	0.86
Identical twins growing up apart	0.72
Non-identical twins growing up together	0.60

Table 8.2 suggests that there is both a genetic and an environmental influence at work:

- **genetic influence**: identical twins who grow up apart are closer in their scores than non-identical twins who grow up together.

- **environmental influence**: identical twins who grow up together are closer in their scores than identical twins who grow up apart.

Statistical evidence from these studies suggests that the influences of genes and the environment are about equal. Our intelligence, or scores on intelligence tests, are determined half by our genes and half by the environment we grow up in.

Other features of our behaviour and personality can be shown through studying twins. One example is schizophrenia. If a non-identical twin has schizophrenia, there is a 10 per cent chance that the other twin will also develop the illness. However, if the twins are identical, the chance of the other twin developing the condition jumps to 40 percent.

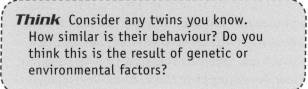

Think Consider any twins you know. How similar is their behaviour? Do you think this is the result of genetic or environmental factors?

The influence of the nervous system on behaviour

The nervous system has two parts: the **central nervous system**, which is made up of the brain and the spinal cord, and the **peripheral nervous system**, comprising the sensory and motor nerves (see Figure 8.10).

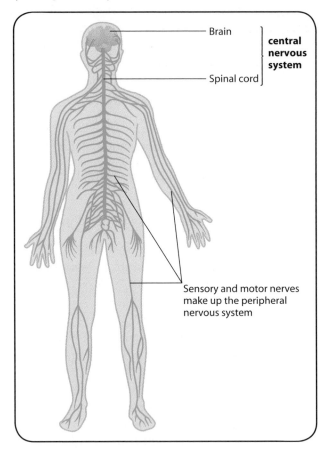

Figure 8.10 Human nervous system

Damage to the brain can have an effect on behaviour, but the nature of the effect depends on which part of the brain is damaged and how serious the damage is.

Damage to the brain can cause major changes in people's behaviour, but very small changes in the nerve cells can also have an effect. The nervous system is made up of nerve cells that carry messages in the form of **nerve impulses** around our bodies and to and from the brain. The impulse travelling along the length of a nerve cell is a tiny electrical charge. When the impulse reaches the **synapse**, the gap between one nerve fibre and the next, the electrical charge can go no further. Instead it releases a tiny amount of chemical, called a **neurotransmitter**. This chemical flows across the synapse and causes the charge to begin in the next nerve cell in the pathway (see Figure 8.11). All of this happens very quickly!

If a person's neurotransmitters are out of balance, they can experience psychological problems. For example, people who have depression have reduced levels of the neurotransmitter serotonin, and people with schizophrenia have an excess of the transmitter dopamine. Drugs can be used to restore or improve the correct balance within the body.

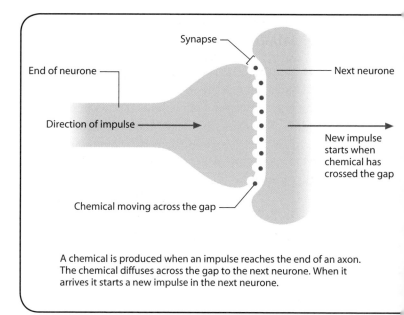

A chemical is produced when an impulse reaches the end of an axon. The chemical diffuses across the gap to the next neurone. When it arrives it starts a new impulse in the next neurone.

Figure 8.11 How a nerve impulse crosses from one nerve cell to another

CASE STUDY: RECOVERING FROM HEAD INJURY

Jamie is 17, and has been involved in a car accident. He has suffered a head injury that has caused serious brain damage.

Six weeks have passed since Jamie's accident. His injury was on the left side of his head and he now has difficulty using his right hand. As Jamie was right-handed before the accident, he is finding it difficult to do simple tasks like washing and dressing, and he also finds eating difficult. He has started working with an occupational therapist, Rehan, who has devised a programme to help Jamie recover the use of his right hand.

Jamie also has difficulty walking. His left-side head injury has affected his control of his right leg. It just doesn't work for him the way it ought to. He also sees a physiotherapist, Carol, who has devised an exercise programme to help him. Both the physiotherapist and the occupational therapist are looking at aids and adaptations he will need around the home. Jamie will eventually recover many of his motor skills, but this may take some time.

The area of the brain responsible for language is on the left side and Jamie is also having problems communicating. He appears to understand what others say to him, but he has real problems putting his own ideas into words and sentences that make sense. A speech and language therapist, Paula, will help him with this. As Jamie is still able to read, she is considering a communication system where Jamie simply has to point to the words he wants to use.

One year after his accident, Jamie's motor skills are very much better. He can communicate well, but a little slowly, as he needs time to think about what he wants to say. He has problems concentrating, and his short-term memory is very poor. These effects are the result of his head injury and are unlikely to get better.

QUESTION

1. What changes to Jamie's life could result indirectly from Jamie's head injury? Think about his self-image, employment prospects and relationships with others.

The influence of the endocrine system on behaviour

The endocrine system uses chemicals to carry messages around the body. These are hormones, which are released from various glands in our bodies. These pass into the bloodstream and act on organs elsewhere in the body. Some, but not all, hormones have an effect on our behaviour (see Table 8.3).

Table 8.3 Some hormones that affect behaviour

Hormone	Secreted by	Located	Effect
Testosterone	male gonads	scrotum	development of male sexual characteristics and sex drive
Oestrogen Proesterone	female gonads	ovaries	development of female sexual characteristics
Adrenalin	adrenal gonads	kidneys	increases our heart and breathing rate and prepares us for 'fight or flight'
Melatonin	pineal body	brain	regulates our sleep-wake cycle

Problems with the endocrine system can affect behaviour, but medication may resolve the problem. For example, shift workers may be given small doses of melatonin to help them cope with disturbed sleep patterns.

8.2 Applying psychological approaches to health and social care

APPLICATION OF PSYCHOLOGICAL PERSPECTIVES

Behaviourist approach

Behaviourists use an ABC approach to understanding behaviour:

- **A** stands for **antecedents**: what is happening just before the behaviour occurs

- **B** stands for **behaviour**: what the person is actually doing

- **C** stands for **consequences**: what happens next.

People who work in health and social care may use adjectives (describing words) like aggressive, unco-operative, antisocial and so on, when they talk about their service users' behaviour. People who take a behaviourist approach find these descriptions unhelpful and call them **fuzzy words**, meaning that they are too general. They believe that to change a person's behaviour, we need to know what the person is actually doing, and how the care workers want things to change.

Table 8.4 shows a range of descriptions that use what a behaviourist would call 'fuzzy words'. A behaviourist would describe what the observed behaviour is and what behaviour we might want to see instead.

Table 8.4 How a behaviourist would record problematic behaviour

Fuzzy words	What we might see	What we might want to see instead
Kuba is unco-operative at home time	Kuba does not comply with staff requests to put on his coat	Kuba will put his coat on when staff ask him to
Sara is aggressive in class	Sara hits other children	Sara will work alongside other children without hitting them
Asha is unsociable	Asha plays on her own	Asha will play effectively with a group
Ali can't concentrate when he's left to work on his own	Ali wanders off when left to work on his own	Ali will complete a four-piece jigsaw without staff support

CASE STUDY: A BEHAVIOUR MODIFICATION PROGRAMME

Joel is three years old and has just started nursery. He seems to enjoy it but rushes around from one thing to another, and never settles to play with other children or work with staff. Nicola is the manager of the nursery. She often uses behaviour-modification programmes with the children. She observes Joel over a number of sessions looking for the antecedents, the behaviour and its consequences.

The most difficult time for Joel is morning break when the children come to the table for their snack. The antecedent seems to be staff telling Joel to stop what he's doing and come to the table for his snack. The behaviour is Joel running off. And the consequence is that staff chase after him. Nicola thinks that Joel is enjoying this attention, and wonders if it might be reinforcing his behaviour.

The nursery staff want Joel to be more settled, so Nicola asks what they would like Joel to do instead of running around, and if he was 'settled', what they would see him doing.

The staff decide to focus on sitting at the table alongside staff and children. Joel sometimes approaches the table, but quickly runs off.

Nicola devises a programme for morning break. Firstly, she will change the antecedents: staff will tell all the children it is time for a drink, but they won't tell Joel separately to come to the table. If Joel approaches the table, a staff member will show him a piece of fruit and point to his seat. If he sits on the seat, she will give him smiles, hugs and a small piece of fruit. Joel likes fruit and this will be rewarding (or reinforcing). The attention he gets for sitting down will also be reinforcing. If Joel stays in his seat for ten seconds, he will be given another piece of fruit and so on.

If Joel doesn't come to the table, the staff will ignore him and not chase after him. This, in a behaviourist approach, is known as **time out** from reinforcement. If his running about is not reinforced by their attention, she thinks it may stop. This process is known as **extinction**. You eliminate an inappropriate behaviour through **planned ignoring**, while reinforcing an **incompatible behaviour**. By ignoring Joel's running around staff will reinforce the incompatible behaviour of sitting down.

Nicola's plan works. Joel starts to sit at the table and gets one piece of fruit every ten seconds. Once this behaviour is established, they change the programme. Now they expect him to sit for 20 seconds, and then they reward him with two pieces of fruit. This technique of building up a response from small beginnings is called **shaping**. The aim is to get Joel to sit at the table for the whole ten-minute session.

They hope eventually to get Joel coming to the table at other times in the day, and staying at the table to get attention (positive reinforcement) from the staff member. They can then involve Joel in activities with the other children.

Key words

Time out – removing someone from anything that might be reinforcing their behaviour

Extinction – eliminating behaviour by not reinforcing it

Planned ignoring – removing social reinforcement in order to extinguish behaviour

Incompatible behaviours – behaviours are incompatible if doing one excludes doing the other; for example, playing co-operatively with other children is incompatible with taking their toys

Shaping – building up a complex piece of behaviour through reinforcing attempts that get closer and closer to it

Understanding challenging behaviour

Behaviourist approaches have been very influential in health and social care practice. They have been used to tackle a wide range of issues with a variety of services users. People use this approach because it works. A behaviourist approach can also be very cost effective, which can be an important consideration in health and social care settings. Services users don't have to go on waiting lists to see highly trained specialists. A care worker with some training can draw up the programme, and others with day-to-day caring responsibilities can carry the programme out. This contributes to the effectiveness of the programme: it can bring about behaviour change in the context where the problem occurs. Service users don't need to go for weekly therapy sessions in a clinic.

Because behaviourists are concerned with observable behaviour, they don't need to label people as 'aggressive' or 'neurotic', for example. Many people see labelling of this sort as unhelpful. It can lead us to deal with people on the basis of their label, not in terms of their own unique strengths and needs. Behaviourist approaches manage to avoid this sort of labelling.

Criticism of the approach

Critics of the behaviourist approach argue that it is wrong to ignore what is going on inside people's heads. For example, if we can help people to understand their fears and feelings, they can bring about change for themselves. Critics also argue that behaviourist programmes only deal with surface behaviour and don't address the underlying issues that people have. Behaviourists might reply that their approach works with people who can't communicate their thoughts or feelings, for example with young children and people with learning difficulties, and other approaches just won't work with these groups.

Critics also say that using reinforcement is simply a form of manipulation. The behaviourist would reply that reinforcement occurs quite naturally. How we respond to people in our day-to-day contact with them reinforces some behaviours and extinguishes others. A behaviour-modification programme simply uses reinforcement more thoughtfully and consistently. Some critics might argue that some of the techniques, such as time out, can be upsetting for children and may not be far short of punishment. The behaviourist would say that they are careful about this and that time out periods are always very short.

The final criticism made against the behaviourist approach is that behaviourists offer us a view of people which has no place for free will. The approach implies that people don't make choices, but are pushed and pulled about by things that happen to them. Skinner would probably have agreed with this. So what, he might have said? Lots of theories are like that – are psychoanalytic theories really any different? At least the behaviourist theory gives health and social care workers some tools with which to make things better for service users.

Evidence activity

P1

1. Work out a behaviour modification programme to help the following service users:

- Wendy wants to stop smoking. She smokes 20 a day, feels breathless and is always short of money.

- Annie is in her 80s and is afraid to leave her house. She never goes out and this has become a problem for her.

- Martin is in his early twenties. He is very shy and finds it difficult to speak to people he doesn't know very well.

- Amir has learning difficulties. He wants to learn to use public transport so that he can go to college. (P1)

2. Use the ABC approach to help you understand what might be happening that is stopping the person changing. In particular, are the consequences reinforcing the problem behaviour in some way? Don't worry if you have to make this up. Describe the behaviour you want to develop, i.e. what we want to see the person doing. Think about how the behaviour might be shaped up, if necessary. Think about how it might be reinforced. (P1)

Social learning theory

The great strength of social learning theory is that it directs our attention to the ways in which other people can influence behaviour. This approach can help us to understand better why service users behave in the way they do: they could be modelling their behaviour on someone else, for example someone with higher status who they look up to.

Social learning theory is less clear about what we might do with this information. The insights it offers us might be used better, for example, in cognitive behaviour therapy which we will look at later in this unit. Social learning theory would be very useful to health workers who are designing a health promotion campaign that will use advertising to reach large numbers of people. It would be important to choose positive role models to appear in the campaign. Attention to cultural factors would allow them to target specific groups more effectively, whether these are age groups, gender, social class or ethnic groups.

When we work in a care role, we need to be very aware of the cultural differences that might exist between ourselves and our service users. For example, a young, white British male care worker needs to be sensitive to the cultural expectations of a service user who is an African or Asian woman. If he does not understand her culture, he might behave in ways that upset or offend her.

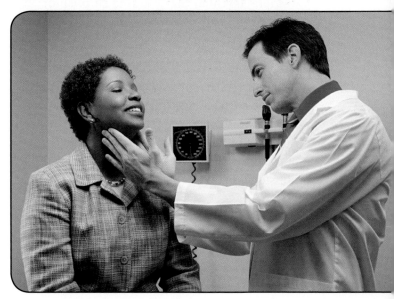

Figure 8.12 It is important to be culturally sensitive when working in a care role

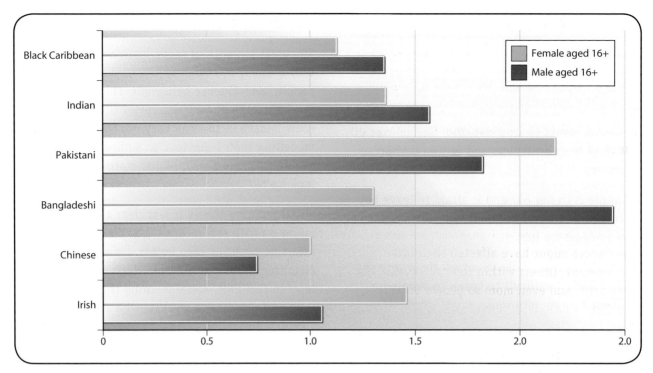

Figure 8.13 How often men and women from different ethnic groups in England consult their GP [Source: Department of Health, 2000, Health Survey for England, 1999, The Stationery Office, London]

Cultural factors also affect how service users view their problems and whether they seek help when they feel unwell. Figure 8.13 shows how often men and women from different ethnic groups in England consulted their GP in 1999. The average for the population as a whole has been set at 1.

> **Think** What does Figure 8.13 tell us? Is there anything that you find surprising? Can you think how to explain it?

These differences could reflect real differences in people's health, but why should Bangladeshi women be so much healthier than their male relatives? This could also reflect cultural differences in how readily different ethnic groups define themselves as 'ill' and then seek professional help.

EVIDENCE ACTIVITY

P2

1. A group of NHS managers is reviewing the provision of health and social care services in their area, and they have identified a number of priorities. Explain how the social learning theory might help them to understand:

- smoking in primary-school-aged children

- teenage pregnancies

- substance abuse in young adults

- cultural differences in the rate of GP consultation. (P2)

2. How could the NHS managers use these insights to promote better health outcomes? (P2)

Evaluating approaches

Psychoanalytic approaches have been very influential in shaping how we think about the way people's personalities develop. They have also had a huge impact on the work of creative people, including artists and writers, who have found a source of inspiration in this approach for their work. The influence of these approaches in health and social care practice, however, has been less than their reputation might suggest.

Freud was concerned with how people's early experiences might have affected their later development. Others within the psychoanalytic movement, and even more so people outside it, would say that our later experiences also have an effect on our behaviour.

Psychodynamic theorists draw attention to people's unconscious thinking, which is a useful concept for the work of health and social care practitioners. Critics would say that Freud makes too much of this. How can you build a theory about human development, they ask, based on the problems that wealthy Austrians took to a psychiatric clinic at the end of the 19th century? How can analysts know that their interpretation, or analysis, of their unconscious is anywhere near the truth? And many people find the theories about infant sexuality and the Oedipus complex just a bit far fetched!

Freud's followers might respond by saying that whatever you think about the theory, the techniques of psychoanalysis work. Critics would argue with this. They would point out that many people just get better by themselves, which is known as spontaneous remission. Psychoanalysis itself is a lengthy process, and practitioners, service users and service managers often need something which is more cost effective. Psychoanalysis is not used often in health and social care practice in the UK. It requires a long specialist training and there are very few people trained to use it.

Evidence activity

P3

Jane is 14, she has an eating disorder and has been referred to the Child and Adolescent Mental Health Service. She meets Pat, a clinical psychologist.

Describe how Pat might use a psychoanalytic approach in working with Jane. You might want to consider:

- what early experiences might have contributed to Jane's problem

- what techniques might Pat use to get the information she needs from Jane. (P3)

Humanistic approaches

How is Maslow's hierarchy of needs relevant to work in health and social care? Unlike some approaches, Maslow's theory doesn't give practitioners any tools that they can use directly with service users. However, the theory can affect the way we look at people's lives and at the issues they face. This may lead us to understand their situation better, and help us find ways to bring about change.

Example

Margaret is 92. Her physical health is good, but she has dementia – her memory is very poor and she gets very confused. Margaret has been finding it very difficult to look after herself. For example, she often leaves the cooker on and there have been a number of fires in her kitchen. Her daughter Jane has been very worried about her and was very relieved when Margaret moved into a residential care home.

However, the move has not gone well for Margaret. She's now not sure where she is. She thinks she is still at home, and that her house is full of people she doesn't know. She wants them to leave, gets upset and angry and has hit out at the staff and other residents.

The staff in the care home have a meeting with Jane to discuss how to handle this. The staff think they need to do something to help Margaret's sense of belonging. One of the staff thinks they should work on Margaret's sense of belonging as a member of the community in the care home. This is where Margaret is now, he says. Another thinks they should emphasise her belonging as part of her family. Margaret still has some memories of this, she argues.

Think What would you do to help Margaret?

Humanistic psychology is the basis for person-centred counselling, and this has had a major influence on practice in health and social care. Most people working in health and social care are not counsellors, however. This requires special training, and counsellors should all have supervision in their work. Nevertheless, person-centred counselling does influence people who are not counsellors.

Firstly, person-centred psychology shows us the

sorts of skills we should try to develop in work with all service users: the skills of acceptance, empathy and genuineness. Some people can do this really well. For example, care workers who address their elderly residents with respect, who try to see the world as they see it, and who bring a little of themselves into their relationships are using some key ideas from humanistic psychology, perhaps without realising it.

Secondly, and closely related to this, person-centred psychology expresses some important principles about the right way to treat people. You will meet these ideas again when you study the value basis of care, but notice for now that this approach involves things like:

- accepting and respecting service users

- creating equality in our relationship with service users

- empowering them to make choices and changes that will work for them.

A person-centred approach means we avoid labelling, stereotyping and unfair discrimination.

Person-centred counselling might not be the best way to help someone who has a problem such as losing weight or stopping smoking. Other more focused approaches might be quicker and more effective for them. Person-centred approaches are more useful for clients who are thinking about making major changes in their lives.

Some clients will find the person-centred approach unusual and hard to understand. For example, they might expect the counsellor to behave like an expert who will tell them what to do. If this is what they expect, then person-centred counselling may not work for them. Person-centred counselling takes time, and so it is expensive, either to the client, if they are paying, or to the organisation providing it. Finally, it is important to remember that no form of counselling will work if the client does not want to change.

Evidence activity

P4

1. Use a range of examples to show how understanding the humanistic approach would help to provide a better service to services users. You could think about:

- the way we work with our service users

- the way we run our services on a day-to-day basis, and

- the way we organise our services. (P4)

2. What is the value of using this approach? (P4)

Cognitive approaches

Cognitive behaviour therapy

Cognitive behaviour therapy (CBT) is a way of looking at how people think about things, so that they can understand and change the ways they feel about them.

When we think about things, we sometimes get it wrong. Our thinking is distorted. A women may think:

> *'That guy on the bus was looking at me. He must think I look weird.'*

This is an example of distorted thinking. Perhaps the man wasn't looking at her at all: he could have been looking at someone behind her. Or if he was looking at her, maybe he thought she was quite interesting, or even attractive.

> *Think* Can you think of similar examples where you, or someone you know, might have drawn the wrong conclusion from what someone else has done?

Distorted thinking often takes place when we use words like 'should' or 'must'. A client, Rosie, says:

> *'I should do what my parents ask me to do.'*

> *'I must lose weight.'*

> *'I need to stay in and study.'*

> *'I ought to be thinking about a gap year.'*

The client might be right in some cases, but perhaps we ought to ask what would happen if she does each of these and what would happen if she doesn't.

Example

Patrick has trained in CBT and decides to use this technique with Claudia. Her biggest worries are about going out and meeting people and Ian asks her to talk about one or two situations where she felt awkward and uncomfortable. Sandra begins with the episode of the man on the bus.

Claudia: Well I was on the bus, going to college. And this guy was, like ... staring at me.

Patrick: Staring at you?

Claudia: Yes. Right at me!

Patrick: And how did you feel about that?

Claudia: Well it's rude, isn't it? I mean, how would you like it?

Patrick: Hmm.

Claudia: And anyway. Did he think I'm some kind of freak, or what?

Patrick: Why do you say that, Sandra?

Claudia: Well, look at me! I mean no one's exactly going to ask me out, are they?

> *Think* How is Patrick using some of the listening and prompting techniques from Rogers' person-centred counselling?

Example

Ian notices that Sandra has some unhelpful beliefs, which are called 'dysfunctional beliefs' in CBT. He will now examine these with her.

Ian: This bloke. Did you catch his eye at all? (Ian has noticed that Sandra tries to avoid eye contact.)

Sandra: Erm, no.

Ian: So can you be really, really sure that he was looking at you, and not at the person behind you?

Sandra: Well, no. But he would be looking at me. 'Cos I look weird and stuff.

Ian will follow this up in a moment, but he decides to try something else.

Ian: Suppose he was looking at you. Maybe he was thinking something different?

Sandra: What? Like he maybe fancied me?

Ian: Hmm. Possible?

Sandra: Possible ... but unlikely. Blokes don't fancy women like me, do they?

> **Think** How is Ian helping Sandra to examine her beliefs? Can you see how what she thinks affects how she feels, and what she does?

Cognitive behaviour therapists often ask their clients to try something different between sessions. They call this homework. This helps the client get more out of their therapy and they can talk about this when they meet next.

Example

Ian has a few ideas in mind.

- Maybe Sandra could look around the bus each morning, quickly, and count up the number of people who are not looking at her. She thinks people stare at her, but what is the evidence for this?
- Perhaps he could ask Sandra to look out for times during the week when someone does look at her, and she feels comfortable about this. Could she make a note of who this was, where it happened, and how she felt about it? They might learn something from this.
- Maybe he could ask Sandra to look up and catch someone's eye, on the bus, for just one second. Could she try this once on her way into work and once on the way home? Perhaps she could choose an older person to begin with. How did the other person respond? And how did that feel for Sandra?

This homework will help Sandra to examine her belief that people stare at her because they think she looks 'weird'. Ian will try to find exceptions: times when Sandra feels OK about people looking at her, and she doesn't think that they think she looks weird.

The following points form the basis of CBT.

- Look at the events that set off a train of thought.

- Examine the thoughts: are they examples of distorted thinking?

- Try out different ways of thinking.

- See how this feels.

We said earlier that Piaget's theories have been used in early-years work and are now an established part of what early-years practitioners know and do. However, developmental psychology has moved on in recent years, and other writers now have more influence on day-to-day practice in nursery settings and in the early years of schooling. Piaget helps us understand children's thinking, whereas Vygotsky gives us a theory which helps us to accelerate their learning.

Personal construct theory has also been very influential. Many psychologists like it because it has some simple tools, like the repertory grid, which help us to see how a service user understands their world, and allows us to work with the words and ideas that have meaning for them. It accepts and respects the service user's experiences and does not try to analyse or reinterpret them. It is also easy to understand!

Cognitive behaviour therapy has become very popular in recent years. It is widely used in health and care settings where people have difficulty coping, where they suffer from stress, depression, and anxiety, and where they have difficulty managing their anger. One of the aims is of CBT is to give the service user techniques that they can use on their own. They should be able to go on to uncover other examples of distorted thinking and dysfunctional beliefs in their lives. This will make them independent of the therapist. The approach is said to work quickly, which makes it cost effective.

CBT is not be suitable for everyone. Clients need to be able to put their thoughts and feelings into words, and they need to have at least some motivation to want to change. Clients also need to have some capacity for logical thinking: we can work with distorted thinking but not with thinking that is just chaotic. CBT may be used to good effect alongside drug treatments with people suffering from depression.

Evidence activity

P5 – M1

1. Think about in what circumstances a cognitive perspective would be helpful in our work in health and social care. Think about the service users who might benefit from this approach, and the sort of issues it might help them with. (P5)

2. Make a copy of Table 8.5, and make some notes in each box to say how each theory might be able to help us understand and respond to the behaviour in question. Some approaches may have little to offer on some of the issues. You can then use these notes as the basis of an essay. (P5)

3. You have looked at five theories so far and should now be able to analyse their contributions to understanding and managing a range of challenging behaviours. (M1)

Behaviour	Psychoanalytic approaches	Behavioural approaches	Social learning theory	Humanistic psychology	Cognitive approaches
Tara has learning difficulties. She bites her hands until they bleed.					
Elena wants help to stop smoking. She's worried about her health.					
Mary is 85. She lives in a nursing home and is now incontinent.					
Peter is 25 and he is agrophobic. He seldom goes out of the house.					

Table 8.5

Biological theories

Biological theories are linked with a medical model of well-being and many psychologists have problems with this. This may seem odd, because there are areas where biological explanations and medical interventions will work well. If melatonin helps shift workers to sleep during daylight hours, and if medication can help people with schizophrenia to live better lives, what could be wrong with that?

Evidence activity

P6

1. Look back to page 29 where we looked at Geseil's Development Schedules. Make a list of the professionals who might use these, and say why they would find them useful. (P6)

2. Look back at the case study of Jamie, the young man recovering from a head injury. Write a short essay explaining how a knowledge of how the brain works would help the various professionals who are working with Jamie. (P6)

People who experience problems are often pleased to have a medical diagnosis. This helps them to understand that the problem is not their fault. Critics of biological theories are concerned, however, when any attempts are made to locate the problem inside the individual. They argue that we also need to consider their environment; believing that diagnosis is just another form of labelling, which creates stereotypes and adds nothing to our understanding of the person and how to help them.

People who take a biological perspective would disagree. They would point to many successful treatments; however their critics would point to the short-term benefits of medication and the long-term side effects of some medication.

There is of course a middle position that involves seeing behaviour as the interaction of our biology and our environment. Most people who work in health and social care are not doctors and can do nothing about their service users' biological make up. They can, however, do something to influence their environment – the experiences they have and how they understand them.

Evidence activity

M2 – D1

1. Your local Strategic Health Authority has set up a working party to look at improving services in the area. Three people have been invited to speak to the working party.

- Dr Forbes is a psychiatrist. She takes a biological perspective.

- Ms Olomaiye is a social worker who takes a social learning perspective.

- Mr Crompton is a counsellor and he takes a humanistic perspective.

What might each of them say to influence the way health and social care services are provided in their community? (M2)

2. You have now studied six psychological perspectives and should be able to evaluate their contributions to work in health and social care. Make a start on this by copying and completing Table 8.6. Now prepare a presentation that evaluates these perspectives. (D1)

Perspective	What it does well	Areas of weakness	Where it might be used
Psychodynamic approaches			
Behavioural approaches			
Social learning theory			
Humanistic approaches			
Cognitive perspective			
Biological perspectives			

Table 8.6

INDEX

abuse, 54, 62, 75, 81, 142 – 3
accidents, 5, 94, 98, 101, 110, 122, 144
Acheson Report, 253
Acheson, Don, 137
Acts of Parliament, 78
acupuncture, 242
adepose tissue, 158
adolescence, 121, 124 – 5, 138, 146, 270, 273
adulthood, 121 – 2, 124 – 5, 144, 270, 275
advertising, 17, 20
advocates, 40, 57, 78
Age Discrimination Act, 69, 72
ageing, 10, 118, 142, 144 – 5, 149
alcoholism, 244
Alzheimer's disease, 130, 244, 246
amniocentesis, 131
anaemia, 131 – 2, 140, 220
anatomy, 150, 153
anthrax, 102
anti-discriminatory practice, 19, 50, 68, 76, 78, 80
anti-harassment, 74 – 5
anxiety, 36, 289
areolar tissue, 158
Arm's Length Bodies, 222
arteries, 167
arthritis, 147
artificial insemination, 120
asphyxia, 102
asthma, 114, 138, 147 – 8
atherosclerosis, 147, 167
attitude, 32 – 3, 52 – 3, 61, 135, 199, 252
autism, 259

bacteria, 95, 156 – 7, 171, 173, 175, 177
Bales, RF, 18
Bandura, Albert, 138, 264 – 6
behaviour, 32 – 4, 52, 64, 72, 75, 77, 105, 127, 205, 231, 234, 236, 239, 244 – 5, 248, 251, 256, 261 – 7, 272, 275, 277 – 8, 280 – 3, 287 – 9
beliefs, 19, 50, 52 – 3, 55, 57, 76, 78, 139, 196, 204, 211, 213 – 14, 216, 231 – 2, 235, 243, 266, 288
Bernard, Claude, 179
best practice, 81
biomedical, 11, 245 – 6
birth, 142, 145, 195, 224

Black report, 253, 256
Black, Douglas, 137
Blaxter, Mildred, 22
blood pressure, 140, 147, 164, 167, 224
blood vessels, 167, 185
body mass index (BMI), 122
bomb scares, 94, 98
bone tissue, 158
Bowlby, John, 125
Braille, 14, 41 – 2
Braille, Louis, 42
breathing rate, 10, 180
British Deaf Association, 40
British Sign Language (BSL), 40, 42
bronchitis, 141, 148
bullying, 62, 74 – 5, 136, 139

caesarean, 120
cancer, 36, 102, 140 – 1, 147, 244, 248, 253 – 4
capillaries, 168, 170 – 1, 177
capitalism, 237 – 8
cardiac muscle, 159
cardiology, 49
cardiovascular, 140, 147, 160 – 1, 164, 178 – 9
Care Commission, 97
Care Standards Act, 71
care workers/practitioners, 20, 46, 55, 57, 262
cartilage tissue, 158
charters, 9, 50, 72
chemical spillage, 94 – 5
childbirth, 119
childcare/protection, 105, 107, 226, 229
childhood, 121, 124, 138, 245, 275
Children Act, The, 70
children's homes, 4, 71
chiropodists, 4
chlamydia, 132
cholera, 251
chromosomes, 127, 131, 144
circulation, 168
clinical iceberg, 250
clothing, 89 – 90
Code of Practice for Social Workers, 43
codes of practice, 9, 50, 72 – 3, 81, 99, 211
collectivism, 240
Commission for Social Care Inspection, 222
Communication Aids for Language and Learning, 29

Communication cycle, the, 17, 35
communication passport, 29
communication, 8, 14 – 22, 24 – 47, 57 – 8, 78 – 9, 83, 89, 125, 136, 198, 201, 208, 210, 259
community resource centres, 51
community, 20, 22, 46, 63, 67, 88, 117, 145, 211, 219, 223 – 4, 240, 244, 253, 256, 290
conception, 119 – 20
confidentiality, 16, 19, 43 – 6, 48, 57 – 9, 74 – 5, 78 – 9
connective tissue, 158
Connexions, 4
conservatism, 241
contamination, 94 – 5, 100 – 1
continuity theory, 145
Control of Substances Hazardous to Health (COSHH), 95, 100, 102, 109
Convention on the Rights of the Child, 70
counsellors, 40, 272 – 3
covert discrimination, 54
criminality, 44, 64
culture, 24, 36, 55 – 6, 64, 66, 76, 139, 231, 234, 241, 244, 266, 283
cystic fibrosis, 130, 220
cytoplasm, 155

Data Protection Act, 44, 69, 75, 100, 102, 110
day centres/care, 4, 51, 58
dementia, 40, 112, 246, 286
dentists, 219, 232
Department of Health, 217 – 18, 222
depression, 36, 130, 246, 289
dermatitis, 102
dermis, 185
diabetes, 114, 129 – 30, 140, 188 – 9, 221
dialect, 22
diaphragm, 183
differentiation, 60, 122, 124
digestive system, 120, 153 – 4, 160 – 1, 164, 173, 176, 178 – 9, 188
Disability Discrimination Act, The, 65, 67 – 9, 79, 107
Disability, 35, 38 – 40, 54, 58, 61 – 2, 65, 67 – 8, 77, 96, 98, 136 – 7, 217, 220, 226, 248
discrimination, 9, 48, 53, 57, 59 – 62, 64 – 7, 69, 75 – 6, 78, 136, 139, 286
disease, 101, 144, 217, 242, 245,

248, 251, 253
disempowerment, 52, 63
diversity, 9, 48, 50 – 2, 55 – 6, 60, 64, 79 – 80, 212, 233
DNA, 144, 155
Doctors/GPs, 4, 47
domiciliary care, 4, 51
Down's Syndrome, 39, 131
drugs, 141
Durkheim, Emile, 237
duty of care, 92
dyslexia, 247

economy, 4
education, 61 – 2, 65 – 7, 70, 138, 218, 221, 224, 231, 247, 254
electronic patient-record system, 21
embryo, 119 – 20
emergency procedures, 99
emphysema, 141, 147 – 8
employment, 61 – 2, 65 – 6, 136 – 7, 206, 254
empowerment, 43, 48, 52, 54, 57 – 8, 76, 78 – 9
endocrine system, 160 – 1, 178, 181, 280
endoplasmic reticulum, 155 – 6
energy, 10, 162 – 4, 169 – 70, 173, 177 – 9, 181, 184, 188, 268
epidemiology, 251
epidermis, 185 – 6
epilepsy, 114
epithelial tissue, 156, 158
equal opportunities, 43, 212
equaliser, 30
Equality Commission, 65
equality, 9, 48, 50 – 2, 56, 58, 60, 65, 67, 73, 76 – 80
equity, 52, 64, 81
Erikson, Erik, 125, 145, 270
European Union, 65
Every Child Matters, 37
evolution, 145
exercise, 138, 140, 142, 178, 181 – 3, 190, 192, 246, 252, 256

family, 231, 237, 241
feminism, 238 – 9, 270
fertilisation, 120
fire, 94, 98, 104 – 5
first aid, 82, 84, 89, 104, 114 – 5
five life factors, 118, 143
foetal alcohol syndrome, 132
foetus, 119 – 20
Food Safety Act, 100
Food Safety Regulations, The, 91, 100

formal communication, 19
Freud, Sigmund, 267 – 70, 285
functionalism, 237

gender, 56 – 7, 60, 62 – 3, 65, 136, 139, 205, 233 – 4, 236, 240, 248, 283
General Social Care Council, 43, 72
genetics, 129 – 30, 143, 220, 238 – 9, 253, 277 – 8
Gesell, Arnold, 275, 277
gestation, 120
glucagon, 188
glucose, 188 – 9
Golgi apparatus, 155 – 6
gonorrhoea, 132
group dynamics, 18
growth, 119, 122, 140

harassment, 62, 75
Havinghurst, 145
Hawking, Professor Stephen, 30
hazards, 84 – 8, 90 – 3, 95, 98, 102 – 4, 106, 108 – 9, 111 – 3, 133
Health and Safety at Work Act, 100, 102
Health and Safety Commission, 92
health and safety, 19, 74, 82 – 4, 88 – 9, 99, 103 – 7, 109 – 10, 113 – 4, 257
Healthcare Commission, 222
hearing aids, 41
heart disease, 128, 140, 147, 253 – 4
heart/heart rate, 10, 164 – 7, 170, 180 – 3, 189, 192 – 3, 205, 221
hepatitis, 102
HIV, 244
homeostasis, 10, 152, 179, 181, 189, 191
homeostatic mechanisms, 10, 180, 183, 192 – 3
homophobia, 54, 80
hormones, 146 – 7, 158, 178 – 9, 188, 280
housing, 61 – 2, 65 – 7, 136 – 8, 221, 243, 245, 256
Human Rights Act, 65, 69, 73
hygiene, 100, 104, 235
hypertension, 129 – 30
hypothalamus, 187
hypothermia, 101, 184

iatrogenesis, 249
identity, 57, 63, 78, 125
Illich, Ivan, 249

immune system, 160 – 1
Improvement Notices, 100
Incident Contact Centre, 101, 110
individuality, 79
Inequalities in Health, 137
inequality, 53, 76 – 8, 81, 234, 237 – 8, 243, 253 – 4, 256 – 7
infancy, 120
infection, 89, 91, 93, 104, 132, 245
infestations, 100
informal communication, 19
ingestion, 173
injury, 110, 142, 217
insulin, 188 – 9
intellectual development, 124 – 5
interactionism, 239 – 40
interdependence, 54
Internet, 103, 199, 201, 209 – 10
interpersonal interaction, 8, 16 – 7, 21, 25, 27, 39, 83
interpreters, 29 – 30, 35, 40, 42, 57 – 8, 78
intruders, 94, 96

Kelly, George, 275 – 6
Key Worker, 77
Kolb, David A, 197

labour, 120, 195, 224
large intestine, 175, 177
Lawrence, Stephen, 67
learning, 11, 22, 26, 197 – 200, 203 – 5, 207, 212
Legionnaire's Disease/Legionella, 95, 102
legislation, 9, 48, 50, 65, 68, 70 – 2, 74, 80, 82, 99, 101, 103, 211, 215, 238, 247
leptospirosis, 102
life expectancy, 123
life stages, 10, 118 – 9, 127, 129, 136
listening, 21, 25, 33
literacy, 200
lung diseases, 102, 141, 244
lymphatic system, 160 – 1

Macpherson Report, 67
Makaton, 42
malaria, 252
malpractice, 53
Management of Health and Safety at Work Regulations, 100, 102, 104
Manual Handling Operations Regulations, 100 – 1, 109
manual handling, 82, 89 – 90, 98,

101, 104, 109
marginalisation, 62 – 4, 78
marriage, 61, 116, 142
Marxism, 237 – 8
Maslow, Abraham, 271, 285
Mason, David, 30
maternity, 66
maturation, 123, 275
Mead, George, 239
measles, 252
Media Trust, 41
medicine, 49, 223, 236, 245
Medulla, 182 – 3
meningitis, 252
menopause, 145 – 6
menstruation, 146 – 7
Mental Capacity Act, 71
Mental Health Act, 40
Mental Health Act, The, 70
Mental Health Foundation, 140
Mental Health Trusts, 38
mental health, 6, 21, 51, 54, 61,
88, 96, 219 – 20, 246, 254, 259,
268, 276
mentors, 41, 203
metabolism, 10, 150, 152, 163
– 4, 169 – 70, 173, 178 – 9, 184
– 6
midwives, 4, 17, 195, 219, 223
– 4
mildews, 95
Millar, Sally, 29
MIND, 38
miscarriage, 224
Misuse of Drugs Act, 141
mitochondria, 155
modelling, 265 – 6
Motor-Neurone Disease, 30, 147
– 8
moulds, 95
MRSA, 249
multi-agency working, 37 – 8
multi-disciplinary working, 54,
223
multiple sclerosis , 130
Multi-Systemic Therapy Pilots, 63
muscle tissues, 158
musculo-skeletal system, 160 – 1

National Care Standards
Commission, 72
nature-nuture, 10, 118, 127 – 9,
143
nervous system, 120, 147 – 9, 160
– 1, 178, 181 – 2, 187, 278
nervous tissue, 160
neuroglia, 160
neurones, 160

New Right, 241, 247
NHS, 5, 21, 37 – 8, 40, 96, 135,
217 – 20, 222 – 3, 225, 232, 236,
253, 256, 259, 284
non-striated muscle, 159
non-verbal communication, 8, 16,
21, 23 – 6, 32 – 3, 35, 45, 47,
208
nucleus, 155
numeracy, 200, 202
nurseries, 4, 111, 274
nursery nurses, 4, 37
Nursing and Residential Care
Homes Regulations, 71
Nursing Midwifery Council, 72
Nursing Sciences, 49
nursing, 4, 38, 46, 49, 51, 54, 59,
94, 195, 219, 221, 225, 233, 244,
259, 262

obesity, 138
occupational therapists, 4, 38 – 9,
46, 219, 223, 259, 262, 277, 279
Oedipus Complex, 270, 285
oesophagus, 174
oestrogen, 146 – 7
oncology, 49
oppression, 63 – 4, 76, 78 – 9,
238
optometrists, 219, 225
organisational policies, 9, 50
orthoptists, 4
osteoporosis, 147 – 8

paediatrics, 37
parenthood, 142
Parkinson's Disease, 148
Pavlov, Ian, 262 – 3
pharmacists, 4, 219
phenylketoneuria, 130, 140
photosynthesis, 162
physiology, 10, 150, 152 – 3, 179,
205
physiotherapy, 4, 38 – 9, 46, 51,
117, 124, 130, 219, 225, 262, 279
Piaget, Jean, 124, 273 – 4, 288
plasma, 170
pneumonia, 95
policies, 64, 74 – 5, 81 – 2, 84,
89, 99, 104, 106, 108, 211, 247
pollution, 134, 137, 243
postmodernism, 240
pregnancy, 66, 119 – 20, 132,
195, 224, 244
prejudice, 53, 61, 66, 79, 81, 135
Primary Care Trusts, 218
private sector, 5, 73
psychoanalysis, 268 – 9, 272, 275,

285
psychodynamics, 11, 260, 285
psychology, 10, 12, 21, 41, 125,
141, 258 – 9, 261 – 2, 271, 273,
277, 286, 288, 290
puberty, 146
public sector/services, 5, 65, 67,
232
Pulse rate, 189 – 90, 224

Quality assurance, 108

rabies, 252
Race Relations NI Order, The, 65
– 7
racism, 54, 66, 79 – 80, 139, 197,
243
radiographers, 4
red blood cells, 158, 169, 171
Red Cross, 27
Registrar General, 136
rehabilitation, 51
religion, 57, 61, 64, 212, 233 – 4,
266
renal system, 160 – 1
Reporting of Injuries, Diseases
and Dangerous Occurrences
Regulations (RIDDOR), 100 – 1,
110
reproductive system, 160 – 1
residential care, 51, 71 – 2, 83,
85, 111, 223, 229, 286
resources, 199
respiration, 155, 162, 168, 170,
177 – 8, 184, 186, 188
respiratory system, 148, 160 – 1,
164, 178 – 9, 183
resuscitation, 101
retirement, 116
risk assessment, 102, 104, 106,
108, 113 – 4
Rogers, Carl, 272 – 3
role theory, 266 – 7
rubella, 132
rules of conduct, 9, 50

sanitation, 133
schizophrenia, 129 – 30, 246, 278
– 9, 290
school, 116
security, 82 – 4, 88, 99, 103 – 7,
109 – 10, 113
self-fulfilling prophesy, 64
self-harm, 57
Sex Discrimination Act, The, 65
– 7, 238
sexism, 54, 79 – 80
sexual harassment, 66

sign language, 14, 28
signs/signers, 28 – 30, 40, 42
skin cancer, 102, 134
Skinner, B.F., 263 – 4, 282
small intestine, 175, 177, 188
smoking, 138, 140, 148, 244 – 5, 247, 252, 286
Snow, John, 251
Social Care Partnership Trusts, 38
Social Exclusion Unit, 63
social learning theory, 264 – 6, 275, 277, 283
Social Services, 37 – 8, 217, 219
social workers, 4, 37, 39, 46, 71, 223 – 4, 226
socialisation, 52 – 3, 61, 78, 80, 138, 235 – 6
sociology, 228, 230, 233, 239, 259
Special Needs and Disability Act, 69
speech and language therapists, 4, 22, 29, 38, 40, 117, 259, 262, 277, 279
state sectors, 73
stereotyping, 36, 53, 61, 79, 81, 286, 290
stomach, 174
Strategic Health Authorities, 217 – 18, 290
striated muscle, 159
support services, 4, 38
surgery, 223, 245

technology, 8, 14, 16, 21, 29 – 30, 40 – 2, 202, 238
temperature, 10, 180, 184, 186 – 7, 189 – 93, 224
terminology, 34, 50, 52, 55, 60, 230, 241
testosterone, 146
tetanus, 102
therapeutic activities, 21
touch, 20, 24, 26, 36
training, 83, 86, 89, 117
translators, 40, 42
treatment, 19, 63, 102, 209, 220 – 1, 223 – 4, 242, 245 – 6, 249 – 50, 289
trisomy, 131
tuberculosis, 102, 252
Tuckman, Bruce, 18

UN General Assembly, 70
United Nations, 70, 243

Veins, 167
Ventilation, 172

Virus, 95

waste products/materials, 82, 90, 93, 106, 109, 161, 168, 170, 177 – 8, 181, 185
Watson, John B, 262
Welfare State, 65, 232, 241, 247
welfare, 81
white blood cells, 158
White Paper, 37, 221, 247
Woltosz, Walt, 30
Work placement/experience, 9, 14 – 5, 25, 84, 88, 104, 195, 214, 216
World Health Organisation, 133, 148, 217, 243, 252
zero tolerance, 96
Zygote, 122

Edexcel
190 High Holborn
London WC1V 7BH

© Edexcel 2007

The rights of Mary Crittenden, Alison Thompson, Douglas Thomson, Elizabeth Shackels and Sam Pope to be identified as authors of this Work have been asserted by them in accordance with the Copyright, Designs and Patents Act, 1988.

All rights reserved. No part of this publication may be reproduced, stored in a retrieval system or transmitted in any form or by any means electronic, mechanical, photocopying, recording, or otherwise, without either the prior written permission of the publishers and copyright owners or a licence permitting restricted copying in the United Kingdom issued by the Copyright Licensing Agency Ltd., 90 Tottenham Court Road, London W1P 9HE

ISBN: 978-1-40586-810-5

Printed in the Great Britain by Scotprint Ltd, Haddington
Illustrations by Pearson Education
Indexed by Richard Howard

Acknowledgments
The Publisher is grateful to the following for their permission to reproduce copyright material:

Stephen Hawking; Robert Fairburn; Walsall Environmental Health and Consumer Services Department; nhs.uk; General Social Care Council; Wales Audit Office; Worcester County Council; Office for National Statistics; Department of the Environment, Transport and the Regions; Department of Health; Martin Jarvis; Makaton Vocabulary Development Project, www.makaton.org.

Wadsworth, a division of Thomson Learning: www.thomsonrights.com, Fax 800-730-225, for permission to include an extract from 'Exercises in Helping Skills', 3rd edition, by EGAN. 1986.

Sally Millar, for permission to use an extract from her book: Millar, S. (2003), Personal Communication Passports: Guidelines for Good Practice, CALL Centre, University of Edinburgh. ISBN 1-898042-21-1. Picture Communication Symbols 1981 – 2002, Mayer-Johnson Inc.

Hansell, Sen, Sufi, McCallum, (September 1998), Journal Communicable Disease and Public Health, Vol 1, No 3, Health Protection Agency.

Auditor General for Wales, Protecting NHS Trust Staff from Violence and Aggression, (September 2005), Wales Audit Office

Kolb, David A., EXPERIENTIAL LEARNING: Experience as a Source of Learning, © 1984, p.42. Adapted with the permission of Pearson Education, Inc., Upper Saddle River, NJ.

© Crown copyright material is reproduced with the permission of the Controller of HMSO and Queen's Printer for Scotland.

Every effort has been made to trace the copyright holders and we apologise in advance for any unintentional omissions. We would be pleased to insert the appropriate acknowledgement in any subsequent edition of this publication.

The publisher would like to thank the following for their kind permission to reproduce their photographs:

(Key: b-bottom; c-centre; l-left; r-right; t-top)

4 Getty Images: Stone / Jonathan Selig; 5 Corbis: Goodshoot (b); Image Point FR / FURGOLLE (t); 14 Corbis: Randy Faris;16 Corbis: Randy Faris;20 Alamy Images: Warren Kovach; 21 PunchStock: Digital Vision; 23 Corbis: Zefa / Jon Feingersh; 24 Alamy Images: ImageState; 27 © Crown Copyright / Office of Public Sector Information; 30 Getty Images: Justin Sullivan; 32 Alamy Images: Janine Wiedel Photolibrary (t). Corbis: Helen King (c); Mike Watson Images (b); 48 iStockphoto: Ethan Myerson; 50 iStockphoto: Ethan Myerson; 53 PunchStock: DesignPics; 56 Corbis: Fabio Cardoso; 62 PunchStock: DesignPics; 68 Alamy; Images: Tom Kidd; 71 Science Photo Library Ltd: Michael Donne; 76 Alamy Images: geogphotos; 79 Alamy Images: Alan Schein; 82 Corbis: Goodshoot; 84 Corbis: Goodshoot; 85 © Crown Copyright / Office of Public Sector Information; 90 Corbis: Image Point FR / FURGOLLE.
91 Rex Features.; 93 Alamy Images: Tom Carter; 110 © Crown Copyright / Office of Public Sector Information; 111 Alamy Images: David Pearson; 112 Corbis: Brand X / Keith Brofsky; 116 Science Photo Library Ltd: Bluestone; 118 Science Photo Library Ltd: Bluestone; 129 Getty Images: Stone / Seth Kushner; 132 Wellcome Trust Medical Photographic Library; 143 PunchStock: Digital Vision; 145 Rex Features; 150 iStockphoto: Kativ; 152 iStockphoto: Kativ; 162 Corbis: Henrik Trygg; 194 Science Photo Library Ltd: Tek Image; 196 Science Photo Library Ltd: Tek Image; 201 PunchStock: Photodisc; 208 Corbis: Ned Frisk Photography; 217 Thanks to www.nhs.uk for their kind permission to reuse this diagram; 226 Alamy Images: PHOTOTAKE Inc.; 228 Corbis: Image Point FR / IMANE; 230 Corbis: Image Point FR / IMANE; 232 iStockphoto; 234 Alamy Images: Hugh Threlfall; 237 Corbis: Bettmann; 239 iStockphoto: Peter Close; 240 iStockphoto: Denise Crew; 258 Getty Images: Stone / Jonathan Selig; 260 Getty Images: Stone / Jonathan Selig; 263 Archives of the History of American Psychology / The University of Akron; 264 Corbis: Laura Dwight.; 265 Albert Bandura: Albert Bandura, D. Ross & S.A. Ross, Imitation of film-mediated aggressive models. "Journal of Abnormal and Social Psychology", 1963, 66. P. 8; 272 Pulse Picture Library; 274 Trevor Clifford; 283 PunchStock: Image Source

Cover images: Front: Corbis: Tom Stewart

All other images © Pearson Education

Picture Research by: Sarah Purtill

Every effort has been made to trace the copyright holders and we apologise in advance for any unintentional omissions. We would be pleased to insert the appropriate acknowledgement in any subsequent edition of this publication